HYPERTENSION: NEW RESEARCH

HYPERTENSION: NEW RESEARCH

Elwood F. Benhagen
Editor

Nova Biomedical Books
New York

For permission to use material from this book please contact us:
Telephone 631-231-7269; Fax 631-231-8175
Web Site: http://www.novapublishers.com

Library of Congress Cataloging-in-Publication Data

Hypertension : new research / Elwood F. Benhagen, editor.
p. ; cm.
Includes bibliographical references and index.
ISBN 1-59454-204-X (hardcover)
1. Hypertension.
[DNLM: 1. Hypertension. WG 340 H9987 2004] I. Benhagen, Elwood F.
RC685.H8H9125 2004
616.1'32--dc22 2004022796

Published by Nova Science Publishers, Inc. ✣ New York

Contents

PREFACE

Hypertension is a major cause of cerebral accidents, cardiac disease and renal failure. Essential or secondary hypertension occur in between 15-20% of the population. The leading risk factors are family history, race, stress, obesity, a high intake of saturate fats or sodium, tobacco use, sedentary lifestyle, and aging. It may also be caused by other diseases, medical events, or taking of drugs of a wide variety. Most cases of hypertension are treatable although prolonged elevated blood pressure can lead to severe consequences including death. This new book gathers leading research from around the world on the etiology, pathogenesis, prevention, diagnosis and treatment of this widespread disease.

Chronic-degenerative diseases, particularly cardiovascular, have a wide prevalence and they are the most frequent cause of mortality in a large number of industrialized communities, occupying a priority place in medical research. There is a frequent association of hypertension, dyslipidemias, obesity and diabetes, called "The deadly quartet". Hypertension is a condition whose causes are multiple. Comparative studies in different rat models have shown that although they share some of the main features, there are others, such as heart or kidney failure and stroke, that only appear in a few subsets of the hypertensive models as discussed in chapter I. As far as treatment is concerned, the same variation is seen in effectiveness: some drugs may reduce blood pressure but do not prevent end-organ damage. Hence the need to choose a model that is the most adequate for the intended purpose.

Aging is determined by a series of morphological and functional changes over time and by the deterioration of the biological functions after an organism has passed its maximum reproductive potential. We do not know whether aging starts from the moment of conception or at maturity, or if it constitutes a process of evolution or involution. Several suggestions have been proposed to explain why we age; they offer partial solutions and indicate possible guide-lines for future investigation. Theories of aging have been grouped either as genetic or evolutionary currents. Many mechanisms that lead to aging have been proposed, although none of them solves all the doubts and gives us a clear answer. These mechanisms are discussed in this article and an example of aging of the cardiovascular system under normal and physiopathological conditions is offered. Although some data on human aging are presented, the review is mainly focused on recent advances made on animal models. Aging in the cardiovascular system is characterized by an increase in blood pressure, a reduction both in cardiac output and in the response to stress. In blood vessels, aging is related to structural and functional changes in the endothelium, smooth muscle and extracellular matrix. Age-related vascular changes vary in different species and in vessels irrigating various organs. Oxidative stress appears to be the primary explanation for aging in the cardiovascular system. Hypertension, which is an age-dependent disorder, and diabetes and insulin resistance, which are associated with aging, contribute to vascular malfunction, altering the aging mechanisms of blood vessels. Several models of hypertension and diabetes have been used to study the alterations produced in the aging processes of the cardiovascular system and are summarized in chapter II.

Idiopathic portal hypertension (IPH) is characterized by a long-standing presinusoidal portal hypertension of unknown etiology and by the definite absence of cirrosis, and obliteration of intrahepatic small portal veins and dense portal fibrosis may be related to its pathogenesis as explained in chapter III. While the etiologies of IPH remains only speculative, some unidentified agent(s) may affect the intrahepatic small vasculatures or portal tracts, or may play a role in the increased portal venous blood flow. Portal fibrosis may be explainable by imbalanced synthesis and degradation of collagen and elastic fiber involving connective tissue growth factor and matrix metalloproteinase-9. During the long clinical course of IPH, several pathological changes may develop secondarily, including subcapsular parenchymal atrophy, atrophy of the liver, focal and mild intralobular fibrosis, and portal venous phlebosclerosis and thrombosis. Subcapsular parenchymal and hepatic atrophy may result from hepatocellular dropout via apoptosis or necrosis due to chronic portal venous blood insufficiency. Portal venous thromboemboli of the larger intrahepatic portal veins may be responsible for segmental or zonal hepatic parenchymal collapse. Increased expression of heme oxygenase-1 and endothelin-1 in the hepatic lobules of IPH livers may be related to the altered sinusoidal hemodynamics. Focal and mild intralobular pericellular fibrosis and thin fibrous septa may be due to activation of hepatic stellate cells. However, liver cirrhosis does not occur eventually. Taken together, a new staging or categorization of IPH with a combination of hepatic parenchymal atrophy and portal venous thrombosis was proposed: non-atrophic liver without subcapsular parenchymal atrophy (stage I), non-atrophic liver with subcapsular parenchymal atrophy (stage II), atrophic liver with subcapsular parenchymal atrophy (stage III), and portal venous occlusive thrombosis (stage IV). IPH livers are likely to progress from stage I to stage III, and stage IV develop rarely in stage I, and more frequently in stage III than in stage II, and means a poor prognosis. This staging is applicable to clinical cases without consideration of histologic sampling errors. Nodular parenchymal hyperplastic changes are also frequently found in IPH liver, resembling nodular regenerative hyperplasia, and partial nodular transformation, or even focal nodular hyperplasia, probably due to heterogeneity of intravascular lesion in the liver. These histopathologic feastuers of IPH livers may be shared in IPH and its equivalents characterized by long-standing presinusoidal portal venous high pressure with reduced portal venous inflow into the hepatic parenchyma, though the etiopathogenesis of such disease complex may be different in the several districts in the world.

For many years it has been accepted that hepatic stellate cells play a key role in the pathogenesis of hepatic fibrosis. Accumulating evidence from *in vitro* and *in vivo* studies suggests that these cells are also implicated in the regulation of intrahepatic blood flow in normal liver, and in the pathogenesis of intrahepatic portal hypertension. The liver is a well perfused organ with dual blood supply by the hepatic artery and the portal vein. The intrahepatic vasculature is made up by a number of discrete components, but the liver sinusoid is the principal site of blood flow regulation in the normal liver. The anatomical location of hepatic stellate cells, which embrace the liver sinusoids, provides a favorable arrangement for perisinusoidal constriction, and control of sinusoidal vascular tone and blood flow. Chapter IV describes that portal hypertension is a major complication of cirrhosis. It is responsible for most of the lethal complications, and is caused by both increased portal blood flow and augmented vascular resistance. In turn, the increased vascular resistance results from anatomical abnormalities and functional vascular alterations which are caused by an imbalance of local concentrations of vasoconstrictors and vasodilators. In chronic liver disease, hepatic stellate cells are activated and transdifferentiate to a myofibroblast-like phenotype. These activated cells have, among many other properties, enhanced contractile properties. Although the contractile apparatus and signaling pathways of contraction and relaxation of hepatic stellate cells are not as well studied as those of skeletal or smooth muscle cells, recent studies have shed light on some aspects of hepatic stellate cell contractility. Activated hepatic stellate cells respond with increased contractility to a number of vasoactive substances, including endothelin-1. In this way they contribute to the increased intrahepatic vascular resistance, characteristic of portal hypertension. On the other hand, several substances which relax activated hepatic stellate cells, and could potentially decrease portal pressure, have been identified. Since hepatic stellate cells contribute to the pathogenesis of both intrahepatic vascular resistance and hepatic fibrogenesis, they are currently regarded as therapeutic targets to prevent and treat different complications of chronic liver disease.

During the pathogenesis of hypertension, blood pressure may rise as a result of genetic or environmental determinants of increased neurohumoral and hormonal drive which is reported in chapter V. The incidental induction of growth and other processes such as oxidative stress, inflammation, mechanosensing, extracellular matrix components deposition and turnover, as well as apoptosis may contribute to vascular fibrosis and remodeling. Importantly, vascular remodeling may perpetuate a cycle in which blood pressure elevation is amplified to further drive these modulators of remodeling (for example, hypertension-induced inflammation). Oxidative stress or excess generation of reactive oxygen species has been described both in animal models of hypertension and in human essential hypertensive patients. Inflammation in the vascular wall likewise plays a major role in the pathogenesis of vascular disease. Vascular cells and inflammatory cells interact leading to increased expression of adhesion molecule, cytokines, chemokines, matrix metalloproteinases, and growth factors. Fibrosis also occurs, where extracellular matrix components such as collagen, elastin, and/or fibronectin accumulate in the vessel wall, whether by increased deposition or by reduced degradation via diminished matrix metalloproteinase/protease activity. Apoptosis or gene-regulated cell death also appears to be a modulator of hypertension-related resistance artery remodeling, whether increased or decreased in various tissues. The combined effect of all of these processes is remodeling of resistance arteries. Initially adaptive, resistance artery remodeling must be addressed therapeutically before it becomes maladaptive, compromises organ function, and contributes to the complications of hypertension. Understanding the mechanisms underlying vascular remodeling provides attractive therapeutic targets to this end.

Chapter VI discusses how the differential diagnosis of lower extremity ulcers is large. Most commonly, lower extremity ulcers are due to vascular disease, both arterial insufficiency and venous disease. Venous ulcers are the most common ulcers of the lower extremity. They are typically on the medial malleolus, at the point of highest venous hydrostatic pressure. Venous ultrasonography usually quickly confirms the presence of clot or venous insufficiency as the etiology of the ulcer. Arterial disease leading to ischemic leg ulcers is primarily from large vessel occlusive disease (atherosclerosis obliterans). The clinical examination and simple testing such as the ankle brachial index (ABI) and transcutaneous oximetry can usually identify ulcers on the basis of large vessel occlusive disease. A reduction in both the ankle brachial index and transcutaneous oximetry is diagnostic of that condition. Ulcers from small vessel (arteriolar) ischemia may also occur. They have a normal ankle brachial index due to normal large vessel perfusion and a reduced transcutaneous oximetry. Small vessel ischemic ulcers may be due to vasculitis, atheroemboli, and smoking (Berger's disease). A unique form of arteriolar ischemic ulcers occurs only in hypertensive patients. First described in the 1940s by Martorell, and by Hines and Farber, these ulcers have a distinct clinical presentation and specific therapy. Several key clinical features define hypertensive leg ulcers. These clinical features include: (1) the location of the ulcers on the medial malleolus, medial to posterior aspect of the thigh, or dorsum of the foot; (2) by their intense pain which is out of proportion of the size of the ulcer; (3) the presence of long-standing poorly controlled hypertension; (4) female predominance; and finally; (5) how refractory these ulcers are to conventional ischemic ulcer therapy. The pathophysiology of these ulcers is inappropriate vasoconstriction accompanying the structural changes arteriolar hypertrophy of the dermal vessels due to long-standing poorly controlled hypertension. Resolution of these ulcers requires that effective blood pressure control be achieved with vasodilatory antihypertensive therapy to reverse the arteriolar vasoconstriction that is the physiologic hallmark of the hypertensive leg ulcers. Two cases are presented to illustrate the cardinal features of Martorell's hypertensive leg ulcers including the painful delay in diagnosis and successful therapy common to this condition. All physicians who deal with lower extremity ischemic vascular disease need to be aware of this entity's unique presentation and therapy to avoid needless suffering by the patient.

High arterial blood pressure (hypertension) is a major health problem that significantly increases the risk of myocardial infarction, heart failure, stroke, renal disease and peripheral vascular disease. There is increasing evidence that gender influences blood pressure and that sex hormones contribute to the pathophysiology of hypertension. For example, on average premenopausal women have lower arterial blood pressures than either age-matched men or age-matched postmenopausal women, and these findings suggest that ovarian hormones modulate blood pressure. Moreover, in aging males, increases in blood pressure correlate with decreases in androgen levels, and these findings imply that testosterone may also influence blood pressure. However, whether sex hormones are responsible for the observed differences in blood pressure in women versus men and premenopausal versus postmenopausal women remains unclear. The chapter VII is to discuss the blood pressure modulating actions of female and male sex hormones, and to describe cellular, biochemical and molecular mechanisms by which sex hormones may modulate the cardiovascular effects of hypertension.

The number of pregnant women receiving immunosuppressants in the context of anti-rejection therapy or autoimmune diseases is constantly increasing and over 80% of these pregnancies result in surviving infants as explained in chapter VIII. Yet, all immunosuppressive drugs cross the placental barrier, raising questions about the long-term outcome of the children exposed *in utero*. Although there is no higher risk of congenital anomalies, an increased incidence of prematurity (from 14 to 83%, as compared to 5-15% in the general population), intrauterine growth retardation (IUGR) and generally low birthweight

(19 to 67% of neonates, as compared to 5-13% in the general population in developed countries) has been reported, along with maternal hypertension (71% with cyclosporine A vs 31.5%) and preeclampsia. Neonatal complications include adrenal insufficiency associated with corticosteroids; immunological disturbances with azathioprine and cyclosporine; hyperkalemia with tacrolimus. However, the most frequent complications are those associated with prematurity, IUGR and low birthweight, mostly respiratory tract diseases and neurological affections such as periventricular leukomalacia and intraventricular hemorrhage. Experimental as well as epidemiological studies have shown that low birthweight is also a predisposing factor for metabolic abnormalities such as atherosclerosis, cardiovascular diseases, renal disease, non-insulin diabetes, hypertension, obesity or the metabolic syndrome. Indeed, the human fetus adapts to undernutrition by redistribution of blood flow, but also by metabolic and endocrine changes in the production of fetal and placental growth hormones. These adaptations may all lead to a programming of the fetus with lifelong effects. The long-term follow-up of infants exposed to immunosuppressants *in utero* is still limited, but experimental studies raise the question whether there could be an increased incidence at adult age of some pathologies including renal insufficiency and hypertension.

Cardiac related morbidity and mortality is as much as 20 times higher in patients suffering from chronic renal failure (CRF), when compared to general population. It is mainly due to exacerbation of atherosclerotic processes in this group of patients. Lipid disturbances play a major role in atherosclerosis development. They also compose a constant feature of CRF. Therefore, they are considered as prime risk factors for cardio-vascular related complications in CRF patients, especially in those with hypertension or diabetes mellitus as their primary disease. HMG-CoA reductase inhibitors (statins) are the most potent drugs lowering plasma cholesterol level. They are also capable of decreasing triglycerides concentration. Numerous trials have shown the effectiveness of statins in slowing down the progression of atherosclerosis and in decreasing number of cardio-vascular incidents. However, the beneficial effects of statins go beyond the simple ability to normalize cholesterol level. Results of many recent studies point to the existence of other, cholesterol – independent mechanisms of statins' actions. These, so called pleiotropic effects include: anti-proliferative, anti-inflammatory and anti-thrombotic actvities. It is of special importance in CRF population, since cell proliferation, inflammatory processes and coagulation disturbances contribute significantly to CRF pathogenesis. Statins, therefore seem not only to decrease cardiac related complications in CRF patients, but also to have the abilities to slow down the progression of CRF itself. Chapter IX aims at presenting studies on pleiotropic activities of statins, with special emphasis on their nephroprotective role.

Essential hypertension is a world-wide disease affecting nowadays approximately 30-40% population in Western countries. The modern medicine limited cardiovascular complications and death rate in this population, and in turn, the mean life time of these patients was prolonged. Otherwise, the systematically increasing rate of kidney injury, another organ complication is observed. The specific lesion of nephroangiosclarosis affects the medium and small-sized arteries up to the interlobular arteries. Arteriolosclerosis denotes lessions of the afferent and/or the efferent glomerular arterioles. The arcuate and interlobular arteries show myointimal hypertrophy, reduplication of the internal elastic lamina and hypertrophy of the media. The arterial/arteriolar wall is also thickened by hyaline, eosinophilic, PAS-positive deposites. In these places smooth muscle cells are atrophic. Intimal and media hypertrophy seems to play the most important role as far as the patient outcome is considered. In morphometric studies, it was demonstrated that glomerulosclerosis, interstitial volume, and creatinine clearance correlated with the presence of arterial muscular hypertrophy, but not with arterial/arteriolar. Along with arterial changes, glomeruli are usally ischaemic, with thickened and folded capillary walls. Numerous glomeruli are completely sclerotic presenting global glomerulosclerosis. Possible pathways to transduce these forces into biochemical signals include ion channels, integrin interaction between cells and extracellular matrix, and activation of tyrosine kinases. In turn, synthesis of growth factors or mitogenic agonists is increased, among which angiotensin II, transforming growth factor (TGF) beta-1, and plasminogen-activator inhibitor type 1 (PAI 1) play the most important roles. Oxidative stress is also involved in this process where reactive oxygen species serve as signaling molecules. According to chapter IX the vascular injury leads to the development of progressive damage of subsequent kidney structures such as glomeruli, tubules and interstitium.

Pulmonary hypertension is a rare disease the characteristic of which is a treacherous progressive course, which almost always leads to a sudden death. It mainly affects middle and younger middle age group. The treatment of this disease is difficult as the actual underlying disorder has not yet been identified into details. After using all the traditional intensive conservative means of treatment, lung/ heart-lung transplantation often remained the only possibility to improve the quality of patient's life. Prostacyclins represent a newest and most important therapeutic approach in treatment of pulmonary hypertension nowadays. Prostacyclin PGI2 (Epoprostenol) is the strongest pulmonary vasodilator with potent aggregation-inhibitory, anti-inflammatory and anti-proliferative properties. Lately more and more reports about successful application of prostacyclin PGI2 in pulmonary hypertension treatment appear in the specialized literature. The objective of chapter X is to offer a review on the current activities and results of pulmonary hypertension treatment by means of prostacyclins, and to introduce Epoprostenol to experts.

In: Hypertension: New Research
Editor: Elwood F. Benhagen, pp. 1-46

ISBN: 1-59454-204-X

Chapter I

Models of Experimental Hypertension

Guadalupe Baños and Mohammed El Hafidi
Department of Biochemistry. Instituto Nacional de Cardiología
"Ignacio Chávez" Mexico, D.F.

Abstract

Chronic-degenerative diseases, particularly cardiovascular, have a wide prevalence and they are the most frequent cause of mortality in a large number of industrialized communities, occupying a priority place in medical research. There is a frequent association of hypertension, dyslipidemias, obesity and diabetes, called "The deadly quartet" [1]. Hypertension is a condition whose causes are multiple.

Comparative studies in different rat models have shown that although they share some of the main features, there are others, such as heart or kidney failure and stroke, that only appear in a few subsets of the hypertensive models. As far as treatment is concerned, the same variation is seen in effectiveness: some drugs may reduce blood pressure but do not prevent end-organ damage. Hence the need to choose a model that is the most adequate for the intended purpose [2].

Abbreviations

1K-1C	one kidney-one clip
2K-1C	two kidneys-one clip
AA	arachidonic acid
ACE	angiotensin converting enzyme
Ang II	angiotensin II
ANGIO II	Angiotensin II
ANP	atrial natriuretic peptide
AT (1A) or (1B)	angiotensin receptor 1A or 1B
BOR	ouabain-resistant rats

BOS	ouabain sensitive rats
BW	body weight
C	control
cGMP	cyclic guanosine monophosphate
COX	cyclo-oxygenase
DOCA	deoxycorticosterone acetate
DOCA	Deoxycorticosterone acetate
DR	Dahl-resistant rat
DS	Dahl-sensitive rat
EDRF	endothelium-derived relaxing factor
ET-	endothelin
FHH	Fawn hooded hypertensive rat
GH	genetically hypertensive rat
HDL-cholesterol	high density lipoprotein cholesterol
HT	Arterial Hypertension
HTG	hypertriglyceridemic rat
L-NAME	nitro-L-arginine monomethyl ester
MI	myocardial infarct
MMF	mycophenolate mofetil
mRNA	messenger RNA
N	normal rats
NEFA	non-esterified fatty acids
NO	nitric oxide
NOS	nitric oxide synthase
OHR	ouabain-hypertensive rats
OP	obesity-prone
OR	obesity-resistant
PGE2	prostaglandin 2
PH	pulmonary hypertension
ROS	reactive oxygen species
S	salt-sensitive
SD	Sprague-Dawley rat
SHHF	hypertensive heart failure rat
SHR	spontaneously hypertensive rats
SHROB	obese SHR
SHRSP	stroke-prone SHR
SNP	sodium nitroprusside
ZDF	Zucker obese rat with metabolic syndrome
ZSF	Zucker obese rat

INTRODUCTION

Chronic-degenerative diseases, particularly cardiovascular, have a wide prevalence and they are the most frequent cause of mortality in a large number of industrialized communities, occupying a priority place in medical research. There is a frequent association of hypertension, dyslipidemias, obesity and diabetes, called "The deadly quartet" [1].

Hypertension is a condition whose causes are multiple. Figure 1 shows some inducing factors, their pathways and target sites. Under these conditions, a large variety of models can be produced, with particular characteristics. Table 1 shows a rough classification of some of the animal models of cardiovascular and renal hypertension used in experimentation and their approximate equivalent in humans.

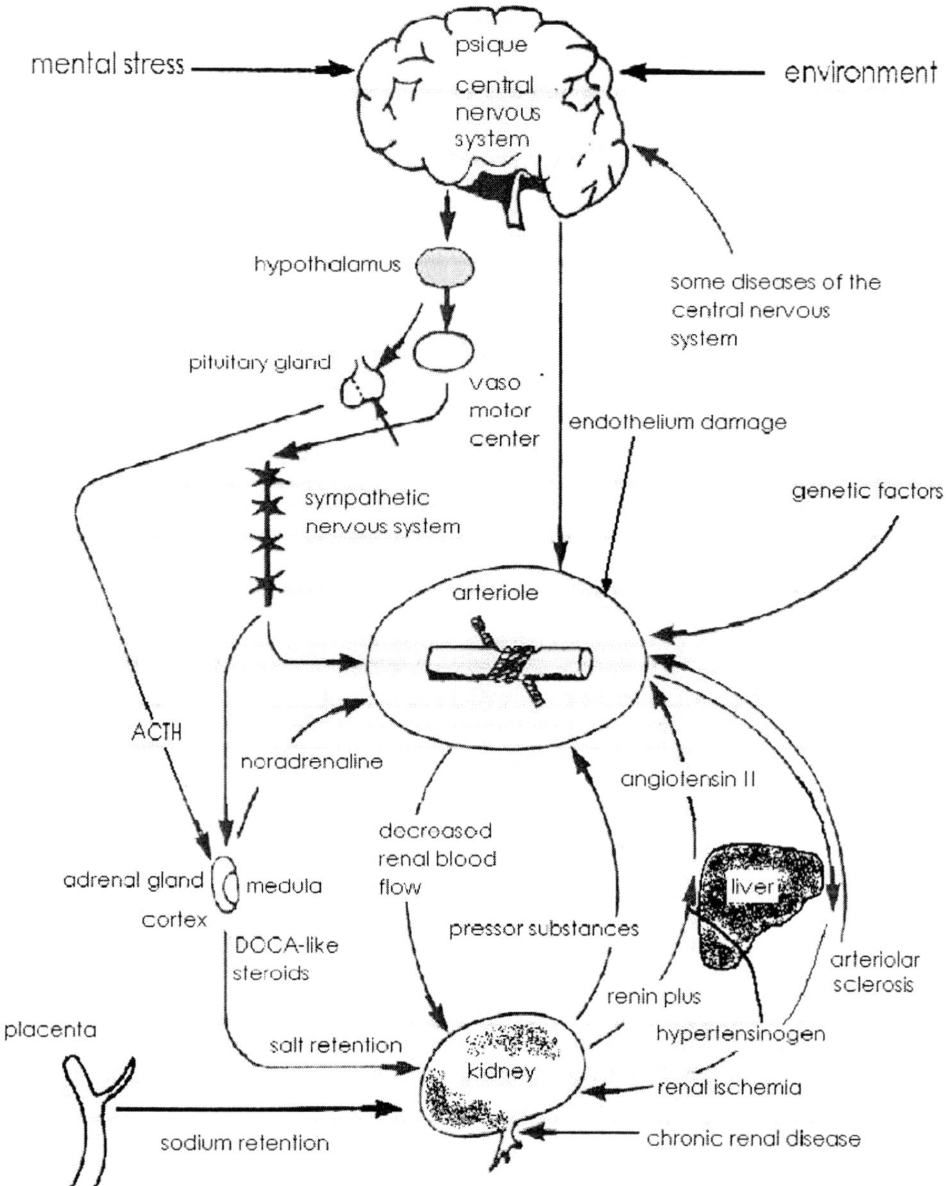

FIGURE 1. Modified from Ref. 1

Figure 1.

Table I

Models	Clinical Equivalent
Genetic:	
Spontaneously Hypertensive Rat (SHR)	Essential Hypertension
Surgical:	
Aortic Coarctation	High BP, Severe Cardiac Failure, Atherosclerosis (in Mice)
5/6 Nephrectomy (Renal Mass Reduction)	HT Due to Nephropathy, Uremia
Goldblatt HT, 2k-1c	HT Due to Aging, Reno-Vascular Nephropathy and ↑ Angio II
Goldblatt HT, 1k-1c	HT Due to Vasoconstrictión, ↑ Angio II and Volume
Pharmacological:	
Admin. Angio II	HT, Nephropathy
Admin. L-NAME	HT, Endothelial Damage
Admin. Endothelin	HT, Endothelial Damage
Admin. Alcohol	HT Due to Chronic Alcoholism
Metabolic:	
Hypertriglyceridemic	Moderate HT, Dyslipidemia
DOCA + Salt	High BP, Sensitivity to Salt
Various Inducers:	
Pulmonary Hypertension	Pulmonary Hypertension
Obesity-Induced Hypertension	Metabolic Syndrome

Although several species have been used, the most widely preferred are rats and mice, on account of the advantages they possess, such as ease of handling, low upkeep costs and, most importantly, the resemblance of the pathologies they develop with those found in humans. More recently, the use of mice for genetic manipulations has prompted a larger preference over other species.

Comparative studies in different rat models have shown that although they share some of the main features, there are others, such as heart or kidney failure and stroke, that only appear in a few subsets of the hypertensive models. As far as treatment is concerned, the same variation is seen in effectiveness: some drugs may reduce blood pressure but do not prevent end-organ damage. Hence the need to choose a model that is the most adequate for the intended purpose [2].

GENETIC MODELS OF HYPERTENSION

Several genetic models have been developed and they are readily available from commercial animal farms; their main characteristics are :

a) New Zealand Genetically Hypertensive Rat (GH)

Probably the best studied model and the earliest produced strain [3]. Its main characteristics are high blood pressure, cardiac hypertrophy and vascular alterations, Genetic variants have been shown to exist that determine some of its features such as heart mass and blood pressure; they are also dependent on the sex of the animal [4].

Further details are given at: http://www.informatics.jax.org/external/festing /rat/docs/GH.shtml).

A large part of the experimental work with this model has involved evaluation of the effects of several antihypertensive drugs, since it possesses characteristics similar to those found in human essential hypertension, the most common variety of the disease. Nevertheless, other areas of interest such as its physiological aspects have also been explored.

In experiments with atrial natriuretic peptide (ANP) infusions in a strain of vasopressin-deficient GH rats, it was found that their responses were different from those of the normotensive ones. Hypotonic saline infusion elicited a significant increase in the level of plasma ANP in GH, but ANP injection elevated it in both. The levels of angiotensin II, already high in GH, were raised in both groups, although there was significant change in the normotensive only. Aldosterone, from a normal plasma level, was decreased by ANP. The response of GH rats to the hypotensive effect of ANP was larger than in the normal animals, and so was the degree of natriuresis. Generally, GH rats seemed to be more responsive to ANP, probably due to their being subjected to high blood pressure for long periods, which in turn would elicit compensatory mechanisms [5].

The endothelial functionality and structure in this strain were studied by means of oral administration of the nitric oxide synthase inhibitor L-NAME for 2-3 months, together with serial measurements of blood pressure, which indicated significant increases in GH and control rats. Histological preparations of mesenteric arteries and left ventricle showed significant alterations in GH rats as a result of the treatment, but not in the control, indicating increased sensitivity in the former [6].

The same group of researchers investigated the effects of nitric oxide synthase inhibition with L-NAME and acetylcholine, as well as sodium nitroprusside (SNP), the non-endothelium dependent vasodilator, on the cardiovascular system. The treatment lasted two weeks, from age 7 to 9, and normal (N) and hypertensive (GH) animals were used. Blood pressure was higher in GH; perfusion pressure increase in hindquarter and left ventricular hypertrophy appeared in GH but not in normal rats. Acetylcholine and SNP had the same effect on both N and GH hindquarters, and was potentiated by L-NAME. The authors concluded that the NO generation system functions normally in the GH rats but also a non-NO- mediated process might be involved in their vascular reactivity [7].

A variant of the genetically hypertensive rat has been developed, based on the fact that a "ouabain-like" circulating substance is found in a large number of essential hypertensive patients. Normal outbred rats received infusions of high doses of ouabain and developed sustained hypertension (OHR); according to their responses two strains of rats were selected, either resistant (BOR) or sensitive (BOS) to the effect of ouabain as inducer of high blood pressure. Breeding pairs were chosen from each group and several generations were produced; the inbreeding induced spontaneous hypertension in BOS animals. The pathological characteristics of OHR and BOS models are similar to those of the SHR, suggesting similar etiopathological mechanisms [8].

b) The Okamoto Spontaneously Hypertensive Rat (SHR)

This strain is characterized by its high blood pressure, accompanied by dyslipidemias (hypercholesterolemia and hypertriglyceridemia), insulin resistance and hyperinsulinemia [9] (see http://www.informatics.jax.org/external/festing/rat/docs/SHR.shtml).

The SHR model is also very much in favor although it has the characteristics of primary hypertension, a not-so-common subtype of human hypertension [2].

Collagen accumulates when cardiac hypertrophy develops as a consequence of hypertension; this phenomenon contributes to myocardial rigidity leading to abnormal ventricular function. In *in vitro* experiments it has been demonstrated that synthesis of collagen in isolated cardiac fibroblasts from SHR is significantly larger than in normal rats. Angiotensin II also increased it, dose-dependently, but more importantly in SHR than in normal animals. Administration of Ang II inhibitors reversed the effects. The expressions of Angio and renin mRNA in ventricle cells and fibroblasts were also higher in SHR, indicating some involvement of the renin-angiotensin system in the increment of collagen synthesis in heart hypertrophy associated with hypertension [10].

A damaged vascular endothelium has been found to be a major contributor to the physiopatology of hypertension, both in humans and in experimental animals, although the tissue itself is a victim of the injurious effect of oxidative stress present in the disease [11]. SHR are more susceptible than normotensive Wistar Kyoto animals to the effect of free radicals on their endothelial cells, that cause more severe damage [12]. Likewise, in the salt-sensitive Dahl hypertensive rat, there is evidence that oxygen free radicals may be important participants in its pathogenesis [13].

A comparative study of vascular reactivity, particularly endothelial function, in normal (N), genetically hypertensive (GH) and spontaneously hypertensive rats (SHR), has demonstrated differences between the strains. SHR do have endothelial alterations and, for comparison, a group of GH (GH+L-NAME) had them induced by administration of L-NAME, an inhibitor of nitric oxide synthase. The behavior of isolated mesenteric arteries was investigated in the three groups. When the vessels were contracted with potassium or noradrenaline, a larger response was observed in SHR, whereas in N and GH they were similar; the same pattern was found when the arteries were relaxed either with acetylcholine (endothelium-dependent) or sodium nitroprussiate (non-endothelium dependent), SHR being less responsive than N or GH. Endothelium-dependent relaxation with acetylcholine increases intracellular cGMP. Basal levels of cGMP were found comparable in all three groups [14].

c) The Hypertensive Heart Failure Rat (SHHF)

A more recently developed model with multiple pathologies, including obesity, congestive heart failure and non-insulin-dependent diabetes [15].

Heyen JR et al [16] have lately undertaken the characterization of this model of heart failure and its complex elements. This model, as its human counterpart, develops multiple and progressive alterations at all levels, from molecular to functional, particularly in the myocardium where anatomical deterioration leads to malfunction associated with an increment in the blood of inflammation markers . The progress of the abnormalities correlates with the aging process in the animals, which were studied from ages 4 to 18 months and the changes are analogous to those present in humans.

d) The Dahl Salt-Sensitive Rat (DSS)

Develops hypertension, insulin resistance, hyperinsulinemia, dyslipidemias (hypertriglyceridemia and hypercholesterolemia), nephropathy. The onset of the pathology is induced by high dietary salt [17,18]. This is one of the more widely studied models because over 50 % of hypertensive patients are salt-sensitive.

These animals show dysfunctional baroreflex control of their cardiovascular system before the appearance of hypertension. While central and efferent pathways are normal, baroreceptor activity is depressed, suggesting that this is a predominant malfunction at the initiation of the pathological condition, rather than the result of later abnormalities, such as hypertension, which in fact might be favored by the pathological condition [19].

Another feature of this model is the presence of a circulating hypertension-inducing component, demonstrated by serum injections from hypertensive salt-sensitive (S) rats into hypertensive or normotensive S rats as well as uninephrectomized S animals. The S serum from hypertensive rats elicited increases in blood pressure and sodium content in the aortic wall and potentiated the responses to Ang II and norepinephrine. These effects were not observed with serum from S normotensive rats, even when these had a high salt diet [20].

Although in some reports it is stated that weanling or very young S rats have normal blood pressure, some groups have found that even at an early age and with a low-sodium diet, the S animals have increased blood pressure, which probably induces a coexisting heart hypertrophy, suggested by an increased heart weight / body weight ratio in S rats [18].

Cardiac remodeling and behavior after myocardial infarct (MI) and hemodynamic overload have been investigated in male and female S rats on a high-salt diet. MI was produced by coronary ligation, which was followed by the salt diet. Hypertrophy developed and although its extent was comparable in the two sexes, its characteristics varied between them. In the females it was concentric without signs of ventricular dilation or change in the scar tissue, whereas in the males it was eccentric, with added left ventricular dilation and thinning of the scar tissue. The contractility was increased in the females but no change was present in the males. The results indicate more favorable responses in the female animals [21]. In the same model, intracellular calcium movement control and calcium-related regulatory proteins were assessed in *in vitro* experiments involving perfused pressure-overload hypertrophic hearts. The organs were tested under different conditions to finally establish that cellular calcium movements and sarcoplasmic reticulum calcium uptake are impaired, accompanied by reduced SERCA2 content [22].

One of the aggravating factors that has been assumed to participate in the development of hypertension, either human or animal, is oxidative stress; the endothelium is particularly sensitive to its deleterious effects. These hypertensives suffer progressive nephropathy and increased generation of free radicals and their antioxidant reserve is reduced. Several animal models of hypertension such as the SHRSP, DOCA-salt and S rat present these alterations, which involve inactivation of nitric oxide by superoxide, with consequent depletion of the antioxidants, accompanied by increased kidney injury [23, 24]. When an Ang II type-1 receptor blocker is given to these rats, some of their abnormalities are reversed, for instance those of superoxide production and vascular reactivity, suggesting upregulation of functional sensitivity to Ang II [25]. The mechanisms involved in the beneficial effects of such blockers appear to include the calcium regulatory proteins, which are possibly modulated by the drug. This is a particularly useful feature in the prevention of cardiac failure, although there is no lowering of blood pressure [26].

Diverse alterations in the cellular handling of ions have been described in human and experimental hypertension and attempts have been made to use them as markers. Unfortunately the problem exists that the same markers are not carried by all hypertensives, but only by a certain percentage of them and the types of marker vary in different populations. In Dahl salt-sensitive rats fed a high-salt diet, sodium, potassium and rubidium erythrocyte transport is abnormal and a dyslipidemia is present in which plasma cholesterol and triglycerides are increased. In this case the rubidium leak could prove a useful marker for salt sensitivity in Dahl and Sabra rats[27]. Further, since the sodium-calcium exchanger modulates the intracellular concentration of calcium, damage to this system can induce changes in calcium levels, which in turn might contribute to aggravating the pathological condition in this model. For example, oxidative stress has been shown to reduce the efficiency of the exchanger in mesangial cells obtained from SHR or normal animals. The injury was more evident in SHR [28].

e) The Hereditary Hypertriglyceridemic, Hypertensive and Diabetic Rat

This model has been developed by selective cross-breeding of Wistar hypertriglyceridemic non-obese rats, which after several generations show hereditary high levels of serum triglycerides, significantly higher blood pressure than controls, as well as diabetes [29]. The same group of researchers has obtained another model of genetic hypertension: the Prague Hypertensive Rat, whose features are high blood pressure (161 ± 14 mmHg at 7 weeks of age) which increases very steeply, ventricular cardiac hypertrophy and high peripheral resistance. Renal functions are unchanged, except that proteinuria is present and the organs are heavier than normal [30].

In a comparative study of ion transport abnormalities and their relationship to blood pressure and plasma lipids in hereditary hypertriglyceridemic, Lyon hypertensive and HTG x Lewis F2 hybrids, it was found that red cell sodium content is positively correlated to the level of triglycerides, the bumetanide-sensitive sodium transport is inversely correlated to plasma cholesterol. In the two genetic strains the sodium leak was positively associated with the blood pressure. The results suggest that the abnormal levels of plasma lipids are involved in the alterations of red cell ion transport [31].

Diminished platelet aggregation is another abnormality present in the hypertriglyceridemic rats, which could be induced, similarly, by the alterations in the lipid metabolism, since the thromboxane pathway is normal [32]. This was demonstrated later by the same authors who found that platelet membrane microviscosity is indeed affected by the high concentration of blood triglycerides [33].

GENETIC MODELS OF HYPERTENSION AND NEPHROPATHY

a) Fawn Hooded Hypertensive Rat (FHH)

A model of pulmonary hypertension, associated with dyslipidemias and nephropathy [34].

This genetic pulmonary hypertension model has been mostly used to study the nephropathy that it develops.

The degree of renal impairment in this model is not uniformly present but its degree depends on some genetic differences found in the animals. The treatment of the hypertensive and normotensive FH varieties with L-NAME reveals the higher susceptibility of the hypertensive strain [35].

The auto regulation of renal blood flow and glomerular capillary pressure in the hypertensive FH rats are abnormally higher than those in the normotensive FH and this impairment is a factor contributing to the renal damage in this model [36,37].

The association of glomerulosclerosis with the expression of nitric oxide synthase-1 and cyclooxygenase-2 in the juxtaglomerular system and thick ascending limb was investigated, comparing two groups of FHH hypertensive rats of different ages (8 and 16 weeks) against an FHL group, normotensive. The histochemical observations indicated that NOS-1 activity is increased in the hypertensive animals, but more so in the younger group. This pattern was also found with regard to COX-2, although higher renin mRNA reactivity and expression in afferent arterioles was present in the older FHH rats. The evidence of glomerulosclerosis appeared at the later stages [38].

Besides the rat models mentioned above, such as the Dahl salt-sensitive, the Fawn hooded and the SHHF, whose alterations include hypertension and nephropathy, the models below are also used for renal studies.

b) The Spontaneously Hypertensive Obese Rat (SHROB)

Obesity has become the new epidemic of the third millennium and the number of research papers on the subject has escalated, adding up to some 17 000 in the last three years. In order to combat the enemy, it is necessary to know it well. The animal models are particularly valuable for this purpose; they can help to devise strategies for prevention or treatment of the condition.

The SHROB develop the metabolic syndrome X, which includes obesity, insulin resistance, hyperinsulinemia, hypertriglyceridemia and hypercholesterolemia, as well as hypertension and nephropathy [39].

Due to a point mutation of the leptin receptor extracellular domain, all leptin receptor isoforms are missing in these animals. Experiments to demonstrate its effects have shown that when muscle insulin-mediated glucose transport in vitro is induced by incubating muscle from SHR and SHROB with recombinant human leptin, glucose transport is reduced by half in SHR but not in SHROB. Therefore, this is a valuable model for the study of the involvement of leptin in energetic metabolism [40].

In a comparative study between the SHROB and non-obese hereditary hypertriglyceridemic (HTg) rats to investigate the correlation between triglyceride levels in muscle with glucose homeostasis and tissue responsiveness to insulin action, it was observed that triglyceride content was highest in SHROB animals, followed by HTg; controls had the lowest. SHROB and HTg showed comparable responses with respect to glucose intolerance and insulin stimulation, suggesting that this behavior was not correlated to the degree of triglyceride accumulation in muscle [41].

The effect of a glucose load on levels of free fatty acid and plasma glucagon was evaluated. Initially SHROB have high levels of both. The glucose load increased glucagon only, in SHROB but not in lean SHR, in which there was a reduction. On the other hand, the effect on plasma free fatty acids was the reverse, i.e. no modification in SHROB and a reduction in SHR. When exogenous glucagon was given to SHR to levels comparable to those of fasting SHROB, a sustained increase in insulin and glucose was induced. The authors concluded that the insulin resistance and glucose intolerance present in SHROB could be partly attributed to the high levels of basal glucagon and the lack of response from glucagon and free fatty acid secretion to the glucose load [42].

c) The Stroke Prone Rat (SHRSP)

This is another of the early bred models. Besides developing nephropathy and metabolic syndrome, the rats become hypertensive. A high percentage (over 80 %) of the male animals is predisposed to stroke, but most of the experimental work has focused on the problems related to the nephropathy [43].

The degree of severity of the nephropathy in these rats varies due to different factors such as gender (in the males it is more pronounced) but more importantly, due to various genetic loci, which have no relation to those responsible for the elevation of blood pressure [44]. Nevertheless, the degree of hypertension is related to the incidence of stroke, although the latter can be avoided with the administration of antihypertensive drugs. Other characteristics include absence of any humoral factor that could be associated with the incidence of strokes, increased vascular permeability, microaneurisms and angionecrosis [45].

A feature of the model is that the hypertension is salt-sensitive and as in other comparable models, such as the Dahl salt-sensitive and DOCA-salt, shows increased release of superoxide with the consequent oxidative stress and significant reduction of the antioxidant reserve. This condition increases the risk of renal damage and nitric oxide inactivation [46].

d) The ZSF Rat

These animals present a multiple pathology model of nephropathy, heart failure, metabolic syndrome, hypertension, diabetes, obesity. This condition is present in a large number of individuals in Western populations and its incidence is increasing. Often this same group consume large quantities of coffee, the effects of which have been investigated by adding caffeine to the dinking water of ZSF rats. It was observed that with the treatment there was a decrease in body weight and food and liquid intake. Insulin sensitivity improved. Also glycosuria diminished and plasma triglycerides and glycerol were unchanged. But cholesterol increased as well as the protein/creatinine clearance ratio; there was decreased creatinine clearance. Caffeine did not modify blood pressure, plasma renin activity, renal blood flow or renal vascular resistance in either controls or ZDF, although there was a tendency for norepinephrine to increase in both. The results show that caffeine can improve insulin sensitivity, while elevating cholesterol levels and deteriorating renal function, and this changes may depend on the state of health of the individual[47,48].

Searching for some means to treat this spreading condition, a group of researchers found that 2-hydroxyestradiol, a metabolite of 17-beta estradiol with hardly any estrogenic activity, had an overall beneficial effect at all levels of the syndrome in ZDF animals, which opens the possibility of effective treatment of this disease [49].

e) The ZDF Rat

Developed from outbred obese Zucker rats, besides obesity, diabetes and metabolic syndrome, they also develop nephropathy and mild hypertension [50].

Research in this model has been focused on diabetes and obesity. Nevertheless, under some regimes the animals easily develop hypertension, acquiring a pathological condition all-too -often encountered in humans. These rats are quite sensitive to mineralocorticoid-induced hypertension, indicating that obesity is thus a risk factor for the onset of hypertension [51].

A means of increasing the blood pressure in animals is the administration of L-NAME, a nitric oxide synthase inhibitor. On the other hand, there is some evidence that insulin can reduce high blood pressure in diabetic patients. A study was conducted in which ZDF rats were treated with insulin alone or insulin plus L-NAME. ZDF weight gain was larger than in controls, but their water intake was smaller. Insulin induced reduced plasma glucose and blood pressure, but increased plasma nitric oxide metabolites and aortic NO synthase activity. L-NAME inhibited the effects of insulin on blood pressure, NO production and NOS activity, suggesting that insulin stimulates NO release and NOS activity, thus inducing a decrease in blood pressure [52].

Later, using immuno-staining techniques, the same researchers demonstrated the presence of inducible NOS in the arteries of several organs from ZDF rats treated with insulin. The density of the synthase was more apparent in the organs of insulin-treated ZDF than in those of controls [53].

Some regional altered NO release exists in this model, and relaxation responses to acetylcholine, histamine and the calcium ionophore A23187 are reduced in pre-contracted arteries, particularly in the basilar artery [54].

Surgically Induced Hypertension Models

Figure 2 shows a diagram of the surgical manipulations that are carried out to induce hypertension in three models.

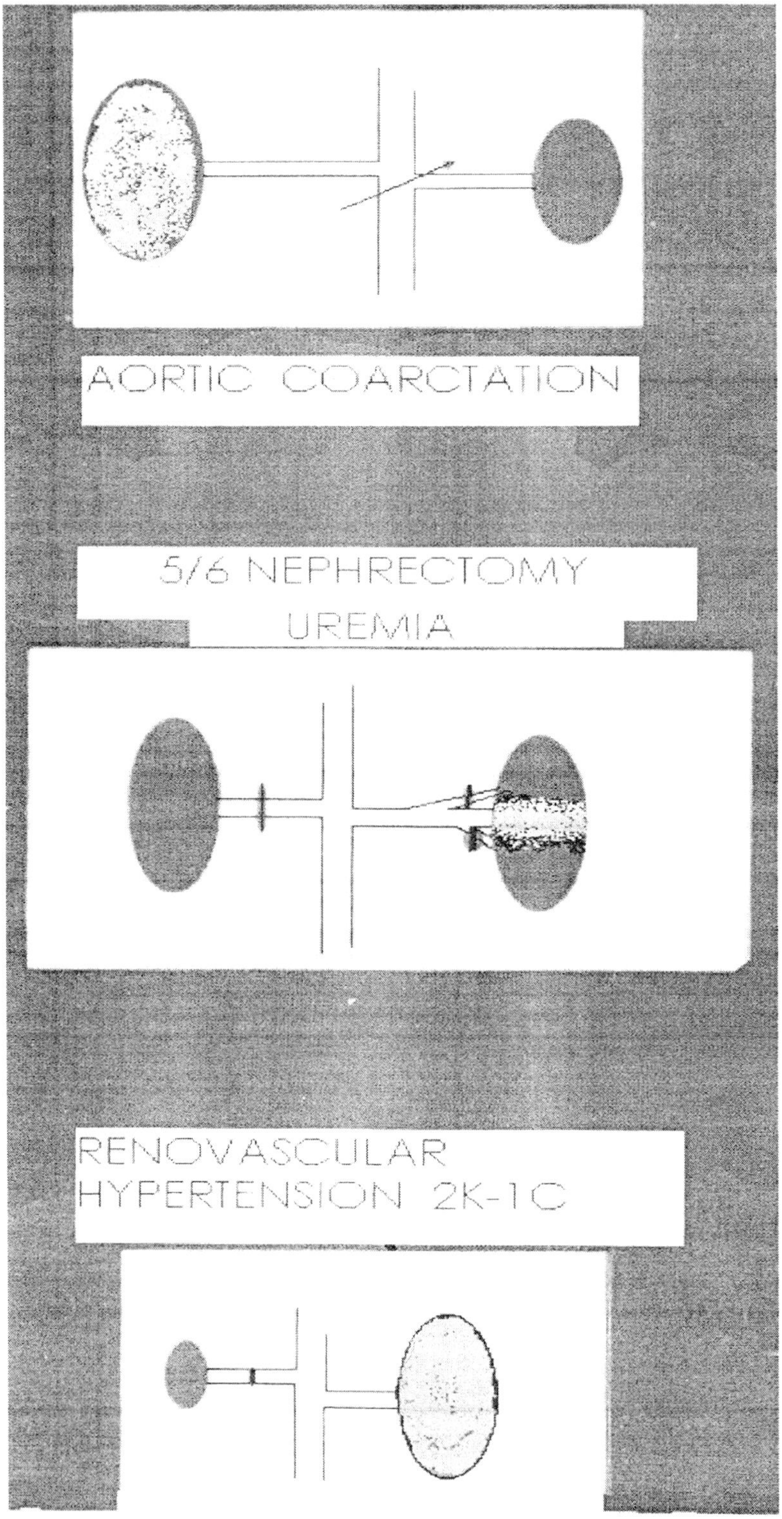
AORTIC COARCTATION
5/6 NEPHRECTOMY
UREMIA
RENOVASCULAR
HYPERTENSION 2K-1C

Figure 2.

a) Aortic Coarctation

The procedure consists in placing a device, such as a clip, to reduce the caliber of the abdominal aorta by about 33 %, at a point between the left and the right renal artery so that the blood supply to the left kidney is diminished. The right kidney becomes hypertrophied and the systemic blood pressure increases significantly. The species preferred for this type of model are the rat and the knock-out mouse; this latter develops atherosclerosis of the vessels proximal to the site of coarctation. In the clinic, the incidence of abdominal coarctation is low, the aortic coarctation being a more frequent occurrence.

Experimentally, in some animal models it has been observed that arachidonic acid and its metabolites can modify the reactivity of some vascular beds and the responses differ from normal. For instance, in perfused kidneys from animals with aortic coarctation and renovascular hypertension, the infusion of arachidonic acid (AA) increases perfusion pressure, an effect that is inhibited by indomethacin or an endoperoxide/thromboxane blocker [55]. The authors, on the other hand, describe that the activity, protein content and mRNA expression of COX-1 are increased in the renal tissue of hypertensive rats, resulting in an increase if vasopressor prostaglandins; in the proximal tubule they found a relationship between endothelin-1 and NO synthase (NOS) with metabolites of AA, particularly with 20-HETE, whose synthesis increases as ET-1 also increases. Treatment with L-NAME, to induce elevation of blood pressure through inhibition of NOS, increased the production of 20-HETE likewise [55].

The inactivation of NO by reactive oxygen species (ROS) in some arteries was measured as tissue nitrotyrosine, in this model. The larger concentrations of nitrotyrosine were localized above the ligature in brain, heart and thoracic aorta, but it was not altered in the segment of abdominal aorta below the coarctation and not subjected to elevated blood pressure. This indicates that regional baromechanical factors are present, whereas circulating plasma components might be operating in areas exposed to the increased blood pressure [56].

b) 5/6 Nephrectomy (Mass Reduction)

In this model, uremia and hypertension are induced by placing a ligature in 3-4 branches of the left renal artery, followed two weeks later by right nephrectomy or clipping.

A component in the serum of these rats was found to produce enhanced vasoconstriction and calcium uptake in isolated aortas [57]. The identity of the factor was unknown at the time, but from studies by another group it seems to be either a prostaglandin or Ang II, both of which are increased in uremia.

When renal failure develops, either by mass reduction or treatment with Ang II, other alterations include, besides high blood pressure, increased expression of COX-2 and concentration of 2. If the animals are treated either with an antagonist of the Ang II converting enzyme or an Ang receptor-1 blocker, the development of pathological changes is avoided. The possible mechanism by which the renal failure develops is that when Ang II level increases, the expression of COX-2 also increases, favoring an increment in the prostaglandin synthesis and, consequently, renal failure [58].

The association of renal pathology with vascular and renal production of NO was investigated in animals with renal mass reduction and saline load. NOS activity in various nephron areas and NO metabolite excretion were higher in normotensive animals, but aortic NOS activity and urinary chemiluminiscence were increased in the hypertensive ones, indicating that a regulatory mechanism had been activated [59].

c) Renovascular Hypertension or Goldblatt Hypertension Models (2 K-1 C or 1K - 1C)

These are achieved by inserting a narrow clip in the right renal artery and preserving both kidneys, thus it is a 2-kidney-1-clip model or by inserting a clip and performing nephrectomy on the left kidney (1clip-1kidney). After the surgery, the model 2K-1C presents three stages of evolution:

I. of approximately 5 weeks, with increase of Ang II level, reversible if the clip is removed or if the rat is treated with low doses of angiotensin-converting enzyme (ACE) inhibitors;
II. lasting about 7 weeks; there is salt retention, reversible by the above treatment;
III. 7-8 weeks duration, independent of renin-Ang II, irreversible; high blood pressure persists even if the clip is removed, although it can be reduced by ACE inhibitor treatment.

It has been suggested that after the III stage irreversible changes to the endothelium have occurred, therefore vasoconstrictors are released, while vasodilators and anti-platelet aggregation factors, such as NO and prostacyclin, decrease. This hypothesis was demonstrated indirectly with platelet aggregation experiments. There is a positive and significant correlation between the percentage of platelet aggregation in hypertensive rats and the evolution time. Besides, crossover experiments were conducted in which normal platelets suspended in hypertensive platelet-poor plasma showed an increase in aggregability. On the other hand, hypertensive platelets suspended in normal plasma aggregated normally. These results indicate that, indeed, a damaged endothelium contributes to the release of pro-aggregating factors, which could also contribute to hypertension, while either normal or hypertensive platelets do not seem to behave abnormally if suspended in normal plasma [60].

The participation of the Ang II receptors AT(1A) and 1B (1B), favoring vasoconstriction, in the development of hypertension in a 2K-1C mice model, was explored by evaluating the role of increased NOS activity and its possible beneficial effect in antagonizing the increase in blood pressure. It was demonstrated that AT(1A) receptors are mediators in the development of high blood pressure, action that tends to be antagonized by stimulated NO release [61].

Pharmacological Models

a) Administration of Angiotensin II

Angiotensin is a polypeptide with vasoconstrictor properties, which belongs to a family of hormones derived from their precursor, angiotensinogen, through the catalytic action of renin. The first product of the reaction renders Angiotensin I, a decapeptide with low potency. The angiotensin-converting enzyme (peptidyl-dipeptidase A), in turn, acts upon Ang I to produce the more potent hormone angiotensin II, an octapeptide with several roles: stimulator of aldosterone secretion in the adrenal cortex, neurotransmitter and vasoconstrictor. It increases systemic blood pressure and decreases diuresis. Its degradation renders Angiotensin III, a less active compound.

The role of angiotensin II in hypertension has been the subject of a large number of studies; both angiotensin-converting enzyme inhibitors or, more recently, angiotensin receptor blockers, have been successfully used as antihypertensive drugs. Gene manipulation has also been widely investigated in different models and in these experiments it has been observed that moderate changes in the gene expression of the Ang converting enzyme (ACE) do not affect blood pressure significantly, although one of the therapeutic approaches for the treatment of hypertension is the administration of inhibitors of ACE. To explain this paradox, a group of researchers [62] developed a novel computer simulation which comprised blood pressure as an explicit variable plus kallikrein-kinin system and feedback control of plasma renin through plasma Ang II levels. The simulation was matched to experimental data and their results indicated that reduced levels of bradykinin increase the risk of diabetic nephropathy that accompanies genetically determined elevated levels of ACE activity.

Ang II and sodium balance influence one another's status and by themselves or in association can modify blood pressure, which in turn may result in vascular and cardiac damage. When reviewing these interactions it is noted that cardiac hypertrophy can be modified by events such as the fact that an increase of blood pressure during sleep but not while awake can induce cardiac hypertrophy in rats. But if the increase is reversed by ACE, the hypertrophy can be reverted in 2K-1C rats. On the other hand, if the animals are given either low or high salt diet, the cardiac hypertrophy is less or more, correspondingly. Paradoxically, rats on low salt diet, receiving an ACE inhibitor together with an Ang type 1 receptor blocker, develop a lethal syndrome, which can be prevented by high salt intake. The hypothesis to explain the phenomenon is based on the handling of ions, which can be altered and produce undesirable results. [63] Since these events can occur in the clinic, the knowledge of possible adverse effects is of great importance.

Although administration of Ang II at low doses only induces blood pressure to increase slowly , it was found that even when the levels of pressure were not significantly elevated, the pressure responses to minimal stress were high; these hypertensive episodes could induce undesirable effects in an apparently normotensive animal [64]

When Ang II is administered to rats, they develop persistent salt-sensitive hypertension after two weeks of treatment. A study in which the immunosupressor mycophenolate mofetil (MMF) was tried on the animals, showed the efficacy of MMF in preventing the elevation of blood pressure. Glomerular hemodynamics was assessed after Ang II treatment, when the rats had developed a pathological condition, including severe hypertension, proteinuria, afferent and efferent vascular constriction and glomerular hypertension; the animals that received MMF as well, had the same symptoms but their proteinuria was lower. After 2 weeks, the Ang II was stopped and the rats were given a high salt diet, with which the alterations persisted and some vascular manifestations worsened. With MMF treatment + Ang II, although the blood pressure remained high, hemodynamic functions returned to normal, indicating that immunosupression by MMF reduced cortical vasoconstriction, which would then be an important factor in the development of salt-induced hypertension [65].

b)Administration of L-NAME

The discovery of the importance of the vascular endothelium in Physiology is due to Furchgott et al [66], who were able to interpret paradoxical experimental results: acetyl choline, which administered in vivo produces vasodilation, induced contraction in isolated aortas in some of their in vitro experiments. The reason is that in the latter preparation the endothelium cell layer had been inadvertently removed. The researchers concluded that, possibly, the endothelial cells produced some substances that induced relaxation of the vessels. The history of nitric oxide (chemical formula NO) began and the authors received the 1998 Nobel Prize in Medicine for their research in this field [67] .Since then many studies have been carried out which have contributed to the knowledge of endothelium characteristics and functions, including the modulation of the vascular contraction and relaxation, on account of its production of vasoactive substances that participate in the maintenance of a delicate balance in the circulatory system. When this balance is disturbed, pathological conditions appear, such as hypertension, which has been called a disease of the endothelium.

Initially, the vasoactive substance responsible for vascular relaxation was called endothelium-derived relaxing factor (EDRF). Almost simultaneously two groups of researchers later identified it as nitric oxide (NO) or a very similar compound. [68, 69].

Soon afterwards, reports about L-arginine being the physiological source of NO were published [70] and the existence of a synthase involved in the process was made known, although later three enzymes were described and called NOS-1, constitutive, found mainly in the nervous system, NOS-2 inducible, and NOS-3, constitutive, located in the endothelial cells. Analogues of L-arginine, such as L-NAME, are inhibitors of NOS-1 and NOS-3 and their administration blocks the generation of NO, producing a rapid and long-lasting increase in arterial blood pressure. Due to this effect, those compounds have been frequently used in models that require high blood pressure and experimental periods of comparatively short duration. The preferred species is the rat, but mice have also been used [71].

Pathological changes such as hypertension and cardiomyocyte and mitochondrial collagen remodeling without hypertrophy are induced when NOS is inhibited. The question is whether they are the result of the hypertension induced by L-NAME or by NO deficiency. Rossi et al [72] demonstrated that in hypertension induced by L-NAME, NO release could regulate mitochondrial biogenesis and tissue function. The presence of discrete interstitial ventricular myocardial fibrosis suggests that a reduced level of NO could be involved in the process.

c) Administration of Endothelin

Furchgott and Zawadski [67] published their leading discovery in 1980, regarding the endothelium and its properties as an endocrine entity capable of generating the most important physiological vasodilator, NO. Eight years later, the group of Masaki published a report of the isolation, sequencing and cloning of another substance derived from endothelial cells, with constricting properties, which they named endothelin (ET). It is the most potent vasoconstrictor known, 10 times more than angiotensin II [73], a 21-amino acid peptide produced in many tissues.

The next year the same group described the three human endothelins, ET-1, ET-2 and ET-3, of which ET-1 is the best studied so far, being the main endothelin produced by the endothelium, although it is also found in tracheal epithelium and neurons; it has positive inotropic effects and the most sensitive organ to its action is the kidney. ET-2 is found in placenta and tumor cells; ET-3 is associated with nervous tissue. They are codified by three individual genes. A fourth ET has recently been found. [74,75].

The infusion of exogenous ET-1 initially induces a decrease in blood pressure and peripheral resistance, possibly by release of NO, prostacyclin or atrial natriuretic factor. Afterwards, it increases both pressure and resistance in a dose-dependant and sustained manner [76].

Two types of receptors have been described for ET-1: ET_A and ET_B (Figure 3) [77,78] They are located in the endothelium and in the vascular smooth muscle, among other places, and their stimulation produces different effects. Thus, in endothelial cells stimulation of ET_A receptors induces vasoconstriction as it does on vascular smooth muscle. On the other hand, stimulation of receptors ET_B in endothelial cells produces a signal that is translated into release of NO, and therefore, relaxation. The regional distribution of ET-1 and its receptors varies in the different vascular beds, suggesting that there are also variations in the local function of ET-1[79].

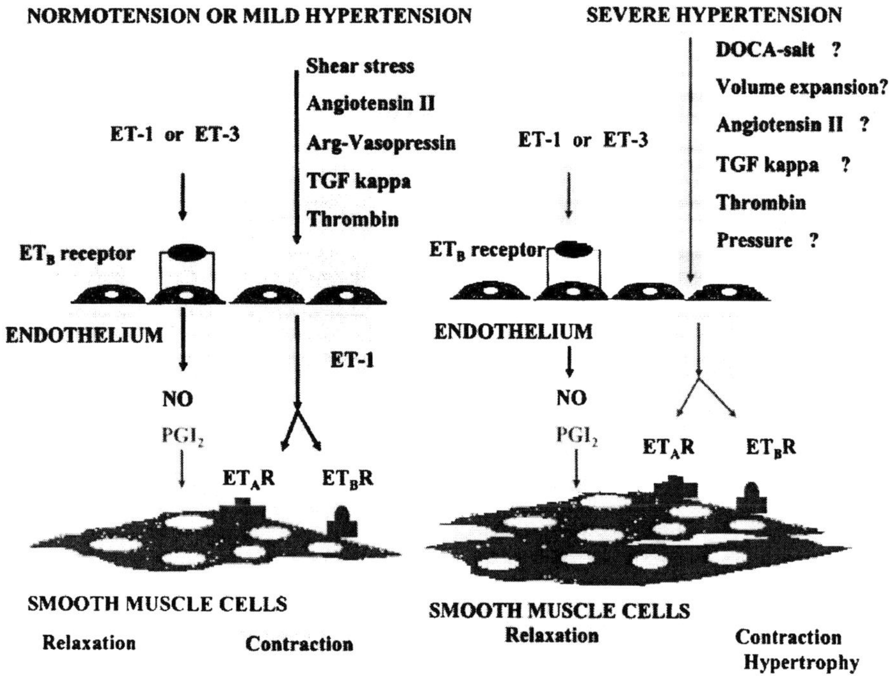

Figure. 3. Progress in Hypertension Research

Endothelins may be involved in a number of pathological conditions, including cardiovascular diseases such as some types of hypertension. This is not only by increasing blood pressure, but also by promoting vasospasms and stroke, coronary artery disease, heart failure, cardiac hypertrophy, and atherosclerosis, since they enhance cell proliferation and hypertrophy [80, 81].

Usually endothelins are not chronically administered to animals, due to their very short half-life of only minutes, but it has been found that they have an important role in the pathology involved in many animal models, particularly of pulmonary hypertension. This is also the case with patients. Endothelin levels are not elevated in some types of human hypertension, but they do increase in malignant and pulmonary hypertension [80].

d) Administration of Alcohol

Alcoholism is frequently associated with hypertension and at the beginning of the XX century Lian [82], an army doctor in World War I, investigated the number of hypertensives among the population of alcoholic soldiers. He found that the degree of alcoholism correlated with the number of hypertensive subjects, which reached about 25 % of the heaviest drinkers. A large number of papers have been published concerning the possible link between the two conditions, although the mechanisms by which alcohol may elevate blood pressure have not been completely elucidated, partly on account of the paradoxical effect that ethanol has on the circulatory system.

Alcohol induces vasodilation in acute experiments in vivo, regardless of the route of administration; its effect is more apparent on terminal arterioles and muscle venules [83]. On the other hand, systemic alcohol administration may induce vasoconstriction or biphasic effects on peripheral blood flow [84,85]. The concentration of alcohol influences its direct effects on isolated rat aortic strips as shown by Altura et al. In their experiments low levels abolished mechanical activity and reduced baseline tension whereas levels above 100 mM produced contractions. Equally, disparate effects are observed in other vascular beds [86].

The species used for the study of alcoholism vary a great deal. Rats and mice are the most common but the former are generally averse to alcohol as a drink. The latter are the preferred animal for genetic manipulations such as knockout, transgenic lines, random mutagenesis, virus-mediated gene transfer and many others. Models also include non-human primates, zebra fish [87] and fruit flies. These latter, when having to deal with comparatively large amounts of alcohol present in fermenting fruits, their natural source of nutrients, offer a very interesting model, since they possess enzymes for the metabolism of alcohol like mammals do and exhibit similar dose-dependent behavioral patterns such as stimulation, relaxation, sedation and tolerance after repetitive exposure [88].

There are also models that typify different features of alcoholism, all of them requiring *ad lib* consumption of alcohol; they include characteristics such as craving, relapse, loss of control, reinstatement, deprivation or point-of-no-return conditions. [89-92].

A rat strain, the Fawn-Hooded, is used as a model for pulmonary hypertension but also for experimental alcoholism, since the animals accept alcoholic drinks [93].

Vascular reactivity in isolated aortas was investigated either by norepinephrine-induced contractility or with norepinephrine and further addition of serum from normal or alcoholic rats. The alcoholic animals received 10 % alcohol in their drinking water for 8-10 weeks; those whose blood pressure had increased significantly above the normal were chosen for the experiment in vitro: the alcohol administration was stopped, they were given tap water for 18 hours and then their blood was collected and their aortas suspended in a chamber for isolated organs. Parallel preparations were made with controls. Contractions induced by alcoholic serum were larger than those induced by normal serum. Relaxation to verapamil was decreased by both sera but more by the alcoholic one. The results suggest the participation of a circulating serum component with pressor activity, independent from alcohol or its metabolites, which at the time the rat blood was obtained would be absent [94]. This had been previously hypothesized by experimental evidence from rats being given alcohol intermittently, by gavage, during 10 weeks. Hemodynamic measurements indicated no alteration in the blood pressure at the time when the alcohol level was highest, but there were increases 24 hours after the last alcohol drink. Therefore, alcoholic hypertension seems to be the result of withdrawal, rather than of the presence of alcohol [95].

Transgenic and knockout techniques are being used to determine genetic factors, which concur with environmental ones in the development of alcoholism. Thus, genetic engineering should prove a very useful tool in the study of this health and social problem [96-99].

METABOLIC MODELS

a) Hypertensive and Hypertriglyceridemic Models. Fructose- or Sucrose-Fed Animals

Hypertension, being a multifactorial disease, imposes a great challenge both for its prevention and for its treatment. Its development might be dependent on environmental factors such as those encountered in industrialized populations. Among those factors, diet can determine the onset of such pathological conditions as obesity, hyperinsulinemia, insulin resistance, dyslipidemias and hypertension, i.e. the metabolic syndrome, which has become particularly interesting on account of the disquieting increase in its prevalence among all populations, even those previously regarded as hunger-stricken. The pathology is frequently the result of an inadequate diet, high in carbohydrates or fat, and lack of exercise, although the genetic factor cannot be excluded.

In genetically transmitted diseases the symptoms may not be apparent, but they can develop under the influence of environmental factors such as high-salt or high-carbohydrate diets [100]. For example, the Zucker obese rat is not hypertensive but it can be easily made so with appropriate treatment.

Reaven et al [101] described a rat hypertension model developed by feeding the animals a sucrose-rich diet (60 % in their chow). There are some variants of this model, such as the original one, where fructose was used, and another one in which sucrose or commercial sugar was given in the drinking water for longer periods (Figure 4). This treatment not only increases their blood pressure but causes hypertriglyceridemia, hyperinsulinemia, insulin resistance, intra-abdominal obesity and nephropathy. The model has the features of the pathology frequently found in humans, the metabolic syndrome, where what is called "The deadly quartet" is present, (which includes diabetes,) and its prevalence has shown some dependence on age, gender and circulating levels of sex hormones [102,103].

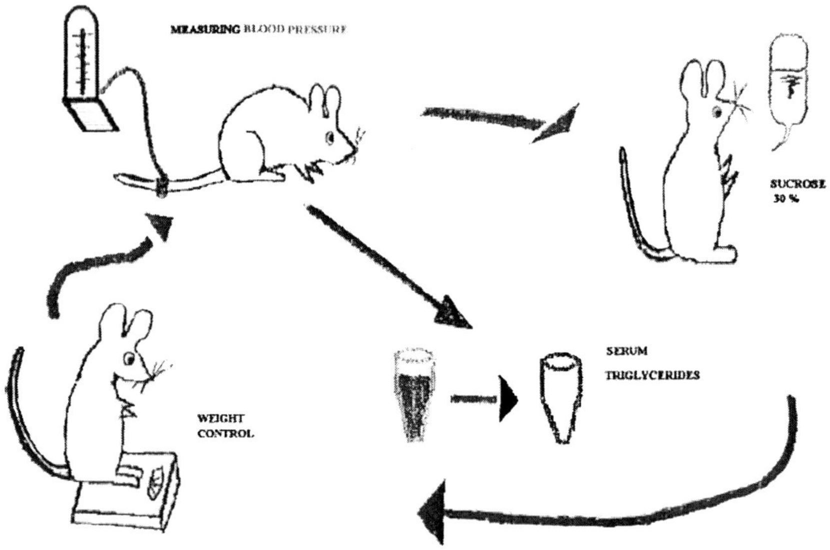

Figure 4.

In the variant in which sucrose is given (HTG), resembling a high-carbohydrate diet, there is no hyperglycemia and cholesterol is normal. The increase in blood pressure is moderate but other pathologies are significant. Vascular reactivity is abnormal and suggests endothelial damage: in isolated aortic or mesenteric rings there is hypercontractility to norepinephrine or phenylephrine and hyporelaxation to acetylcholine. When normal or HTG serum is added to the preparation of either vessel, contraction is observed, but it is larger with HTG serum; if norepinephrine is added after the serum the response is potentiated, more with the HTG serum; the largest effect is seen in HTG arteries. These serum effects indicate the presence of some circulating serum component(s), possibly the altered lipids that induce increased contractility [104].

The infusion of serum produces alterations in the cardiac function in isolated heart preparations (Langendorff), increasing perfusion and ventricular pressures. Normal serum induces a larger response in HTG hearts than in controls and HTG serum induces significantly higher pressures than control serum in both control and HTG hearts, that of the HTG being the highest of all [105].

Differences in the lipid composition of plasma HTG have been found associated with gender. In the HTG rat, the proportion of arachidonic acid is much higher in the female (this acid is very sensitive to lipoperoxidation, given the number of double bonds it possesses). When oxidative stress is induced by iron-dextran injections, the lipoperoxidation index becomes lower in the control female as compared to the control male, probably due to the protective effect of antioxidants in the female, but in HTG females the sugar treatment makes the difference disappear [106-108].

It has been observed that obese hypertensive patients have high levels of non-esterified fatty acids, including oleic acid. These are not fully susceptible to degradation by insulin, suggesting that they might be involved in the pathological condition, since oleic acid interferes with the synthesis of nitric oxide and, consequently, with endothelium-dependent vasodilation. This was confirmed by experiments on healthy human volunteers who received high doses of non-esterified fatty acids, to equal levels found in patients. It was demonstrated that the treatment impaired vascular reactivity. In experiments in vitro, addition of oleic acid to cultured vascular smooth muscle cells proved that the acid induces mitogenesis and release of reactive oxygen species [109].The lipid profile in HTG rats shows alterations comparable to those found in patients with metabolic syndrome, i.e. high levels of unsaturated fatty acids and a reduced proportion of arachidonic acid, a pattern that could be a risk factor for the pathological features in this model [106-108].

In general, the changes induced by the treatment in HTG rats are more numerous and unfavorable in males. In females the estrogens are a likely source of protection against cardiovascular pathological events. The vascular reactivity response patterns become altered when the levels of sex hormones are modified by castration or by castration and subsequent treatment with estradiol or testosterone. Indomethacin reverses some of the abnormal vascular responses in HTG, indicating the participation of components of the arachidonic acid metabolism [110]. In this respect, a group of researchers studying the fructose-fed model, a variant of HTG, which received the treatment for one month, found that the addition of an inhibitor of the thomboxane synthase prevented the animals from developing the characteristic hypertension [111].

As in several models of hypertension, in HTG there is an involvement with endothelin release. In isolated aortas and femoral arteries contracted with potassium chloride, the addition of moderately high doses of insulin evoked a potentiation of the contractile response in both control and HTG vessels, but it was larger in the latter; the largest was that of the femoral artery. The addition of specific ETA and ETB blockers inhibited the response, to a larger extent in the HTG, suggesting that endothelin is indeed released by HTG vessels, probably under physiological stimulation by insulin. Since the HTG are moderately hyperinsulinemic, the stimulus would be larger than under normal conditions [112]. The association of insulin and endothelin in hypertriglyceridemia had been previously observed [113].

The use of an inhibitor of ET receptors, bosentan, has proved useful as a pressure-lowering drug in the fructose-fed rat [114] and in some cases of human hypertension [115].

The important participation of endothelin in the condition, i.e. the metabolic syndrome, particularly the increase in blood pressure and possibly vascular hypertrophy, has prompted a large number of investigations in this subject [116].

The main features of the nephropathy present in HTG, are oliguria, proteinuria and histological changes, particularly in the arterioles. (Figures 5A: control rat kidney vessel and glomerulus , 5B: transversal section HTG kidney vessel, 5C: longitudinal section HTG kidney vessel).

In fructose-fed animals given also a high-salt diet, there is insulin-induced sodium retention, the result of a down-regulation of renal insulin receptors [117].

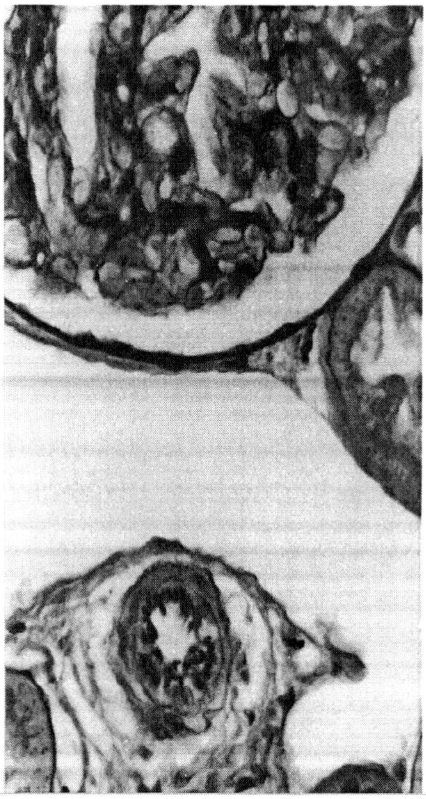

Figures 5A. Control rat kidney vessel and glomerulus.

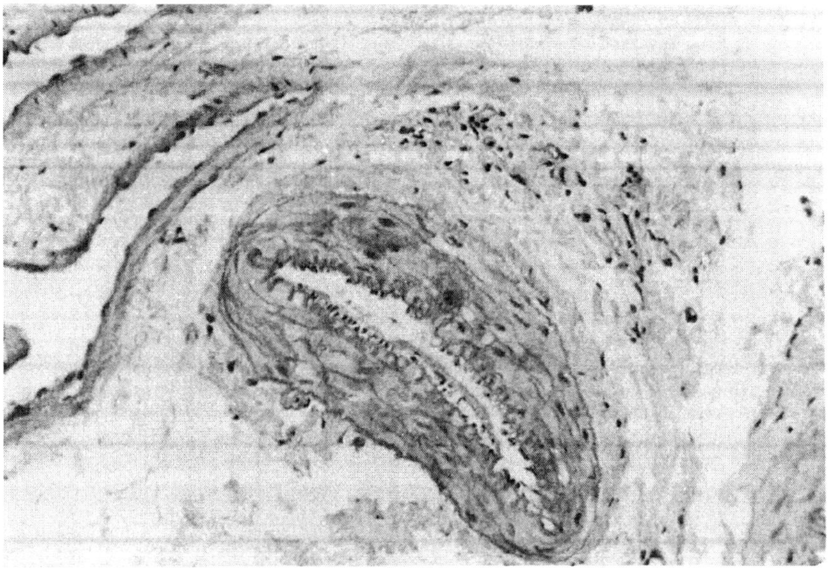

Figure 5B. Transversal section HTG kidney vessel.

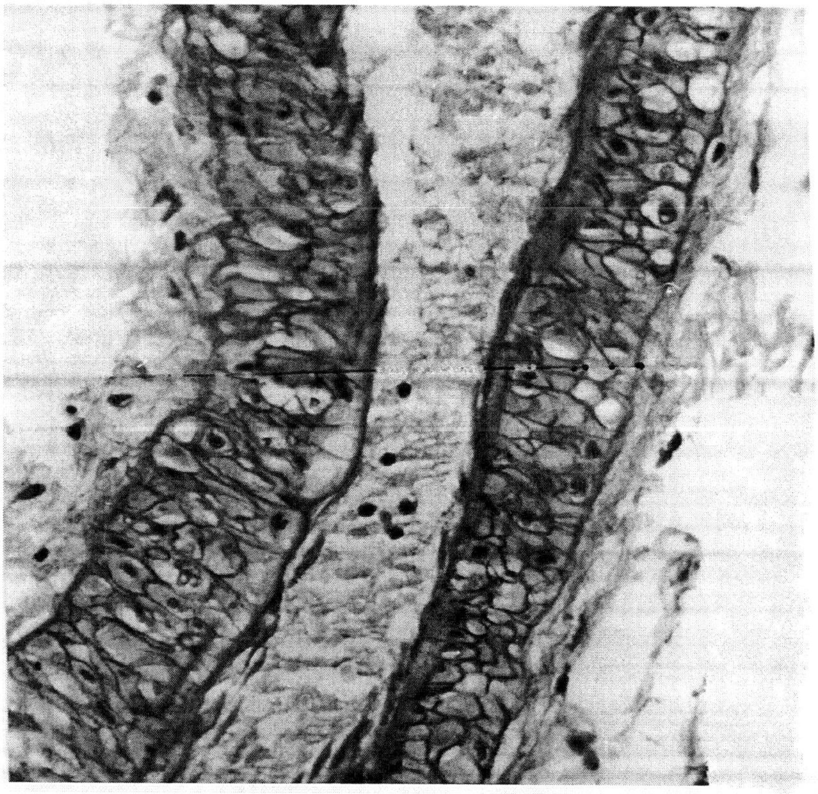

Figure 5C. Longitudinal section HTG kidney vessel

b) Salt- Sensitive Models. Dahl and DOCA (Deoxycorticosterone Acetate) + Salt Treated Animals

Dahl and collaborators were the first to observe that the development of genetic hypertension in the inbred strain of Dahl rats would take place more rapidly and acutely in some of the animals when given a high salt diet, whereas in others, receiving the same treatment, this did not occur [118,119]. The strain that developed malignant hypertension was called Dahl salt sensitive (DS) strain and the one that remained normotensive was named Dahl salt resistant (DR) strain (see Genetic models).

A few years later the same group hypothesized that a natriuretic circulating substance could be responsible for the increase in blood pressure in the DS rats [120]. Tobian et al demonstrated that there is a genetic alteration responsible for the disparity in responses between the two strains and it is to be found in the kidney [121].

Corticoids have been found to induce or potentiate high blood pressure and they have been used alone or in combination with high-salt treatments in some models, such as the dexamethasone-induced hypertension [122], the DOCA + salt treated rats, or DOCA + salt treated spontaneously hypertensive rats [123].

c) Obesity-Related Hypertension (Fat Diet)

Obesity is an important contributor to essential hypertension in humans. Data from the Framingham Heart Study suggest that essential hypertension in 78% of men and in 65% of women can be directly attributed to obesity [124]. However, the mechanism that link obesity with high blood pressure has not been fully understood.

One problem in the study of the mechanisms of obesity hypertension has been the lack of a suitable animal model. The ideal model would not only have the features of human hypertension but also allow the study of sequential changes in cardiovascular and kidney function that occur with weight gain. The genetic models of obesity do not mimic the changes observed in humans. For example, Zucker rats have decreased plasma renin activity (PRA) [125] as opposed to the high PRA observed in humans [126]. In contrast, diet-induced obese animal models appear to be the most relevant with regard to human obesity. Some of these models, such as dogs fed high fat diet that induces obesity-related hypertension [127, 128], obese rabbits [129,130] fed a high-fat diet, or rats with a chronic consumption of a high-fat and refined-carbohydrate diet [131], are used extensively to study obesity hypertension because they closely mimic some of the altered cardiovascular and renal systems found in obese humans.

A particularly interesting model of diet-induced obesity is Sprague-Dawley (SD) rats fed a purified moderately high-fat diet, which exhibit a bimodal pattern in body weight (BW) gain similar to that observed in humans [131, 132]. Approximately half the rats gain weight rapidly compared with chow-fed rats (obesity prone [OP]), whereas the other half gain BW at a rate similar to or lower than that of the chow-fed animals (obesity resistant [OR])[132]. This model enables one to distinguish between the factors related to a high-fat diet and obesity per se. In addition, when fat diet in this model was supplemented with salt (NaCl at 2 to 4 %), it induced an early increase in systolic blood pressure in OP but not in OR or C rats. In summary, high-salt diet accelerates the development but does not increase the severity of hypertension [133].

A rat model of fat diet-induced obesity also develops a close similarity to human obesity hypertension, namely activation of renin-angiotensin system, dyslipidemia, increased oxidative stress, and associated vascular and renal pathology. It also provides the ability to dissociate between the effect of moderately high fat diet (specific differences between OP, OR, and chow-fed C rats) and other factors specifically related to obese state (differences between OP and OR rats).

Another type of fat-diet supplemented with carbohydrate induces obesity-related hypertension in female Fischer rats through a mechanism involving an increased nitric oxide (NO) inactivation by reactive oxygen species (ROS) and functional NO deficiency [134]. Thus chronic consumption of a high fat diet supplemented with carbohydrate results in hypertension, which may be in part due to a combination of ROS-mediated NO inactivation and depressed renal nNOS protein expression.

Obesity hypertension is also associated with dyslipidemia, indicating low levels of HDL-cholesterol and higher levels of triglycerides [135]. Dyslipidemia occurring in the model of fat diet-induced obesity, is a common feature of obesity in humans and is frequently associated with hypertension [136]. In addition, hyperlipidemia combined with hypertension is associated with an increase in the level of circulating non-esterified fatty acids (NEFA), which has been postulated to contribute to increased blood pressure in obese hypertensive subjects [137]. Obese hypertensive patients have high fasting plasma NEFA concentrations, approximately double those of normotensive subjects, and raising NEFA acutely increases vascular reactivity to alpha-adrenergic agonists [138]. High levels of NEFA also enhance reflex vasoconstrictor responses in the peripheral circulation [138].

In addition to enhancing the acute pressor responses to adrenergic stimuli, it has been suggested that fatty acids activate the sympathetic nervous system indirectly through afferent pathways originating in the liver. Grekin et al. [139] found that acute infusion of free fatty acids into the portal or systemic veins increased blood pressure and heart rate in rats, and that these effects were abolished by adrenergic blockade.

Pulmonary Hypertension Models

The etiopathology of primary pulmonary hypertension (PH) is unknown, but many models exist that mimic some of its features. The species used are a large number, such as dogs, rabbits, calves, steers, sheep, pigs, broilers, and more frequently, rats and mice.

The means of inducing PH are quite varied, such as:

1. surgical procedures: pulmonary artery coarctation, inducing hypoxia [140], arteriovenous shunt [141];
2. mechanical: vascular obstruction with beads or some particles (microembolism) [142,143];
3. injection of toxic agents: monocrotaline [144], bacterial preparations (*E. Coli* endotoxin);
4. administration of vasoconstrictors: arginine-vasopressin;
5. environmental changes: hypoxia at high altitudes or induced by means of artificial atmospheres.

The involvement of endothelin in pulmonary hypertension was investigated in rats with medial hypertrophy and perivascular fibrosis of pulmonary arteries. The main pathological findings were elevated ET-1 levels and mRNA expression and type V collagen increase; the progression of hypertension seems associated with such pathological changes [145]. In this regard, in experiments carried out in pigs, it was observed that severe pulmonary hypertension developed after cardiopulmonary bypass, a situation that is encountered in patients undergoing such intervention. The hypertension was avoided by administration of bosentan, an endothelin receptor blocker [146].

In hypoxia-induced pulmonary hypertension, paradoxically, while lung angiotensin converting enzyme (ACE) activity is diminished in chronic hypoxia, ACE inhibitors also reduce it. The participation of Ang II, ACE and the type 1 receptor (AT1) expression in the development of the condition has been explored by hemodynamic tests and estimates of whole lung ACE activity and local pulmonary vascular ACE expression. [147]. The experimental results showed that by the fifth day of evolution only 50 % of ACE total lung activity remained, although the effect was not generalized. There was an increase in ACE mRNA in alveolar ducts and walls of small pulmonary arteries.

Environmentally- Induced Hypertension

There are other models, less frequently used, in which hypertension is induced in rats by means of stressful environmental conditions such as mild cold temperatures (5 ^{0}C) or crowding.

Models of Experimental Gene-Manipulated Hypertension

Genetically Hypertensive Mice

With the advances in mouse molecular genetics and physiology during the last decade, the mouse has become the animal model of choice for studying the genetic basis of many diseases. Terms such as "transgenic" and "knockout" have become part of the language used in most research laboratories that are investigating human diseases [147]. These terms are related to the two most commonly used methods for analyzing the function of a gene in vivo: overexpression (transgenic mouse) and disruption (knockout mouse). Hypertension is a cardiovascular disease and many factors contribute to its development, including environment, diet, daily stress and genetics. Several candidate genes for manipulation which are associated with hypertension in animal models or in man have been discovered in recent years. To study the function of these genes in vivo, transgenic animals have been shown to be very useful models.

Molecular and physiological evaluations of transgenic and knockout animals have provided a great quantity of information about the mechanisms of blood pressure regulation and the development and maintenance of hypertension. The choice of genes being investigated in relationship to hypertension was governed by the knowledge of systems regulating vascular and renal physiology. Thus, most of the focus was given to the renin-angiotensin system (RAS). Apart from the RAS, other systems known to regulate vascular tone and/or electrolyte and fluid homeostasis were also analyzed, using transgenic and knockout approaches. The experience of using drugs for the control and treatment of hypertension for many years, has facilitated the identification of which genes must be targeted for studying hypertension, such as a gene coding for angiotensin 1 receptors (AT1R), angiotensinogen (AGT), angiotensin converting enzyme (ACE) and adrenergic receptors implicated in the regulation of blood pressure.

Experimental Design to Identify a Candidate Gene

The experimental design to identify a candidate gene that participates in high BP, was elaborated by looking at the separation patterns of genetic markers in correlation with BP [148]. Another type of analytic approach is to look directly for gene variations that correlate with the phenotype as described for renin gene variation in rats [149] and polymorphism in the human angiotensinogen (methionine *versus* threonine at position 235). Subjects who inherit the threonine variety are prone to develop higher BP and higher plasma angiotensinogen than those who inherit the methionine variety [150]. In general, analytic experiments demonstrate a correlation between specific genetic variants and BP. However, it is not easy to prove that the observed change in a candidate gene is the cause of high BP. To prove causation in a complex system requires experiments designed to detect the effect of changing only one variable at a time. Properly designed synthetic experiments in the mouse with a targeted gene meet this requirement and allow proof of genetic causation. In carrying out a synthetic experiment of this type, it is first necessary to pick a test gene based on previously acquired data from physiological or analytical experiments. For example, in the case of angiotensinogen, the previous analytic experiments suggested that it would be a valuable test to generate mice with threonine at position 235 instead of methionine. However, in practice, a simple experiment of this type is not possible in the mouse because there is no methionine at position 235 in mouse angiotensinogen.

Gene Titration

A "gene titration" method was performed to alter the plasma level of angiotensinogen by genetic manipulation, because of the association with the difference in the plasma concentration of angiotensinogen and the methionine/threonine difference [151]. Gene titration enables one to vary the expression of a gene by generating animals which have different numbers of copies of the gene. To generate animals having different gene copy numbers for a gene titration experiment, both gene-disrupted and gene duplicated animals are needed. In a gene duplication experiment, the DNA fragments used to make the targeting construct are assembled in a different arrangement, and the result is different. Thus, during homologous recombination with this type of construct, the gap between the 59 and 39 ends of the gene fragments that were used for making the targeting construct is first filled, and the crossover then continues in a manner that generates two copies of the gene in one chromosome. Animals with one gene copy are the heterozygotes for gene disruption. Animals with two copies are the wild type. Animals with three and four copies are heterozygotes and homozygotes for gene duplication.

Gene Disruption (Zero Copy)

The generation of animals homozygous for gene disruption ("knockout" animals) consists in determining the effects of complete absence of a gene product . A great deal of information on gene function has been obtained from zero-copy animals. They can also be obtained as a by-product from one-copy animals made in the course of a gene titration experiment.

Candidate Gene

Several genes related to BP control have been disrupted, and some others have also been duplicated. The genes can be divided into three groups, according to the changes in BP, which accompany quantitative changes in their expression. In the first group of genes, BP changes are observed when expression of the gene or the number of gene copies is changed. In the second group of genes, changes in gene copy number do not change BP unless another environmental factor is changed. BP increases in the heterozygotes for disruption, but only when the animals are fed a high salt diet. In the third group of genes, changes in their expression did not induce any difference in BP with or without additional environmental factors, because their function is not directly related to cardiovascular or renal functions.

Natriuretic Peptide System

Gene Titration of the Natriuretic Peptide Receptor 1

The natriuretic peptide receptor 1 (Npr1; also referred to as Npra or GC-A), induces the biologic functions of both the atrial natriuretic peptide (ANP) and the type B natriuretic peptide (BNP). Ligand binding activates the guanylate cyclase (GC) activity of the receptor. As the natriuretic peptide receptor 1 (*Npr1*) gene copy number is increased, a linear progressive increase in GC activity is noted [153]. The BP of mice having one copy of the *Npr1* gene averaged 9 mmHg above normal and mice having three copies of the *Npr1* gene had BP 5 mmHg below normal [152]. These results establish a clear causation and prove that a decrease in the expression of the *Npr1* gene causes BP to rise while increasing expression causes a decrease in BP.

Gene "Knockout" of Npr1

Hearts from *Npr1* zero-copy animals show severe cardiac hypertrophy, being nearly twice as large as those of wild type animals [153]. Although hypertension is a known risk factor for ventricular hypertrophy, the degree of hypertrophy in the *Npr1* zero-copy animals is greater than that expected from their high BP, because other mouse models with a similar degree of hypertension do not show this degree of cardiac hypertrophy; comparable models include endothelial-type nitric oxide synthase zero-copy mice and angiotensinogen four copy mice. The mechanism leading to the cardiac hypertrophy of the *Npr1* zero-copy animals is under investigation. These observations suggest that it would be useful to look for any unique variations of the natriuretic peptide receptor gene in human patients with cardiac hypertrophy.

Atrial Natriuretic Peptide

Changes in the amount of ANP, one of the ligands of *Npr1*, were also studied by gene disruption. The BP levels of heterozygote and wild-type animals did not vary when they were fed regular chow (0.5% NaCl) [154]. However, when the animals were fed a high salt diet (8% NaCl), the BP of heterozygote animals was increased by 28 mmHg, while the BP of wild-type animals was not changed [154]. These results demonstrate that a genetic reduction in ANP expression can cause salt-sensitive hypertension. Conversely, transgenic mice over-expressing ANP or BNP show lower BP [155, 156].

Renin-Angiotensin System

Gene Titration of Angiotensinoge

Angiotensinogen (AGT) is produced in the liver and secreted into the blood where it is broken up by renin. This reaction yields the inactive peptide angiotensin I, from which angiotensin II is formed by the action of angiotensin-converting enzyme. Angiotensin II, the active peptide, is a potent vasoconstrictor that is also able to stimulate the synthesis and secretion of aldosterone in the adrenal glomerulosa. The levels of AGT in the plasma progressively increase with the increase in the gene copy number in a gene titration experiment [151]. In this case, BP rises linearly as the number of copies of the *Agt* gene increases [151]. So this experiment demonstrates that different levels of the functions of the *Agt* gene will directly cause significant changes in BP. Subsequent to this work, a base pair difference was found between the promoter of the human 235 threonine type of *AGT* gene and the 235 methionine type, which changes the effectiveness of the promoter in the expected direction [157]. Tanimoto and coworkers have also disrupted the *Agt* gene, but they did not observe any differences in BP between the wild type and the heterozygous animals [158]. The genetic heterogeneity inherent in this scheme might have made the detection of the subtle difference between the wild-type mice and the heterozygotes difficult.

Kidney from Angiotensinogen Zero-Copy Mice

Homozygotes for disruption of the *Agt* gene not only have reduced BP, but also have thickened arterial walls in their kidneys accompanied by an increased number of smooth muscle cells, atrophy of the cortex with interstitial fibrosis, and an infiltration of chronic inflammatory cells [151, 159]. Similar observations have been reported in the kidneys from angiotensin-converting enzyme zero-copy mice [160] and double knockout mice for type 1A and 1B receptors for angiotensin II [161], indicating that the renin-angiotensin system is indispensable for preserving normal kidney form, including post-natal development and function.

Renin

Some strains of mice (including C56BL/6) have one copy of renin gene (*Ren-1*c) per haploid genome, and other strains (including 129) naturally have two closely linked renin genes (*Ren-1*d and *Ren-2*). Clark and coworkers have disrupted the *Ren-1*d gene and found that this decreased BP in heterozygote females and homozygote females, respectively, by 8 and 13 mmHg compared to wild type [162]. However, they did not find any difference in BP of the males. Disruption of the *Ren-2* gene did not lead to any changes in BP [163].

Angiotensin-Converting Enzyme

The angiotensin-converting enzyme (*Ace*) gene consists of two homologous regions and codes for two isozymes: somatic ACE and testis ACE [14-166]. The testis-specific form of ACE has its own promoter in intron 12 and is encoded by the 3'- half of the gene; it is found only in postmeiotic spermatogenic cells and sperm [167]. When the *Ace* gene was disrupted so as to prevent the synthesis of both isozymes, the BP levels of heterozygotes were not different from wild type, despite the reduction of plasma ACE levels to 50% normal [22]. Similarly, when the *Ace* gene was duplicated, BP levels of three-copy heterozygotes and four-copy homozygotes were normal, despite their increased plasma ACE (150, 200% normal) [168]. Thus, the gene titration experiment shows that changes in the copy number of the *Ace* gene do not affect BP. This result suggests that the genetically determined quantitative changes in ACE known to be prevalent in the general human population are unlikely to affect BP.

Angiotensin II Receptors

Three different receptors for angiotensin II have been identified: type 1A, type 1B, and type 2. Each of these receptors is encoded by a different gene in different chromosomes. The majority of the known physiological effects of angiotensin II are mediated by the type 1A receptor. The gene coding for the angiotensin II type 1A receptor (*Agtr1a*) has been disrupted by two groups, and both male and female heterozygotes show about a 12-mmHg decrease in BP compared with wild-type animals [169, 170]. Disruption of the type 1B receptor gene alone did not show any change in BP [171]. The type 2 receptor of angiotensin II is encoded on the X chromosome. The gene (*Agtr2*) has been disrupted by two groups: Ichiki and coworkers found a 13-mmHg increase in BP in their zero-copy animals, rather than the expected decrease [172].

Adrenergic Receptors

Mice with altered α2-adrenergic receptor genes have also become important tools in elucidating the subtype-specific functions of the three α2-adrenergic receptor subtypes, because of the lack of sufficiently subtype-selective pharmacological agents. Mice with a deletion (knockout) of the α2A-, α2B-, or α2C-gene as well as a point mutation of the α2A-gene (α2A-D79N) and a 3-fold over-expression of the α2C-gene have been generated [173]. α2-Adrenergic agonists activate α2- receptors in the rostral ventrolateral medulla, decreasing sympathetic outflow, which causes a reduction in arterial blood pressure and heart rate [174]. In addition to these centrally mediated responses, there is a transient hypertensive response caused by α2-adrenergic receptor-mediated vasoconstriction of vascular smooth muscle. The hypotensive response to administration of α2-adrenergic receptor agonists was abolished, demonstrating that the α2A-subtype plays a principal role in this response [175]. Furthermore, the hypertensive response was eliminated in α2B-KO mice, and the hypotensive effect was immediate and accentuated. The α2A-subtype appears to play a role in vasoconstriction at least in some vascular compartments, because the hypertensive response in α2A-D79N mice was absent when the agonist was administered through the femoral artery [175]. In contrast, the α2B-adrenergic receptor appears to be the main mediator of the pressor response that results from α2-adrenergic agonist administration.

Dopamine Receptors

The dopaminergic system in the central nervous system (CNS) may participate in the regulation of systemic blood pressure. Dopamine 'D2-like' (D2, D3 and D4) receptors, rather than 'D1-like' (D1 and D5) receptors, are involved in the CNS regulation of blood pressure; post-synaptic D2-like receptors increase blood pressure, while presynaptic D2-like receptors (the predominant action) produce the opposite effect. Thus, increased blood pressure occurs after either blockade of D1-like receptors or of dopamine production in rats or after disruption of the D1 receptor or the D3 receptor gene in mice [176].

Nitric Oxide Synthase

There are three types of nitric oxide synthase (NOS), 1 (neuronal), 2 (inducible) and 3 (endothelial). The endothelial type of NOS expressed in endothelial cells produces nitric oxide, which reduces vascular tone. Heterozygotes for the *Nos3* gene disruption show a tendency toward higher BP, but the data does not reach significance [177]. Homozygotes for inactivation of the *Nos3* gene have 18 mmHg higher BP levels compared with wild-type animals [177, 178]. In contrast, disruption of either the neuronal [179] or the inducible type of NOS does not cause significant changes in BP.

Targeted disruption of eNOS gene results in mice with increased susceptibility to hypoxic-induced PH [180]. These studies conclude that eNOS-derived nitric oxide is an important modulator of the pulmonary vascular response to chronic hypoxia, and more than 50% of eNOS expression is required to maintain normal pulmonary vascular tone [180].

Endothelin-1

Interesting unexpected results following disruption of the gene coding for endothelin-1 have been reported by Kurihara and co-workers [181]. Homozygotes as a result of disruption of the endothelin-1 gene died soon after birth because of craniofacial abnormalities. Heterozygotes had 11 mmHg higher BP levels compared with wild-type animals instead of the lower BP anticipated. This observation that reduction of endothelin leads to an increase in BP was unexpected, because of the known potent pressor effects of endothelin-1.

B2 Receptor for Bradykinin

Bradykinin modulates water and electrolyte metabolism by increasing intracellular calcium activity via the bradykinin B2 receptor, which leads to activation of the endothelial type of NOS and also to prostaglandin synthesis. These changes lower BP. The results of de-activating the *Bdkrb2* gene have been reported by two groups. Madeddu and co-workers reported that heterozygotes for disruption of this gene did not show significantly higher BP compared with wild-type animals, whereas the homozygotes had 15 to 19 mmHg higher BP than wild-type mice or heterozygotes [182]. If the animals were fed a high salt diet, they showed much higher BP, and then even the heterozygotes had higher BP than wild-type. Alfie *et al.* observed higher BP in homozygotes and only when they were fed a high salt diet [183].

5-Lipoxygenase

Mice with targeted disruption of 5-lipoxygenase (Knockout) were exposed to chronic hypoxia [184]. These mice developed less right ventricular hypertrophy than matched controls, supporting the hypothesis that 5-lipoxygenase is involved in pulmonary vascular tone in rodent hypoxia models. Pulmonary hypertension (PH) refers to a spectrum of diseases where the pulmonary artery pressure is elevated [185]. Familial primary pulmonary hypertension has been undoubtedly associated with mutations in the gene coding for bone morphogenetic protein type II receptor (BMPR2) [186, 187]. This has generated extreme interest in investigating the alterations of vasoactive related genes. Animal models, using transgenics, or targeted disruption of genes involved in PH, have been developed. Genomic approaches to the investigation of PH in animals are useful to elucidate the complex mechanism of the pathobiology of pulmonary hypertensive diseases.

Prostacyclin-Synthase (PGIS) and Prostacyclin Receptor

Transgenic mice (PGIS+) and non-transgenic littermates (PGIS–) were subjected to a simulated altitude of 17,000 feet for 5 weeks. After exposure to chronic hypobaric hypoxia, PGIS+ mice have lower right ventricular systolic pressure than do PGIS – mice. The PGIS+ mice were thus protected from the development of PH after exposure to chronic hypobaric hypoxia. PGIS plays a major role in modifying the pulmonary vascular response to chronic hypoxia. Additional data, investigating the prostacyclin receptor knockout mice, support the important role of these receptors in the modulation of PH [188].

11-Hydroxysteroid Dehydrogenase Type 1 (11-HSD1)

Obesity is closely associated with the metabolic syndrome, a combination of disorders including insulin resistance, diabetes, dyslipidemia, and hypertension. The enzyme 11®-hydroxysteroid dehydrogenase type 1 (11®-HSD1) regenerates active cortisol from inactive 11-keto forms, and aP2-HSD1 mice, with relative transgenic overexpression of this enzyme in fat cells, develop visceral obesity with insulin resistance and dyslipidemia. aP2-HSD1 mice have high arterial blood pressure (BP). The mice have increased sensitivity to dietary salt and increased plasma levels of angiotensinogen, angiotensin II, and aldosterone. This hypertension is eliminated by selective angiotensin II receptor AT-1 antagonist at a low dose that does not affect BP in non-Tg littermates. The longterm hypertension is further reflected by an appreciable hypertrophy and hyperplasia of the distal tubule epithelium of the nephron, resembling salt-sensitive or angiotensin II–mediated hypertension. Taken together, our findings suggest that over-expression of 11®-HSD1 in fat is sufficient to cause salt-sensitive hypertension mediated by an activated RAS. [189]

Leptin

The interest in leptin focused initially on appetite, metabolism, and adiposity, but there is mounting evidence that leptin participates in sympathetic and arterial pressure regulation and in vascular biology and that it increases sympathetic activity in the kidney and extremities [190]. This sympatho-excitatory action would be expected to increase arterial pressure. Leptin-deficient *ob/ob* mice have delayed and unstable thrombus formation after arterial injury [191, 192]. Leptin normalizes this phenotype. So leptin, like insulin, has emerged as a metabolic hormone that contributes importantly to regulation of vascular biology. Given that leptin produces both pressor (sympathetic activation) and depressor (increased NO) actions, the integrated actions of leptin on arterial pressure are not predictable. In acute doses leptin does not consistently increase arterial pressure, [190] but chronic infusion of leptin increases arterial pressure in rats despite weight loss, which would be expected to lower arterial pressure [193]. In addition, transgenic mice over-expressing leptin have significantly higher arterial pressure than wild-type control mice despite decreases in body fat. [194]. These increases in arterial pressure are accompanied by increased urinary norepinephrine and are normalized after acute alpha adrenergic or ganglionic blockade [194]. These observations suggest an integrated sympathetically mediated pressor response to leptin. Leptin-deficient, obese *ob/ob* mice have slightly lower arterial pressure than their wild-type controls, despite marked obesity, that would be expected to increase arterial pressure [195]. Administration of leptin to the *ob/ob* mice (so-called leptin reconstitution) increases arterial pressure despite decreases in food intake and body weight [194]. This suggests a physiological role for leptin in arterial pressure regulation. In contrast to the leptin-deficient *ob/ob* mice, agouti yellow obese mice have partial leptin resistance, compensatory hyperleptinemia, and elevated arterial pressure [195] There is evidence that the elevated leptin contributes to the increase in arterial pressure [194].

Uncoupling Proteins (UCP)

Uncoupling proteins cause energy derived from metabolism of food to be dissipated as heat rather than stored as high-energy phosphates. Uncoupling protein-1 (UCP-1) is normally expressed only in brown adipose tissue where it regulates thermogenic metabolism. A recent study by Li et al [196] demonstrated that transgenic overexpression of mitochondrial UCP-1 in skeletal muscle increased skeletal muscle oxygen consumption (metabolic rate) without altering food intake. This was accompanied by weight loss, increased insulin sensitivity, and resistance to high-fat diet–induced obesity. Transgenic overexpression of human UCP-3 in skeletal muscle also promoted weight loss despite hyperphagia [197]. These studies suggest that enhancing respiratory uncoupling in skeletal muscle could potentially reduce obesity and its metabolic consequences. In the present study, Bernal-Mizrachi et al [198] again report that transgenic over-expression of UCP-1 in skeletal muscle of agouti yellow obese mice increased metabolism, promoted weight loss, and increased insulin sensitivity. The major new finding was that skeletal muscle over-expression of UCP-1 decreased arterial pressure, serum leptin, and urinary catecholamines. In the transgenic agouti mice over-expressing UCP-1, superimposed administration of leptin increased arterial pressure. This was not observed with leptin administration in the non-transgenic agouti obese mice. Based on this constellation of findings, it was concluded that "skeletal muscle respiratory uncoupling lowers blood pressure through a leptin-dependent mechanism and prevents insulin resistance in genetic obesity."

Transgenic Hypertensive Rats

Transgenic techniques can be applied in many species and most frequently transgenic mice have been used. Since hypertension is not well defined in the mouse, the use of transgenic rats has been very helpful in the investigation of hypertension.

The production of transgenic rats by DNA micro-injection into fertilized ova has also become an established procedure, although fewer than 20 lines have been described [199]. Overall, transgenic rats remain more difficult to produce than transgenic mice, but satisfactory yields have been obtained by several laboratories. One of the first applications was to transfect the *Ren-2* mouse renin gene into Sprague-Dawley rats. These rats developed a severe form of renin-dependent hypertension and were used for the study of the mechanisms and consequences of this monogenic hypertension.

Because rats are more suitable than mice for a number of experimental settings often employed in cardiovascular research, transgenic rat strain TGR(mREN2)27 harboring the murine Ren-2 gene was developed [200]. These transgenic rats develop fulminant hypertension at an early age, despite low levels of renin in plasma and kidney. In addition, high expression of the transgene in a number of extrarenal tissues is associated with increased local formation of angiotensin II. Thus the TGR(mREN2)27 rat represents a model of hypertension with a defined genetic background. These rats develop severe hypertension, which reaches 200 mm Hg and higher at 8 weeks of age in the heterozygous animal. Homozygous rats develop even higher blood pressures than heterozygous animals and have a higher mortality rate. They develop pathomorphologic alterations which are characteristic of systemic hypertension. The transgenic rats are characterized by unchanged or even suppressed concentrations of active renin, angiotensin I (ANG I), ANG II, and angiotensinogen compared to transgene-negative littermates. In contrast, plasma levels of inactive renin (prorenin) are much higher in TGR (mREN)27 rats than in control animals. [201].

Treatment with ACE inhibitors or angiotensin II receptor antagonists such as losartan is extremely efficient, which could mean that hypertension in this model is mediated through ANG II.

Conclusion

Many common kidney diseases as well as hypertension arise from different combinations of genetic variants and gene–environment interactions. Animal models allow controlled matings to be used leading to the detection of synergistic or antagonistic interactions between mutant genes free from all other genetic variations and unintentional variations in environmental factors. Yet the effects of intentional variations in environmental factors such as dietary salt can easily be determined, thus providing opportunities to evaluate the interaction between gene variation and environment. These types of study help us to understand the pathophysiology of common diseases with complicated patterns of inheritance, to develop useful genetic screening tests, and identify potential targets for therapies. Indeed gene therapy for hypertension is needed for the next generation of antihypertensive drugs. Current drugs, although effective, have poor compliance, are expensive and short-lasting (hours or one day). Gene therapy offers a way to produce long-lasting antihypertensive effects (weeks, months or years). Strategies to use antisense oligodeoxynucleotides (AS-ODN), and antisense DNA delivered in viral vectors, to inhibit genes associated with vasoconstrictive properties, are under intense investigation. AS-ODNs are short, single-stranded DNA that can be injected in pure form or in liposomes. AS-ODNs, targeted to AT1 receptors (AT1R), angiotensinogen (AGT), angiotensin converting enzyme (ACE) and beta 1-adrenergic receptors effectively reduce high blood pressure in rat models of hypertension (SHR, 2K-1C and cold-induced) [202]. The effects can last up to one month when delivered with liposomes. No side effects or toxic effects have been detected and repeated injections can be given.

REFERENCES

[1] Kaplan NM. The deadly quartet. Upper. body obesity, glucose intolerance, hypertriglyceridemia, and hypertension. *Arch Intern Med.* 1989; 149 (7): 1514-1520.

[2] Pinto YM, Paul M, Ganten D. Lessons from rat models of hypertension: from Goldblatt to genetic engineering. *Cardiovasc Res.* 1998; 39(1): 77- 88.

[3] Phelan EL. The New Zealand strain of rats with genetic hypertension. New Zealand Med. J. 1968; 67: 334- 344.

[4] Harris EL, Phelan EL, Thompson CM, Millar JA, Grigor MR. Heart mass and blood pressure have separate genetic determinants in the New Zealand genetically hypertensive (GH) rat. *J Hypertens.* 1995 ;13(4):397- 404.

[5] al-Barazanji KA, Balment RJ. Renal, endocrine and vascular effects of atrial natriuretic peptide in a novel vasopressin-deficient genetically hypertensive strain of rat. *Exp Physiol.* 1995;80(2):275 - 284.

[6] Ledingham JM, Laverty R. Nitric oxide synthase inhibition with N omega. nitro. L. arginine methyl ester affects blood pressure and cardiovascular structure in the genetically hypertensive rat strain. *Clin Exp Pharmacol Physiol.* 1997 ;24(6): 433- 435.

[7] Orange SJ, Ledingham JM, Laverty R. Cardiovascular effects of chronic nitric oxide synthase inhibition in genetically hypertensive rats. *Clin Exp Pharmacol Physiol* 2000; 27 (7): 488- 493.

[8] Hamlyn JM. Acquired and inherited forms of ouabain. induced hypertension: significance and relationship to other models. *Clin Exper Hypertens* 2003; 25 (5): 289-290.

[9] Okamoto K. Spontaneous hypertension in rats. *Int. Rev. Exp. Pathol.* 1969; 7: 227- 270.

[10] Sano H, Okamoto H, Kitabatake A, Iizuka K, Murakami T, Kawaguchi H. Increased mRNA expression of cardiac renin. angiotensin system and collagen synthesis in spontaneously hypertensive rats. *Mol Cell Biochem.* 1998;178(1. 2):51. 58.

[11] Baños G, El Hafidi M, Franco M. Oxidative stress and cardiovascular physiopathology. *Curr Topics Pharmacol.* 2000; 5: 1-17.

[12] Ito H, Torii M, Suzuki T. Comparative study on free radical injury in the endothelium of SHR and WKY aorta. *Clin Exp Pharmacol Physiol Suppl.* 1995; 22(1): S157- S159.

[13] Swei A, Lacy F, DeLano FA, Schmid. Schonbein GW. Oxidative stress in the Dahl hypertensive rat. *Hypertension.* 1997; 30(6):1628-1633.

[14] Liu H, Ledingham JM, Mullaney I, Laverty R. Endothelial function in mesenteric resistance arteries from the genetically hypertensive rat. *Clin Exp Pharmacol Physiol.* 2002 ;29(5. 6):405- 411.

[15] Hohl CM, Hu B, Fertel RH, Russell JC, McCune SA, Altschuld RA. Effects of obesity and hypertension on ventricular myocytes: comparison of cells from adult SHHF/Mcc-cp and JCR:LA- cp rats.*Cardiovasc Res.* 1993;27(2):238- 242.

[16] Heyen JR, Blasi ER, Nikula K, Rocha R, Daust HA, Frierdich G et al. Structural, functional, and molecular characterization of the SHHF model of heart failure. *Am J Physiol Heart Circ Physiol.* 2002;283(5):H1775- H1784.

[17] Rapp JP, Dene H. Development and characteristics of inbred strains of Dahl salt-sensitive and salt. resistant rats. *Hypertension* 1985; 7 : 340-349.

[18] Kurtz TW, Morris RC Jr. Hypertension in the recently weaned Dahl salt- sensitive rat despite a diet deficient in sodium chloride. *Science.* 1985 Nov 15;230(4727):808- 810.

[19] Gordon FJ, Mark AL. Mechanism of impaired baroreflex control in pre-hypertensive Dahl salt- sensitive rats.*Circ Res.* 1984;54(4):378- 387.

[20] Hirata Y, Tobian L, Simon G, Iwai J. Hypertension-producing factor in serum of hypertensive Dahl salt-sensitive rats. *Hypertension* 1984 ;6(5):709- 716.

[21] Jain M, Liao R, Podesser BK, Ngoy S, Apstein CS, Eberli FR. Influence of gender on the response to hemodynamic overload after myocardial infarction. *Am J Physiol* 2002; 283 (6): H2544-H2550.

[22] Seki S, Nagai M, Takeda H, Onodera T, Okazaki F, Taniguchi M et al. Impaired Ca2+ handling in perfused hypertrophic hearts from Dahl salt-sensitive rats. *Hypertens Res.* 2003; 26(8):643-653.

[23] Manning RD, Meng S, Tian N. Renal and vascular oxidative stress and salt-sensitivity of arterial pressure. *Acta Physiol Scand.* 2003 ;179(3):243-250.

[24] Meng S, Cason GW, Gannon AW, Racusen LC, Manning RD Jr. Oxidative stress in Dahl salt-sensitive hypertension. *Hypertension.* 2003 ;41(6):1346-1352.

[25] Zhou MS, Adam AG, Jaimes EA, Raij L In salt-sensitive hypertension, increased superoxide production is linked to functional upregulation of angiotensin II. *Hypertension.* 2003 ;42(5):945- 951.

[26] Zhou MS, Adam AG, Jaimes EA, Raij L In salt-sensitive hypertension, increased superoxide production is linked to functional upregulation of angiotensin II. *Hypertension.* 2003 ;42(5):945- 951.

[27] Vokurkova M, Dobesova Z, Kunes J, Zicha J. Membrane ion transport in erythrocytes of salt- hypertensive Dahl rats and their F2 hybrids: the importance of cholesterol. *Hypertens Res.* 2003 ;26(5):397-404.

[28] Unlap MT, Bates E, Williams C, Komlosi P, Williams I, Kovacs G, et al. Na+/Ca2+ exchanger: target for oxidative stress in salt-sensitive hypertension. *Hypertension.* 2003;42(3):363-368.

[29] Stolba P, Dobesova Z, Husek P, Opltova H, Zicha J, Vrana A et al. The hypertriglyceridemic rat as a genetic model of hypertension and diabetes. *Life Sci.* 1992;51(10):733-740.

[30] Heller J, Hellerova S, Dobesova Z, Kunes J, Zicha J. The Prague Hypertensive Rat: a new model of genetic hypertension. *Clin Exp Hypertens.* 1993;15(5):807-818.

[31] Zicha J, Dobesova Z, Kunes J. Plasma triglycerides and red cell ion transport alterations in genetically hypertensive rats. *Hypertension.* 1997; 30(3 Pt 2):636-640.

[32] Kunes J, Mazeaud MM, Devynck MA, Zicha J. Platelet hypoaggregability in hereditary hypertriglyceridemic rats: relation to plasma triglycerides. *Thromb Res.* 1997; 88(4):347-353.

[33] Kunes J, Devynck MA, Zicha J. Chronic changes in plasma triglyceride levels do modify platelet membrane microviscosity in rats. *Life Sci.* 2000;67(8):959-967.

[34] Brown DM, Provoost AP, Lander ES, Jacob HJ. Renal disease susceptibility and hypertension are under independent genetic control in the Fawn-Hooded rat. *Nature Genet.* 1996; 12: 44-51.

[35] Van Dokkum RP, Jacob HJ, Provoost AP. Genetic differences define severity of renal damage after L-NAME-induced hypertension in rats. *J Am Soc Nephrol.* 1998; 9(3):363-371.

[36] van Dokkum RP, Sun CW, Provoost AP, Jacob HJ, Roman RJ. Altered renal hemodynamics and impaired myogenic responses in the Fawn-hooded rat. *Am J Physiol.* 1999 ; 276(3 Pt 2):R855-R863.

[37] Van Dokkum RP, Alonso-Galicia M, Provoost AP, Jacob HJ, Roman RJ. Impaired autoregulation of renal blood flow in the Fawn-hooded rat. *Am J Physiol.* 1999; 276(1 Pt 2):R189-R196.

[38] Weichert W, Paliege A, Provoost AP, Bachmann S. Upregulation of juxtaglomerular NOS1 and COX-2 precedes glomerulosclerosis in Fawn-hooded hypertensive rats. *Am J Physiol Renal Physiol.* 2001; 280(4):F706-F714.

[39] Koletsky S. New type of spontaneously hypertensive rats with hyperlipidemia and endocrine gland defects. In: K. Okamoto ed. Spontaneous Hypertension: its Pathogenesis and Complications,Tokyo: Igaku Shoin Ltd. 1972: 194-197.

[40] Ishizuka T, Ernsberger P, Liu S, Bedol D, Lehman TM, Koletsky RJ, et al. Phenotypic consequences of a nonsense mutation in the leptin receptor gene (fak) in obese spontaneously hypertensive Koletsky rats (SHROB). *J Nutr.* 1998;128(12):2299-2306.

[41] Divisova J, Kazdova L, Hubova M, Meschisvili E. Relationship between insulin resistance and muscle triglyceride content in nonobese and obese experimental models of insulin resistance syndrome. *Ann N Y Acad Sci.* 2002; 967:440-445.

[42] Velliquette RA, Koletsky RJ, Ernsberger P. Plasma glucagon and free fatty acid responses to a glucose load in the obese spontaneous hypertensive rat (SHROB) model of metabolic syndrome X. *Exp Biol Med.* 2002 ;227(3):164-170.

[43] Okamoto K, Yamori Y, Nagaoka A. Establishment of stroke-prone spontaneously hypertensive rat (SHR). *Circ. Res.* 1974; 34-35 (suppl.): I 143-I 153.

[44] Gigante B, Rubattu S, Stanzione R, Lombardi A, Baldi A, Baldi F. et al. Contribution of genetic factors to renal lesions in the stroke. prone spontaneously hypertensive rat. *Hypertension* 2003; 42(4):702-706.

[45] Okamoto K, Hazama F, Yamori Y, Haebara H, Nagaoka A. Pathogenesis and prevention of stroke in spontaneously hypertensive rats. *Clin Sci Mol Med Suppl.* 1975; 2: 161s-163s.

[46] Manning RD, Meng S, Tian N. Renal and vascular oxidative stress and salt-sensitivity of arterial pressure. *Acta Physiol Scand.* 2003;179(3):243-250.

[47] Tofovic SP, Kusaka H, Jackson EK, Bastacky SI. Renal and metabolic effects of caffeine in obese diabetic hypertensive ZSF Rats. *Renal Failure.* 2001; 232: 159-173.

[48] Tofovic SP, Jackson EK Rat models of the metabolic syndrome. *Methods Mol Med.* 2003; 86: 29-46.

[49] Tofovic SP, Dubey RK, Jackson EK. 2. Hydroxyestradiol attenuates the development of obesity, the metabolic syndrome, and vascular and renal dysfunction in obese ZSF1 rats. *J Pharmacol Exp Ther.* 2001; 299(3): 973-977.

[50] Clark J, Palmer CJ, Shaw WN. The diabetic Zucker fatty rat. *Proc. Soc. Exp. Biol. Med.* 1983; 173: 68-75.

[51] Morrison RG, Carpenter AB, Moore SK, Mangiarua EI, Valentovic MA, Walker EM Jr, et al. Increased sensitivity of the obese Zucker rat to deoxycorticosterone-salt-induced hypertension. *J Hypertens.* 2002; 20(11): 2247-2255.

[52] Kawaguchi M, Koshimura K, Murakami Y, Tsumori M, Gonda T, Kato Y. Antihypertensive effect of insulin via nitric oxide production in the Zucker diabetic

fatty rat, an animal model for non-insulin-dependent diabetes mellitus. *Eur J Endocrinol.* 1999; 140(4): 341-349.

[53] Kawaguchi M, Koshimura K, Sohmiya M, Murakami Y, Gonda T, Kato Y. Effect of insulin on nitric oxide synthase-like immunostaining of arteries in various organs in Zucker diabetic fatty rats. *Eur J Endocrinol.* 2001;145(3):343-349.

[54] Karagiannis J, Reid JJ, Darby I, Roche P, Rand MJ, Li CG. Impaired nitric oxide function in the basilar artery of the obese Zucker rat. *J Cardiovasc Pharmacol.* 2003; 42(4): 497-505.

[55] Vazquez-Cruz B, Lopez P, Talamas-Rohana P, Escalante B. Increased renal vasoconstriction and gene expression of cyclooxygenase-1 in renovascular hypertension. *J Cardiovasc Pharmacol.* 2000; 36 (5): 577-583.

[56] Barton CH, Ni Z, Vaziri ND. Enhanced nitric oxide inactivation in aortic coarctation. induced hypertension. *Kidney Int.* 2001;60(3):1083-1087.

[57] Baños G, Franco M, Bobadilla NA, Lopez-Zetina P, Ceballos G et al. Effect of circulating factors on vascular smooth muscle contraction and its calcium uptake in uremia. *Clin Exper Hyper* 1991; A13 (3): 383-400.

[58] Hernandez J, Astudillo H, Escalante B. Angiotensin II stimulates cyclooxygenase-2 mRNA expression in renal tissue from rats with kidney failure. *Am J Physiol Renal Physiol.* 2002; 282 (4): F592-F598.

[59] Arranz C, Tomat A, Fellet A, Garcia J, Balaszczuk AM, de los Angeles Costa M. Renal and vascular nitric oxide system in reduced renal mass saline hypertension. *Nephron Physiol.* 2003; 95(2):36-42.

[60] Baños G, Franco M. Platelet aggregation and experimental renovascular hypertension in rats. *Med Sci Res.* 1996; 24: 127-128.

[61] Cervenka L, Horacek V, Vaneckova I I, Hubacek JA, Oliverio MI, Coffman TM, Navar LG. Essential Role of AT(1A) Receptor in the Development of 2K-1C Hypertension. *Hypertension* 2002; 40(5): 735-741.

[62] Takahashi N, Hagaman JR, Kim HS, Smithies O. Minireview: computer simulations of blood pressure regulation by the renin- angiotensin system. *Endocrinology.* 2003;144(6): 2184-2190.

[63] Morgan T. Renin, angiotensin, sodium and organ damage. *Hypertens Res.* 2003; 26(5): 349-354.

[64] Pelaez LI, Manriquez MC, Nath KA, Romero JC, Juncos LA. Low-dose angiotensin II enhances pressor responses without causing sustained hypertension. *Hypertension.* 2003 ; 42(4): 798-801.

[65] Franco M, Tapia E, Santamaria J, Zafra I, Garcia-Torres R, Gordon KL, et al. Renal cortical vasoconstriction contributes to development of salt- sensitive hypertension after angiotensin II exposure. *J Am Soc Nephrol.* 2001;12(11):2263-2271.

[66] Furchgott R. F.The discovery of endothelium- dependent relaxation. *Circulation.* 1993; 87 (suppl. V): V-3-V-8.

[67] Furchgott RF, Zawadzki JV. The obligatory role of endothelial cells in the relaxation of arterial smooth muscle by acetylcholine. *Nature.* 1980; 288(5789): 373-376.

[68] Ignarro L. J., Byrns R.E., Buga G.M. y Wood K.S. Endothelium. derived relaxing factor (EDRF) released from artery and vein appears to be nitric oxide (NO) or a closely related radical species. *Fed. Proc. Fed. Am. Soc. Exp. Biol.* 1987; 46: 644 P.

[69] Palmer R.M.J., Ferrige A.G. y Moncada S. Nitric oxide release accounts for the biological activity of endothelium. derived relaxing factor. *Nature.* 1987; 327: 524-526.
[70] Palmer RM, Rees DD, Ashton DS, Moncada S. L-arginine is the physiological precursor for the formation of nitric oxide in endothelium-dependent relaxation. *Biochem Biophys Res Commun.* 1988;153(3):1251-1256.
[71] Peotta VA,Vasquez EC, Meyrelles SS. Cardiovascular Neural Reflexes in L-NAME–Induced Hypertension in Mice. *Hypertension.* 2001;38:555.
[72] Rossi MA, Ramos SG, Prado CM. Chronic inhibition of nitric oxide synthase induces hypertension and cardiomyocyte mitochondrial and myocardial collagen remodeling in the absence of hypertrophy. *J Hypertens* 2003; 21(5): 993-1001.
[73] Yanagisawa M, Kurihara H, Kimura S, Tomobe Y, Kobayashi M, Mitsui Y, Yazaki Y, Goto K, Masaki T. A novel potent vasoconstrictor peptide produced by vascular endothelial cells. *Nature* 1988; 332: 411-415.
[74] Inoue A, Yanagisawa M, Kimura S, Kasuya Y, Miyauchi T. The human endothelin family: three structurally and pharmacologically distinct isopeptides predicted by three separate genes. *Proc Natl Acad Sci U S A.* 1989; 86: 2863-2867.
[75] Lüscher T.F., Noll G. The endothelium as a regulator of vascular tone and growth. In: The Endothelium in Cardiovascular Disease *;* Heidelberg ; Lüscher T. F. (ed) Springer. *Verlag,* 1995 ,171-183.
[76] Krämer BK, Ittner, KP, Beyer ME, Hoffmeister HM, Riegger GA. Circulatory and myocardial effects of endothelin. *J Mol Med* 1997; 75:886-890.
[77] Devadason PS, Henry PJ. Comparison of the contractile effects and binding kinetics of endothelin-1 and sarafotoxin-S6b in rat isolated renal artery. *Brit J Pharmacol* 1997; 121: 253-263.
[78] Ortega-Mateo MA, de Artiñano AA. Highlights on endothelins: a review. *Pharmacol. Res.* 1997; 36: 339-351.
[79] Dashwood M. R., Timm M., Muddle J. R. et al. Regional variations in endothelin-1 and its receptor subtypes in human coronary vasculature: pathophysiological implications in coronary disease. *Endothelium.* 1998; 6(1):61-70.
[80] Schiffrin EL, Intengan HD, Thibault G, Touyz RM. Clinical significance of endothelin in cardiovascular disease. *Current Opinion in Cardiology* 1997; 12: 354-367.
[81] Schiffrin EL. Role of endothelin. 1 in hypertension. *Hypertension* 1999; 34 (part 2): 876-881.
[82] Lian C. L'alcoolisme cause de hypertension arterielle. Bull Acad Med. 1915; 74: 525-528.
[83] Altura BM, Ogunkoya A, Gebrewold A, Altura BT. Effects of ethanol on terminal arterioles and muscular venules: direct observations on the microcirculation. *J Cardiovasc Pharmacol* 1979; 1: 97-113.
[84] Altura BM, Edgarian H, Altura BT. Differential effects of ethanol and mannitol on contraction of arterial smooth muscle. *J Pharmacol Exp Ther.* 1976; 197: 352-361.
[85] Fewings JD, Hanna MJD, Walsh JS, Whelan RF. The effects of ethyl alcohol on the blood vessels of the hand and forearm in man. *Br J Pharmacol.* 1966; 27: 93-106.
[86] Altura BM, Altura BT. Microvascular and vascular smooth muscle actions of ethanol, acetaldehyde, and acetate. *Fed Proc.* 1982; 41: 2447-2451.

[87] Gerlai R, Lahav M, Guo S, Rosenthal A. Drinks like a fish: zebra fish (Danio rerio) as a behavior genetic model to study alcohol effects. *Pharmacol Biochem Behav.* 2000 ;67(4):773- 782.

[88] Guarnieri DJ, Heberlein U. Drosophila melanogaster, a genetic model system for alcohol research. *Int Rev Neurobiol.* 2003;54:199-228.

[89] Phillips T. Animal models for the genetic study of human alcohol phenotypes. *Alcohol Res Health.* 2002;26(3):202-207.

[90] Spanagel R. Recent animal models of alcoholism. Alcohol Res Health. 2000;24(2):124-131. 91. Tabakoff B, Hoffman PL. Animal models in alcohol research. *Alcohol Res Health.* 2000;24(2):77-84.

[91] Spanagel R. Alcohol addiction research: from animal models to clinics. *Best Pract Res Clin Gastroenterol.* 2003 ;17(4):507-518.

[92] Lodge DJ, Lawrence AJ. Comparative analysis of hepatic ethanol metabolism in Fawn. Hooded and Wistar. Kyoto rats. *Alcohol.* 2003 May;30(1):75-79.

[93] Baños G, Lopez. Zetina P, Franco M. A vasoactive serum component and reactivity of isolated rat aorta after chronic alcohol administration. *Toxicology Lett.* 1995; 76: 1-9.

[94] Crandall DL, Ferraro GD, Lozito RJ, Cervoni P, Clark LT. Cardiovascular effects of intermittent drinking: assessment of a novel animal model of human alcoholism. *J Hypertens.* 1989;7 (8):683-687.

[95] Wehner JM, Bowers BJ. Use of transgenics, null mutants, and antisense approaches to study ethanol's actions. *Alcohol Clin Exp Res.* 1995;19(4):811-820.

[96] Browman KE, Crabbe JC. Alcohol and genetics: new animal models. *Mol Med Today.* 1999; 5(7): 310-318.

[97] Bowers BJ. Applications of transgenic and knockout mice in alcohol research. *Alcohol Res Health.* 2000; 24(3):175-184

[98] Tabakoff B, Hoffman PL. Animal models in alcohol research. *Alcohol Res Health.* 2000; 24(2): 77-84.

[99] Rupp H, Brilla CG. Experimental types of hypertension--models for essential hypertension in the human? *Herz.* 1995; 20(5): 315-321.

[100] Reaven GM and Ho H. Sugar-induced hypertension in Sprague. Dawley rats. *Am J Hypertens.* 1991; 4: 610-614.

[101] Bohnen N, Degenaar CP, Jolles J. Influence of age and sex on 19 blood variables in healthy subjects. *Z Gerontol* 1992; 25:339-345.

[102] Kaplan NM. The deadly quartet and the insulin resistance syndrome: a historical overview. *Hypertens Res* 1996; 19 (Suppl. 1):S9-S11.

[103] Baños G, Carvajal K, Cardoso G, Zamora J, Franco M. Vascular reactivity and effect of serum in a rat model of hypertriglyceridemia and hypertension. *Am J Hypertens* 1997;10: 379- 388.

[104] Carvajal K, Baños G Myocardial function and effect of serum in isolated heart from hypertriglyceridemic and hypertensive rats. *Clin Exper Hypertens.* 2002; 24 (4): 235-248.

[105] El Hafidi M, Baños G. In vivo plasma lipid oxidation in sugar-induced rat hypertriglyceridemia and hypertension. *Hypertension.* 1997; 30: 624-628.

[106] Perez I, El Hafidi M, Sanchez C, Baños G. Effect of sugar-induced hypertension in rats on the pattern of serum arachidonic, dihomo. gamma. linoleic and linoleic acids. *Med Sci Res.* 1999; 27: 847-848.

[107] El Hafidi M, Valdez R, Baños G. Possible relationship between altered fatty acid composition of serum, platelets and aorta, and hypertension induced by sugar feeding in rats. *Clin Exp Hypertens.* 2000; 22(1): 99-108.
[108] Egan BM, Lu G, Greene EL. Vascular effects of non-esterified fatty acids: implications for the cardiovascular risk factor cluster. *Prostaglandins Leukot Essent Fatty Acids.* 1999;60(5- 6):411-420.
[109] Perez I. MSc thesis. Unpublished results.
[110] Galipeau D, Arikawa E, Serikov I, McNeill JH. Chronic thromboxane synthase inhibition prevents fructose-induced hypertension. *Hypertension* 2001; 38: 872-876.
[111] Nava P, Guarner V, Posadas R, Perez I, Baños G. Insulin. induced endothelin release and vasoreactivity in hypertriglyceridemic and hypertensive rats. *Am JPhysiol* 1999; 277:H399- H404.
[112] Piatti PM, Monti LD, Conti M, Baruffaldi L, Galli L, Phan CV. Hypertriglyceridemia and hyperinsulinemia are potent inducers of endothelin-1 release in humans. *Diabetes.* 45(3):316- 321, 1996.
[113] Verma S, Bhanot S, McNeill JH. Effect of chronic endothelin blockade in hyperinsulinemic hypertensive rats. *Am J Physiol.* 1995; 269:H2017-H2021.
[114] Schiffrin EL, Intengan HD, Thibault G, Touyz RM. Clinical significance of endothelin in cardiovascular disease. *Curr Opinion Cardiol.* 1997; 12:354-367.
[115] Schiffrin EL. Role of endothelin. 1 in hypertension. *Hypertension* 1999; 34: 876-881.
[116] Catena C, Cavarape A, Novello M, Giacchetti G, Sechi LA. Insulin receptors and renal sodium handling in hypertensive fructose. fed rats. *Kidney Int.* 2003;64(6):2163-2171.
[117] Dahl LK, Heine M, Tassinar L. Effects of chronic excess salt ingestion: Evidence that genetic factors play an important role in susceptibility to experimental hypertension. *J Exp Med* 1962; 115: 1173-1190.
[118] Dahl LK, Schackow E. Effects of chronic excess salt ingestion: Experimental hypertension in the rat. *Can Med Assoc J* 1964; 90: 155-160.
[119] Dahl LK, Knudsen KD, Iwai J. Humoral transmission of hypertension: evidence from parabiosis. *Circ Res* 1969; 1 (suppl 24, 25): 21-33.
[120] Tobian L, Coffee K, McCrea P. Evidence for a humoral factor of non-renal and non-adrenal origin which influences renal sodium excretion. *Trans Assoc Am Physicians.* 1967; 80: 200-206.
[121] Handa M, Kondo K, Suzuki H, Saruta T. Dexamethasone hypertension in rats: role of prostaglandins and pressor sensitivity to norepinephrine. *Hypertension* 1984; 6: 236-241.
[122] Dahl LK, Heine M, Tassinari L. Effects of chronic excess salt ingestion. Further demonstration that genetic factors influence the development of hypertension: evidence from experimental hypertension due to cortisone and to adrenal regeneration. *J Exp Med.* 1965 ;122(3):533-545.
[123] Kannel WB, Brand N, Skinner JJ Jr, Dawber TR, McNamara PM. The relation of adiposity to blood pressure and development of hypertension: the Framingham Study. *Ann Intern Med.* 1967; 67:48–59.
[124] Alonso-Galicia M, Brands MW, Zappe DH, Hall JE. Hypertension in obese Zucker rats: role of angiotensin II and adrenergic activity. *Hypertension.* 1996; 28:1047–1054.

[125] Tuck ML, Sowers J, Dornfeld L, Kledzik G, Maxwell M. The effect of weight reduction on blood pressure, plasma renin activity, and plasma aldosterone levels in obese patients. *N Engl J Med.* 1981; 304:930–933.

[126] Philip. Couderc P, Smih F, Pelat M, Vidal C, Verwaerde P, Pathak A, et al. Cardiac transcriptome analysis in obesity. related hypertension. *Hypertension* 2003; 41:414-421.

[127] Pelat M, Verwaerde P, Tran MA, Montastruc JL, Senard JM. Comment in: Alpha2 . adrenoceptor function in arterial hypertension associated with obesity in dogs fed a high-fat diet. *J Hypertens.* 2002 20: 957-964.

[128] Carroll JF, Dwyer TM, Grady AW, Reinhart GA, Montani JP, Cockrell K,et al. Hypertension, cardiac hypertrophy, and neurohumoral activity in a new animal model of obesity. *Am J Physiol* 1996; 271:H373–H378.

[129] Carroll JF, Braden DS, Cockrell K, Mizelle HL. Obese hypertensive rabbits develop concentric and eccentric hypertrophy and diastolic filling abnormalities. *Am J Hypertens* 1997; 10:230-233.

[130] Levin BE, Triscari J, Sullivan AC. Relationship between sympathetic activity and diet-induced obesity in two rat strains. *Am J Physiol.* 1983; 245:R364–R371.

[131] Lauterio TJ, Bond JP, Ulman EA. Development and characterization of a purified diet to identify obesity-susceptible and -resistant rat populations. *J Nutr.* 1994;124:2172–2178.

[132] Dobrian AD, Schriver SD, Lynch T, Prewitt RL Effect of salt on hypertension and oxidative stress in a rat model of diet- induced obesity. *Am J Physiol* 2003; 285:F619-F628.

[133] Roberts CK, Vaziri ND, Sindhu RK, Barnard RJ. A high. fat, refined-carbohydrate diet affects renal NO synthase protein expression and salt sensitivity. *J Appl Physiol.* 2003; 94(3):941-946.

[134] Glueck CJ, Taylor HL, Jacobs D, Morrison JA, Beaglehole R, Williams OD. Plasma high. density lipoprotein cholesterol: association with measurements of body mass: the Lipid Research Clinics Program Prevalence Study. *Circulation.* 1980; 62:IV-62–IV-69.

[135] Van Itallie TB. Health implications of overweight and obesity in the United States. *Ann Intern Med.* 1985; 103:983–988.

[136] Sclafani A. Dietary obesity models. In: Bjorntorp P, Brodoff BN, eds. *Obesity.* Philadelphia, Pa: JB Lippincott; 1992:241–248.

[137] Stepniakowski KT, Goodfriend TL & Egan BM. Fatty acids enhance vascular □-adrenergic sensitivity. *Hypertension* 1995; 25:774-778.

[138] Grekin RJ, Dumont CJ, Vollmer AP, Watts SW & Webb RC. Mechanisms in the pressor effects of hepatic portal venous fatty acid infusion. *Amer J Physiol* 1997; 273: R324-R330.

[139] Pfeifer M, Wolf K, Blumberg FC, Elsner D, Muders F, Holmer SR et al. ANP gene expression in rat hearts during hypoxia. *Pflugers Arch.* 1997; 434(1):63-69.

[140] Chou TF, Chen YS, Yu CC, Chien CT, Chen CF. Simple methods to elevate pulmonary arterial pressure by pre- and post-tricuspid shunts in rats. *Chin J Physiol.* 2002 ;45(3):131-135.

[141] Mahesree ML, Chakravarti RN, Wahi PL. Packed cells, platelet-rich plasma, and adenosine diphosphate in the production of occlusive vascular changes in lungs of rabbits. *Am Heart J.* 1975; 89(6):753-758.

[142] Drummond WH, Bissonnette JM. Persistent pulmonary hypertension in the neonate: development of an animal model. *Am J Obstet Gynecol.* 1978;131(7):761-763.
[143] Nishimura T, Faul JL, Berry GJ, Vaszar LT, Qiu D, Pearl RG, et al. Simvastatin attenuates smooth muscle neointimal proliferation and pulmonary hypertension in rats. *Am J Respir Crit Care Med.* 2002;166(10):1403-1408.
[144] Mansoor AM, Honda M, Saida K, Ishinaga Y, Kuramochi T, Maeda A, et al. Endothelin induced collagen remodeling in experimental pulmonary hypertension. *Biochem Biophys Res Commun.* 1995 ;215(3): 981-986.
[145] Carteaux JP, Roux S, Siaghy M, Schjoth B, Dolofon P, Bechamps Y et al. Acute pulmonary hypertension after cardiopulmonary bypass in pig: the role of endogenous endothelin. *Eur J Cardiothorac Surg.* 1999;15(3): 346-352.
[146] Morrell NW, Atochina EN, Morris KG, Danilov SM, Stenmark KR. Angiotensin converting enzyme expression is increased in small pulmonary arteries of rats with hypoxia-induced pulmonary hypertension. *J Clin Invest.* 1995; 96(4):1823-1833.

[147] Cvetkovic B, Sigmund CD. Understanding hypertension through genetic manipulation in mice. *Kidney Int.* 2000; 57: 863-874.
[148] Jacob HJ, Lindpaintner K, Lincoln SE, Kusumi K, Bunker RK, Mao YP, et al. Genetic mapping of a gene causing hypertension in the stroke-prone spontaneously hypertensive rat. *Cell* 1991; 67: 213-224.
[149] Rapp JP, Wang SM, Dene H. A genetic polymorphism in the renin gene of Dahl rats cosegregates with blood pressure. *Science* 1989; 243: 542-544.
[150] Jeunemaitre X, Soubrier F, Kotelevtsev YV, Lifton RP, Williams CS, Charru A, et al. Molecular basis of human hypertension: Role of angiotensinogen. *Cell* 1992; 71: 169-180.
[151] Kim HS, Krege JH, Kluckman KD, Hagaman JR, Hodgin JB, Best CF, et al. Genetic control of blood pressure and the angiotensinogen locus. *Proc Natl Acad Sci* USA 1995; 92: 2735–2739.
[152] Oliver PM, John SW, Purdy KE, Kim R, Maeda N, Goy MF, et al. Natriuretic peptide receptor 1 expression influences blood pressures of mice in a dose-dependent manner. *Proc Natl Acad Sci USA* 1998; 95: 2547-2551.
[153] Oliver PM, Fox JE, Kim R, Rockman HA, Kim HS, Reddick RL, et al. Hypertension, cardiac hypertrophy, and sudden death in mice lacking natriuretic peptide receptor A. *Proc Natl Acad Sci* USA 1997; 94: 14730-14735.
[154] John SW, Krege JH, Oliver PM, Hagaman JR, Hodgin JB, et al. Genetic decreases in atrial natriuretic peptide and salt-sensitive hypertension. *Science* 1995; 267: 679-681.
[155] Steinhelper ME, Cochrane KL, Field LJ. Hypotension in transgenic mice expressing atrial natriuretic factor fusion genes. *Hipertensión* 1990; 16: 301-307.
[156] Ogawa Y, Itoh H, Tamura N, Suga S, Yoshimasa T, Uehira M, et al. Molecular cloning of the complementary DNA and gene that encode mouse brain natriuretic peptide and generation of transgenic mice that overexpress the brain natriuretic peptide gene. *J Clin Invest* 1994; 93: 1911-1921.
[157] Inoue I, Nakajima T, Williams CS, Quackenbush J, Puryear R, Powers M, et al. A nucleotide substitution in the promoter of human angiotensinogen is associated with essential hypertension and affects basal transcription in vitro. *J Clin Invest* 1997; 99: 1786-1797.

[158] Tanimoto K, Sugiyama F, Goto Y, Ishida J, Takimoto E, Yagami K, et al. Angiotensinogen-deficient mice with hypotension. *J Biol Chem* 1994; 269: 31334-31337.

[159] Niimura F, Labosky PA, Kakuchi J, Okubo S, Yoshida H, Oikawa T, et al. Gene targeting in mice reveals a requirement for angiotensin in the development and maintenance of kidney morphology and growth factor regulation. *J Clin Invest* 1995; 96: 2947-2954.

[160] Krege JH, John SW, Langenbach LL, Hodgin JB, Hagaman JR, Bachman ES, et al. Male-female differences in fertility and blood pressure in ACE-deficient mice. *Nature* 1995; 375: 146-148.

[161] Tsuchida S, Matsusaka T, Chen X, Okubo S, Niimura F, Nishimura H, et al. Murine double nullizygotes of the angiotensin type 1A and 1B receptor genes duplicate severe abnormal phenotypes of angiotensinogen nullizygotes. *J Clin Invest* 1998; 101: 755-760.

[162] Clark AF, Sharp MGF, Morley SD, Fleming S, Peters J, Mullins JJ. Renin-1 is essential for normal renal juxtaglomerular cell granulation and macula densa morphology. *J Biol Chem* 1997; 272: 18185-18190.

[163] Sharp MG, Fettes D, Brooker G, Clark AF, Peters J, Fleming S, et al. Targeted inactivation of the Ren-2 gene in mice. *Hypertension* 1996; 28: 1126-1131.

[164] Bernstein KE, Martin BM, Edwards AS, Bernstein EA. Mouse angiotensin-converting enzyme is a protein composed of two homologous domains. *J Biol Chem* 1989; 264: 11945-11951.

[165] Soubrier F, Alhenc-Gelas F, Hubert C, Allegrini J, John M, Tregear G, Corvol P: Two putative active centers in human angiotensin I-converting enzyme revealed by molecular cloning. *Proc Natl Acad Sci* USA 1988; 85: 9386-9390.

[166] Sibony M, Gasc JM, Soubrier F, Alhenc-Gelas F, Corvol P. Gene expression and tissue localization of the two isoforms of angiotensin I converting enzyme. *Hypertension* 1993; 21: 827-835.

[167] Langford KG, Zhou Y, Russell LD, Wilcox JN, Bernstein KE. Regulated expression of testis angiotensin-converting enzyme during spermatogenesis in mice. *Biol Reprod* 1993; 48: 1210-1218.

[168] Krege JH, Kim HS, Moyer JS, Jennette JC, Peng L, Hiller SK, et al. Angiotensin-converting enzyme gene mutations, blood pressures, and cardiovascular homeostasis. *Hypertension* 1997; 29: 150-157.

[169] Ito M, Oliverio MI, Mannon PJ, Best CF, Maeda N, Smithies O, et al: Regulation of blood pressure by the type 1A angiotensin II receptor gene. *Proc Natl Acad Sci* USA 1995; 92: 3521–3525.

[170] Sugaya T, Nishimatsu S, Tanimoto K, Takimoto E, Yamagishi T, Imamura K, et al. Angiotensin II type 1□ receptor-deficient mice with hypotension and hyperreninemia. *J Biol Chem* 1995; 270: 18719-18722.

[171] Chen X, Li W, Yoshida H, Tsuchida S, Nishimura H, Takemoto F, Okubo S, et al. Targeting deletion of angiotensin type 1B receptor gene in the mouse. *Am J Physiol* 1997; 272: F299-F304.

[172] Ichiki T, Labosky PA, Shiota C, Okuyama S, Imagawa Y, Fogo A, et al. Effects on blood pressure and exploratory behaviour of mice lacking angiotensin II type-2 receptor. *Nature* 1995; 377: 748-750.

[173] MacDonald E, Kobilka BK, Scheinin M. Gene targeting-homing in on □2-adrenoceptor-subtype function. *Trends Pharmacol Sci* 1997; 18:211–219.

[174] Guyenet PG. Is the hypotensive effect of clonidine and related drugs due to imidazoline binding sites? *Am J Physiol* 1997; 273: R1580-R1584.

[175] Macmillan LB, Hein L, Smith MS, Piascik MT, Limbird LE. Central hypotensive effects of the □2A-adrenergic receptor subtype. *Science* 1996; 273: 801-803.

[176] Jose PA, Eisner GM, Felder RA. Role of dopamine in the pathogenesis of hypertension. *Clin Exp Pharmacol Physiol Suppl* 1999; 26:S10-S13.

[177] Shesely EG, Maeda N, Kim HS, Desai KM, Krege JH, Laubach VE, et al. Elevated blood pressures in mice lacking endothelial nitric oxide synthase. *Proc Natl Acad Sci* USA 1996; 93: 13176-13181.

[178] Huang PL, Huang Z, Mashimo H, Bloch KD, Moskowitz MA, Bevan JA, et al. Hypertension in mice lacking the gene for endothelial nitric oxide synthase. *Nature* 1995; 377: 239-242.

[179] Huang Z, Huang PL, Panahian N, Dalkara T, Fishman MC, Moskowitz MA Effects of cerebral ischemia in mice deficient in neuronal nitric oxide synthase. *Science* 1994; 265: 1883-1885.

[180] Kurihara Y, Kurihara H, Suzuki H, Kodama T, Maemura K, Nagai R, et al. Elevated blood pressure and craniofacial abnormalities in mice deficient in endothelin-1. *Nature* 1994; 368: 703-710.

[181] Madeddu P, Varoni MV, Palomba D, Emanueli C, Demontis MP, Glorioso N, et al. Cardiovascular phenotype of a mouse strain with disruption of bradykinin B2-receptor gene. *Circulation* 1997; 96: 3570–3578.

[182] Alfie ME, Sigmon DH, Pomposiello SI, Carretero OA: Effect of high salt intake in mutant mice lacking bradykinin-B2 receptors. *Hypertension* 1997; 29: 483-487.

[183] Rich S: Executive summary from the World Symposium on primary pulmonary hypertension. 1998.

[184] Deng Z, Morse JH, Slager SL, Cuervo N, Moore KJ, Venetos G, et al. Familial primary pulmonary hypertension (gene PPH1) is caused by mutations in the bone morphogenetic protein receptor-II gene. *Am J Hum Genet* 2000; 67: 737-744.

[185] Lane KB, Machado RD, Pauciulo MW, Thomson JR, Phillips JA III, Loyd JE, et al. Heterozygous germline mutations in *BMPR2*, encoding a TGF-□receptor, cause familial primary pulmonary hypertension. *Nat Genet* 2000; 26: 81-84.

[186] Voelkel NF, Tuder RM, Wade K, Hoper M, Lepley RA, Goulet JL, et al. Inhibition of 5-lipoxygenase-activating protein (FLAP) reduces pulmonary vascular reactivity and pulmonary hypertension in hypoxic rats. *J Clin Invest* 1996; 97:2491-2498.

[187] Fagan KA, Fouty BW, Tyler RC, Morris KG Jr, Hepler LK, Sato K, et al. The pulmonary circulation of homozygous or heterozygous eNOS-null mice is hyperresponsive to mild hypoxia. *J Clin Invest.* 1999; 103: 291-299.

[188] Hoshikawa Y, Voelkel NF, Gesell TL, Moore MD, Morris KG, Alger LA, et al. Prostacyclin receptor-dependent modulation of pulmonary vascular remodeling. *Am J Respir Crit Care Med* 2001; 164: 314-318.

[189] Masuzaki H, Yamamoto H, Kenyon CJ, Elmquist JK, Morton NM, Paterson JM, et al. Transgenic amplification of glucocorticoid action in adipose tissue causes high blood pressure in mice J. *Clin. Invest* 2003; 112: 83–90.

[190] Haynes WG, Morgan DA, Walsh SA, Mark AL, Sivitz WI. Receptor mediated regional sympathetic nerve activation by leptin. *J Clin Invest* 1997; 100; 270-278.

[191] Konstantinides S, Schafer K, Koschnick S, Loskutoff DJ. Leptin-dependent platelet aggregation and arterial thrombosis suggests a mechanism for atherothrombotic disease in obesity. *J Clin Invest* 2001; 8:1533-1540.

[192] Bodary PF, Westrick RJ, Wickenheiser KJ, Shen Y, Eitzman DT. Effect of leptin on arterial thrombosis following vascular injury in mice. *JAMA* 2002; 287: 1706-1709.

[193] Shek EW, Brands MW, Hall JE. Chronic leptin infusion increases arterial pressure. *Hypertension* 1998; 31: 409-414.

[194] Aizawa-Abe M, Ogawa Y, Masuzaki H, Ebihara K, Satoh N, Iwai H, et al Pathophysiological role of leptin in obesity-related hypertension. *J Clin Invest.* 2000; 105: 1243-1252.

[195] Mark AL, Shaffer RA, Correia MLG, Morgan DA, Sigmund CD, Haynes WG. Contrasting blood pressure effects of obesity in leptin-deficient ob/ob mice and agouti yellow obese mice. *J Hypertens* 1999; 17: 1949-1953.

[196] Li B, Nolte LA, Ju J-S, Han DH, Coleman T, Holloszy JO, Semenkovich CF. Skeletal muscle respiratory uncoupling prevents diet-induced obesity and insulin resistance in mice. *Nat Med* 2000; 6: 1115-1120.

[197] Clapham JC, Arch JR, Chapman H, Haynes A, Lister C, Moore GB, et al. Mice overexpressing human uncoupling protein-3 in skeletal muscle are hyperphagic and lean. *Nature* 2000; 406: 415-418.

[198] Bernal-Mizrachi C, Weng S, Bing L, Nolte LA, Feng C, Coleman T, et al. Respiratory uncoupling lowers blood pressure through a leptin-dependent mechanism in genetically obese mice. *Arterioscler Thromb Vasc Biol* 2002; 22: 961-968.

[199] Charreau B, Tesson L, Soulillou JP, Pourcel C, Anegon I. Transgenesis in rats: technical aspects and models. *Transgenic Res* 1996; 5: 223-234.

[200] Lee MA, Bohm M, Paul M, Bader M, Ganten U, Ganten D. Physiological characterization of the hypertensive transgenic rat TGR(mREN2)27. *Am J Physiol* 1996; 270: E919-929.

[201] Langheinrich M, Lee MA, Bohm M, Pinto YM, Ganten D, Paul M. The hypertensive Ren-2 transgenic rat TGR (mREN2)27 in hypertension research. Characteristics and functional aspects. *Am J Hypertens* 1996; 9: 506-512.

[202] Phillips MI. Gene therapy for hypertension: sense and antisense strategies. *Expert Opin Biol Ther* 2001; 1: 655-662.

In: Hypertension: New Research
Editor: Elwood F. Benhagen, pp. 47-68
ISBN: 1-59454-204-X

Chapter II

AGING OF THE CARDIOVASCULAR SYSTEM

V. Guarner[1], *R. Carbó*[1*], *M.E. Rubio*[1], *G. Baños de MacCarthy*[2]
[1]Departamento de Fisiología y [2]Departamento de Bioquímica,
Instituto Nacional de Cardiología "Ignacio Chávez"

ABSTRACT

Aging is determined by a series of morphological and functional changes over time and by the deterioration of the biological functions after an organism has passed its maximum reproductive potential. We do not know whether aging starts from the moment of conception or at maturity, or if it constitutes a process of evolution or involution. Several suggestions have been proposed to explain why we age; they offer partial solutions and indicate possible guide-lines for future investigation. Theories of aging have been grouped either as genetic or evolutionary currents. Many mechanisms that lead to aging have been proposed, although none of them solves all the doubts and gives us a clear answer. These mechanisms are discussed in this article and an example of aging of the cardiovascular system under normal and physiopathological conditions is offered. Although some data on human aging are presented, the review is mainly focused on recent advances made on animal models. Aging in the cardiovascular system is characterized by an increase in blood pressure, a reduction both in cardiac output and in the response to stress. In blood vessels, aging is related to structural and functional changes in the endothelium, smooth muscle and extracellular matrix. Age-related vascular changes vary in different species and in vessels irrigating various organs. Oxidative stress appears to be the primary explanation for aging in the cardiovascular system. Hypertension, which is an age-dependent disorder, and diabetes and insulin resistance, which are associated with aging, contribute to vascular malfunction, altering the aging mechanisms of blood vessels. Several models of hypertension and diabetes have been used to study the alterations produced in the aging processes of the cardiovascular system and are summarized.

* Send correspondence to: Dra. Verónica Guarner, Departamento de Fisiología, Instituto Nacional de Cardiología, "*Ignacio Chávez*", Juan Badiano 1, Colonia Sección 16, 14080, Tlalpan, México, D.F. Tel: 55 73 29 11 ext 1278 o 1222, Fax: 55 73 09 26, Email: vguarner@yahoo.com

Abbreviations

ATP	adenosine triphosphate
DNA	Deoxyribonucleic Acid
EDHF	endothelium derived hyperpolarizing factor
EDRF	endothelium derived relaxing factor
eNOS	endothelial nitric oxide synthase
ET-1	endothelin 1
GH	growth hormone
H_2O_2	hydrogen peroxide
IDDM	insulin dependent diabetes mellitus
IGF-1	insulin growth factor 1
KCl	potassium chloride
LDL	low density lipoproteins
Maxi K	voltage and calcium activated potassium channels
mRNA	messenger ribonucleic acid
NA	norepinephrine
NIDDM	non insulin dependent diabetes mellitus
NO	nitric oxide
O_2^-	superoxide
OH^-	hydroxyl
PDGF	platelet derived growth factor
PKG1	protein kinase G-1
SHR	spontaneously hypertensive rats
TGF-β1	transforming growth factor beta 1
TNF-alpha	tumor necrosis factor alpha

Introduction

Aging is defined as a series of morphological and functional changes which take place over time [1]. The term also refers to the deterioration of the biological functions after an organism has attained its maximum reproductive potential [2]. Although the process of aging is universal and irreversible, its meaning and the biological mechanisms leading to it are still disputed and numerous methods tending to delay its appearance, however briefly, are proposed. We do not know yet whether organisms start to grow old from the moment of conception or from maturity, or if aging constitutes a process of evolution or involution [3]. Theories of aging have been grouped either as genetic or evolutionary currents and many mechanisms that could lead to aging have been proposed. These general mechanisms are discussed in this review.

The rate of deterioration during aging is determined by the species, the individual, environmental factors and life style [4]. Although aging occurs in the organism as a whole, not all the anatomical systems age at the same rate [4]. When changes are moderate, aging is normal or physiological, while exaggerated alterations determine abnormal or physiopathological aging [4]. Arbitrarily, the beginning of old age has been fixed at 65 years in developed countries and at 60 in the underdeveloped world. Approximately at 80, changes that diminish functionality are easily observed and a distinction can be made between the young elderly and the old elderly. At this age the number of weak individuals compared to strong ones increases.

With the exception of tortoises from the Galapagos islands, human beings have the longest life expectancy of all known animals [5]. The maximum life span for human beings is approximately 100 to 110 years [6]. It has increased through infectious disease prevention and treatment improvement as well as through better knowledge of early causes of death [4,6]. This fact has been related to basal metabolism and body temperature [7]. It has also been related to brain/body weight ratio, which is higher in humans than in other species.

In the present review, in addition to analyzing the general mechanisms of aging, an example of aging of the cardiovascular system under normal and patophysiological conditions (hypertension and diabetes) is presented. Aging in the cardiovascular system is characterized by an increase in blood pressure, a reduction in cardiac output and in the response to stress. Oxidative stress appears to be the primary explanation for aging in this system. The data are discussed of altered aging mechanisms induced by hypertension and diabetes in several animal models of hypertensive and diabetic rats. Although some data on human aging are presented, the review is mainly focused on recent advances made on animal models.

Why do Organisms Age?

We still do not have an answer to this question. Nevertheless, several explanations have been proposed that offer partial solutions and indicate possible guide-lines for future investigation. Signs of old age appear at different levels of biological organization and therefore most of the theories proposed must have some truth to them and, most probably, our final explanation will include them in some way [3]. Theories of aging have been grouped either as genetic or evolutionary currents and are ennumerated in Table 1.

Table 1 Theories of the mechanisms leading to aging

Genetic Current

1. Somatic mutations theory.
2. Theory of wear and tear.
3. Theory of the catastrophic accumulation of errors.
4. Theory of the genetic regulation of aging.
5. Theory of the free radicals.
6. Theory of mitochondrial and nuclear DNA loss or inactivation.
7. Calorie restriction theory.
8. Integrative theory.

Evolutionary Current

1. Disposable soma theory.
2. Antagonistic pleiotropy theory.

Genetic Current

This current proposes that longevity is analogous to differentiation and development and is therefore regulated by the sequential expression of genes which dictate the cellular life span. According to evolutionary biology, and contrary to the widespread belief that has led to an extensive search for aging genes, they probably do not exist, and natural selection would work on genes for somatic maintenance[8]. Organisms that are regularly exposed to unpredictable environments have evolved systems that regulate their metabolic allocations to make the best of varying conditions. They usually privilege the competing priorities of metabolic investments in growth and reproduction and can afford only limited investments in maintenance. The result is that aging is linked to the progressive accumulation of late-acting deleterious genes that irreversibly disconnect synthetic processes throughout evolution, through the gradual accumulation of a host of subtle molecular faults [8]. There would be therefore multiple mechanisms and many different genes affecting the rate of aging. Genes similar to those encoding insulin/IGF-1 and sexual hormones, known as pleiotropic genes, which help survival and reproduction in early stages, but which favor aging during the latter part of life, would increase the lifespan. These genes control the switch into the allocation of metabolic resources, increasing the importance of maintenance processes [2,3,9]. Further evidence supporting the role of genes in aging is the fact that many tumoral cells and those into which a viral oncogene is introduced become immortal. Genes make only a 25% contribution to human longevity.

Hormones that regulate gene expression can alter the aging rate. Some of the hormones proposed as participating in this process are insulin and insulin growth factor 1 (IGF-1) [5,8,10-12], growth hormone (GH) [11,12], melatonin [13] and an insect steroid hormone named ecdysone[14]. The intracellular signalling pathways of these hormones could regulate longevity.

In support of this theory, it has been demonstrated that fetal fibroblasts are able to divide 50 ± 10 times before they cease to proliferate. If fibroblasts from a 40 year old person are extracted, their divisions stop after 40 cycles; however if we extract fibroblasts from an 80 year old person, proliferation will stop after 30 cycles [15]. The decline in the proliferative capacity correlates with telomere shortening.It has been reported that the fusion of young and old cells or the injection of mRNA from old cells to young ones delays their capacity to initiate mitosis, by inhibiting the synthesis of DNA. This effect is mediated by a proteic factor. DNA from old fibroblasts has shown that senescent genes are often methylated, amplified or reorganized, due to the action of activated oncogenes or the suppression of anti-oncogenes [3].

-Theories that Support Environmental Effects on the Genetic Program for Aging

The theory of wear and tear proposes that different parts of the organisms waste as they are repeatedly used. It supposes that normal cellular activity leads to a series of disorders. This theory explains why adult organs gradually degenerate with age. However, biological waste is not equivalent to physical waste and often the repeated use of cells and organs does not debilitate them but rather fortifies them. For example, the maintainance of certain mental activities has a favourable effect on the cognitive functions of elderly people [3].

The free radical theory of aging suggests that the production of these species causes deterioration of the organs and cells as they are repeatedly used. Under normal conditions, mitochondrial respiration produces most of the free radicals derived from oxygen, that are responsible for cellular disorganization. Free radicals are efficiently reduced by cellular stores of antioxidants. Approximately 1% of the oxygen used by the mitochondria is transformed to superoxide (O_2^-) and 107 molecules of O_2^- are produced by each mitochondrion per day. This free radical is highly toxic and when reduced by the enzyme Superoxide Dismutase, yields hydrogen peroxide (H_2O_2). This molecule is converted by the enzyme Catalase and intramitochondrial peroxidases to Hydroxyl (OH^-). Hydroxyl, together with O_2, which is also liberated by the respiratory chain, produces the peroxidation of the membrane lipids, causing membrane fluidity changes that alter cellular function [3,16]. Mitochondrial membranes are also peroxidated and this process induces organelle functional alterations [3,,16]. Free radicals become more toxic as organisms age because enzymes that defend the cell against them are expressed at lower levels.

The calorie restriction theory to delay aging suggests that this process is caused as a side effect of metabolism and that when metabolism is reduced, life is prolonged [5,17]. This could be due to a down-regulation of free radicals and lipid peroxide production. Aerobic metabolism controls the rate of senile disorganization and there is a decrease in the number of mitochondria in the older cells. Some nutrients, including excess glucose, induce glycosylation of proteins inside the cells and in the extracellular matrix, diminishing their functionality [18].

The free radical theory does not explain why spermatogonias and the cells of the Lieberkhun crypts of the gut are immune from free radical attacks and therefore are apparently immortal. It is also important to note that free radicals are not always damaging and that they play an important role in microsomal detoxification and fagocytosis.

Theories of the Catastrophic Accumulation of Errors and of Somatic Mutations postulate that DNA and enzymatic systems would be damaged as a consequence of use. These theories suggest that senescence in tissues is the result of the amassing of errors or mutations produced as a result of chemical mutagens, ionizing agents or free radicals. These errors would autopropagate during the transcription or translation of the message from mRNA. Evidence in favor of these theories is the shortening of the life span in organisms that undergo irradiation. However, this theory cannot explain: 1) why some chemical mutagens (clorambucyl and methanosulphonate) do not shorten the length of life, 2) why some animals (the fruit fly) live longer when exposed to high doses of radiation, 3) why some relatively radiation-resistant species have shorter life spans than other radiosensitive ones, 4) why germinal cells or even some ordinary somatic cells maintained under adequate conditions are able to proliferate indefinitely [2,3].

These theories are not supported by other facts such as the proposed (as yet unproven) inactivation of DNA with the passage of time, even in the absence of errors or mutations. This proposal is not favored by the identical physicochemical properties of DNA in cells from old and young individuals. Furthermore, recent investigations also suggest that it is not a failure in the transmission process of information, but rather a decline in the availability of energy (ATP) necessary for synthesis, which produces aging.

Theories of the Catastrophic Accumulation of Errors and Somatic Mutations have also been applied to mitochondrial DNA. This is more vulnerable to disorganization during aging than nuclear DNA, because of its proximity to the internal membrane where free radicals are produced as a result of cellular respiration and also because it lacks histones and repair mechanisms present in the nucleus [3,19]. Observations in mutant mice lacking the mitochondrial form of the Superoxide Dismutase-2, have shown the enormous dependency on optimal mitochondrial function of the brain and heart. Similarly, mutants of the adenine nucleotide translocator have shown that there is a clear correlation between oxidative stress and mutations in mitochondrial DNA. These changes have been shown in several species, including humans [20].

Evolutionary Current

The evolutionary current proposes that aging is a positive or negative consequence of evolution. Two possible reasons can be visualized: 1) senile involution increases survival possibilities of the younger members of the species. This explanation implies that elderly and sick individuals are not harmless for the survival of the species but rather damaging, because they reduce the resources needed for the survival of the young. Natural selection will favor a limited number of old individuals supporting the simultaneous existence of young individuals, according to the disposable soma theory. Although it could be argued that if aging did not exist there would be no need for a substitution of old and sick individuals, variability within the species would be dangerously reduced [4,9]. 2) Aging is a secondary effect of physiological characteristics that have positive effects in earlier stages of life. This explanation supposes that aging is a non-planned and irrelevant consequence of a positive adaptation to the environment. In favor of this current, the antagonistic pleiotropy theory proposes that sexual hormones have secondary effects during the later part of life, inducing or repressing the expression of genes that lead to diseases and old age [2,9,21-23].

MANIFESTATIONS OF AGING IN ORGANISMS

The most characteristic manifestations of aging in an organism are listed in Table 2. The surplus capacity of physiological functions, which is usually used during stress, diminishes during aging, rendering the organisms more vulnerable to illnesses. Oxidative stress tolerance is also reduced [24]. The capacity to react to changes in the environment gets slower and loses precision and the return to basal conditions becomes slow. These changes appear as a consequence of intracellular alterations including increases in glycogen and lipids, a reduced number of mitochondria and a decrease in cellular permeability.

Table 2 Manifestations of aging in the whole organism

1. Reduction of the surplus capacity of physiological functions used during stress.
2. Modification of connective tissue reducing elasticity and flexibility.
3. Reduction of the regenerative capacity.
4. Deterioration of immune mechanisms.

Connective tissue is also modified and there is a reduction in the intercrossing of elastin and collagen fibers, causing loss of tendon, ligament and articular capsule elasticity and flexibility. These restrict articular movements and lead to blood vessel sclerosis [25].

Regenerative capacity diminishes because of the difficulty of parenchimal cells to divide, and tissues so that organs atrophy [24]. At the age of 80 the number of hepatocytes is about 30% of those in the young. The number of brain, lung, muscle and kidney cells is also reduced. Immune mechanisms also deteriorate. Each organ has its own specific aging pattern.

The beneficial effect of exercise against oxidative stress, and therefore against the manifestations of aging, has been demonstrated by several researchers. In a comparative study with young and old rats, either active or sedentary, the authors found an increase in the level of hydroxyl radicals in all the tissues of the young and active rats, except in plasma. In old rats, the level increased in plasma, heart and skeletal muscle, but decreased with exercise. Also in young rats which took exercise, there was more evidence of an elevation of reduced glutathione level in plasma, heart and skeletal muscle. When the animals were allowed to run freely for 5 weeks, the effects were more noticeable than in the sedentary rats. There were elevations in the ratio of reduced glutathione/total in plasma, heart and soleus muscle of young rats, whereas in elderly animals there was more evidence of elevated reduced glutathione levels in plasma, heart, liver and brain, although the total decreased. Such results indicate that exercise can be beneficial not only to delay the onset of aging but also in old rats [26].

AGING IN THE CARDIOVASCULAR SYSTEM

Aging in the cardiovascular system is characterized by an increase in blood pressure, a reduction in cardiac output and in the response to stress. Blood circulation suffers alterations also, since the decrease in the efficiency of the heart to pump blood, as well as the thickening and rigidity that can occur in the vessels, all contribute to produce areas where blood supply is deficient. The most important changes in the cardiovascular system induced by aging are listed in Table 3.

Table 3. Manifestations of aging in the cardiovascular system

Heart

1. Reduction of cardiac output.
2. Increased susceptibility to damage by oxidative stress.
3. Loss of myocytes through necrosis and apoptosis.
4. Mitochondrial deterioration.

Blood Vessels

1. Increased blood pressure.
2. Reduced vasodilator response due to changes in the secretory function of endothelial cells.
3. Increased sensitivity of endothelial cells to oxidative stress.
4. Decreased number of endothelial cell replications and of circulating endothelial cells.
5. Increased proliferation of vascular smooth muscle cells.
6. Change in cellular phenotype of vascular smooth muscle cells from contractile to synthetizing.
7. Changes in sensitivity of vascular smooth muscle cells to mediators secreted by the endothelial cells.

The decreased blood supply to tissues due to cardiovascular changes during aging is conducive to cellular hypoxia and, in more acute cases, ischaemia or, if there are endothelial lesions, thrombosis. In experimental reperfusion an excess of free radicals is produced, followed by a series of phenomena such as mast cell degranulation, neutrophil infiltration in the endothelium, constriction of arterioles with reduction in tissue perfusion, and increased vascular permeability resulting in inflammation and edema. Neutrophil functioning appears to be deficient in old animals, but when these cells are eliminated from the circulation, the beneficial effects are only observed in young rats. This suggests that in the older animals there are alternative mechanisms capable of inducing inflammation [27].

Although many experiments could be planned to test the diverse theories for aging, most of the experimental work has explored the participation of free radicals in the aging process of the cardiovascular system and most of its manifestations have been explained by oxidative stress. Aging associated with oxidative stress produces a series of functional, metabolic and anatomical alterations which finally become irreversible. Although some controversial data exist, the pathogenesis of several cardiovascular diseases is possibly related to abnormally elevated levels of superoxides.

Aging of the Heart

Cardiac function suffers deterioration with aging. One of the alterations is the increased susceptibility to damage by oxidative stress. In experiments in rats in which hydrogen peroxide as a free radical precursor was infused, this susceptibility was evident at various levels, such as increase in blood pressure, more pronounced in animals aged 6 and 12 months than in those aged 3 months. At 6 and 12 months arrhythmias were also more important, while the enzyme levels were compatible with a reduction in the antioxidant reserve [28].

A comparative study was made of isolated hearts from rats aged 4, 16 or 24 months, in which different variables were investigated, including activity of antioxidant enzymes and post-reperfusion syndrome. The activity of catalase decreased, more noticeably in rats aged 16-months than in those aged 24-months. These latter showed more resistance to post-reperfusion damage, which could be explained by natural selection, rendering this group less susceptible to oxidative stress [29].

Myocardial aging leads to a reduction of beta adrenergic-induced metabolic and contractile responsiveness. These changes are associated with modifications in the profiles of gene expression that may contribute to reduced adrenergic signalling [30].

In the aged heart there is an increased loss of myocytes through necrosis and also through apoptosis, which is propitiated by greater oxidative stress. The organ suffers a decrease in various mitochondrial components, among them the antiapoptotic protein Bcl-2 and cytochrome-c, and this facilitates apoptosis [31,32]. As a compensatory mechanism for the cellular loss, hypertrophy of cardiomyocytes occurs. Nevertheless, the phenomena truly associated with aging are rather of a biochemical and structural nature, consequent to oxidative stress, such as accumulation of lipofucsine, increase in the generation of hydrogen peroxide and other oxidation products (although the activity of mitochondrial antioxidant enzymes is also stimulated) [33].

Measurements of cardiac glycogen levels in two subspecies of mice, one prone to accelerated aging and the other normal, showed that in the first there was a 50 % deficiency in the level in animals aged 4-8 weeks, which was not found in adult animals, suggesting that early damage is a causal agent of premature aging in susceptible species [34].

With regard to the cellular components, measurements have been made of the concentration of water and various chemical elements in the cytoplasm, nucleus, mitochondria and lipofuscine granules in rat cardiomyocytes, after being cultured for two weeks in atmospheres containing from 5 % to 40 % oxygen. At the end of the experimental period the lipofuscine granules contained lower concentrations of cations but more phosphorus than the mitochondria [35].

Aging in the heart is characterized by mitochondrial deterioration which can be prevented by alimentary supplementation [36]. Under oxidative stress conditions, dehydration was apparent in the mitochondria, but their cation content did not vary. This pattern is characteristic of in situ cells from old rats, indicating that the dehydration is a consequence of the damage induced by the oxygen free radicals [35]. On the other hand, in pathological cases, when there is a surplus of reactive species (particularly those of oxygen), the risk increases, since in the majority of cells mitochondria do not contain catalase [37].

A model of oxidative stress-induced aging has been developed in mice, using inhaled ozone, which increases the levels of malondialdehyde in various organs, including the heart [38]. In this respect, a group of researchers has demonstrated that oxidative stress is possibly just one of several factors, such as environmental pollutants, therapeutic drugs or transitory hypoxia, that contribute to modify mitochondrial functions through continuous impacts during the lifetime of the animals; this was proved when adult animals were subjected to environmental stress conditions, and their mitochondria behaved like those of old animals [39].

There is a clear disadvantage in elderly organs as compared with young animals under stress conditions such as exhaustive exercise, which is manifested as a larger increase in oxidative stress. Nevertheless there are significant differences depending on the organ, with the heart showing more damage factors than the liver [40].

Aging in Blood Vessels

Few studies have been undertaken of the ontogeny and aging of vascular contractility. Aging in blood vessels is related to structural and functional changes in the endothelium, smooth muscle and extracellular matrix [41]. The most important changes are listed in Table 3. Age related vascular changes vary among different species and in vessels irrigating various organs [42].

Atherosclerosis frequently occurs in the main arteries of the heart, brain and lower limbs, which leads to deficient blood supply. Its pathogeny is associated with oxidative stress, which in turn favors alterations in lipoproteins as well as glyco-oxidation, all contributing to vascular damage [25].

Therapies geared to retard the vascular aging process are of great clinical importance. In fact, there are numerous studies in process, aiming at determining the etiology of cardiovascular aging, as well as the prevention of its more noxious aspects. One of the strategies consists in increasing the antioxidant reserve, which has been found in rats which do not develop atherosclerosis and where a physiological mechanism exists that increases the levels of vitamin E. In one such study, measurements of the vitamin in major organs and plasma of 3-year old animals were carried out. The largest increase, 70 times the normal, was localized in the aortic wall. This observation suggests the existence of adaptative mechanisms, conducive to protecting the organism from possible oxidative stress associated with aging [43].

The Aging Endothelium

One of the most important discoveries in recent decades in cardiovascular physiology has been the role of the endothelium as a generator of vasoactive substances [44]. This concept originated from the studies of Furchgott and his collaborators [45,46] who demonstrated the presence of the endothelium derived relaxing factor (EDRF), which was later identified as nitric oxide (NO) [47]. Other factors described afterwards were the endothelium derived hyperpolarizing factor (EDHF) and prostacyclin, both derived from the arachidonic acid metabolism [48]. These findings have stimulated an enormous interest in this area, since a large number of other endothelium derived factors have been identified and their importance proved, both in normal physiology and in pathological processes.

During aging the vasodilator response to agonists in resistance and capacitance in rat arteries is reduced, and this change has been related to alterations in the secretion equilibrium of vasoconstrictor and vasodilator substances. A decrease in the NO or the endothelium-derived hyperpolarizing factor-induced vasodilation or an increase in vasoconstriction induced by cycloxygenase products, such as thromboxane A2, probably occur during aging [46-48].

Oxidative stress plays a key role in the aging of endothelial cells, which is characterized by an accelerated destruction of NO due to free oxygen radicals. The importance of this response depends on the species and the vascular bed involved [33]. Besides, it has been found that endothelium-dependent vasodilation in arterioles of skeletal muscle deteriorates with age. However its magnitude depends on the vascular bed and in the functionality of the muscle, which is shown in the fact that most damage is found in the resistance arterioles of the skeletal muscle, whereas in the smooth muscle aging does not modify vascular reactivity [49].

It has been demonstrated that endothelial cells are a very sensitive target of oxidative stress, particularly to superoxide radicals, which can damage considerably both the system responsible for the production of NO, and the factor itself. This it transforms into pro-oxidant elements, such as peroxynitrates, which have been associated with aging of the vascular system [43,50,51].

It is well known that NO is synthesized from L-arginine through the action of the NO synthases, particularly the endothelial synthase, in the case of the vessels (eNOS) [52]. Paradoxically, in rats the expression of eNOS increases significantly with age, but the levels of NO diminish, suggesting that this reduction is due to the rapid conversion of NO to peroxynitrates, through the action of superoxide radicals [53]. Vascular and renal mRNA for inducible NO synthase, as well as for proendothelin, increases with age and favors functional and anatomic changes leading to age-related pathologies, including atherosclerosis [54]. The activation of vascular endothelin and inducible NO synthase are important independent factors promoting increase in blood pressure and thereby contributing to structural and functional anomalies during aging [54].

Cellular age, calculated *in vitro* on the number of cellular replications, has been correlated with a decrease in NO synthase and an increase in the number of monocytes adhering to the endothelial cells. The stable expression of telomerase induces a younger endothelial cell phenotype with an increase of NO synthase and higher NO activity. Therefore, telomerase transfection has important functional consequences in the endothelial cells [55].

Aging has been associated with an anatomical heterogeneity of endothelial dysfunctions, increases in the expression of vascular mRNA of preproendothelin, (precursor of the potent endothelium derived vasoconstrictor endothelin-1) as well as vascular superoxide dismutase activity. This alteration can induce functional and anatomical changes conducive to pathologies typical of aging [56].

The number of circulating endothelial cells increases with age, reflecting an increased cellular turnover in rats. This alteration in endothelial function could contribute to a higher risk of pathological processes in the arterial wall [57]. There is an up-regulation of the trophic effect of endothelin with age. Age can increase the sensitivity of the endothelium to apoptotic stimuli. Thus, oxidized low density lipoproteins (LDL) and tumor necrosis factor- alpha (TNF-alpha) increase the caspase-3-like activity more than three times in old cells, in comparison with young ones. Besides, the levels of nitrosilated S-proteins are reduced, indicating that the protection exerted by NO against S-nitrosilating caspases is not achieved efficiently. This effect is reversed when over-expression of endothelial NO synthase (eNOS) is induced [58].

The Aging Vascular Smooth Muscle

When vascular smooth cells from donors of different ages are cultured, the cells of individuals whose lives are ending show characteristics of elderly cells and a deterioration of their replicative potential [59]. However, some situations such as atherosclerosis and restenosis have revealed that age increases the proliferation of vascular smooth muscle [60-62]. An increase in c-fos activity during aging elevates cyclin A expression, enhancing proliferation. This phenomenon may contribute to an increased prevalence and worsening of atherosclerosis in aged animals [1,63]. Nevertheless, in old rats there is no difference in the intima thickness/lumen diameter relation in any vascular region [64]. The rise of smooth muscle proliferation with age might be related to a calcium homeostasis imbalance or a platelet derived growth factor (PDGF) gene over-expression [60]. Also the oxidative response determines the rate of smooth muscle cell proliferation [63]. It has also been proposed that an increase in the sympathetic autonomous nervous system tone activity towards the vessels might play an important role in renovation and proliferation of the muscle [61].

During the aging of the vascular smooth muscle, the cellular phenotype changes from contractile to synthetizing. Old cells do not respond to some inhibiting factors such as transforming growth factor β-1(TGF-β1). They cease to interact normally with the extracellular matrix, due to changes in the expression of integrins or to changes in the extracellular matrix composition [65].

The responses of the vascular smooth muscle to the contracting or relaxing mediators secreted by the endothelium also change with age. Aging does not significantly alter the vascular resistance, contractility or smooth muscle sensitivity [65]. However, vasoreactivity is slightly increased at low pressures, which may be a consequence of geometric changes caused by the intima-interstice increase [66].

Reduced relaxation during aging in rats may be due to a decreased activation of protein kinase G-1 (PKG-1) [67]. Some authors have found that adenosine mediates nitric oxide-dependent relaxation as well as relaxation mediated by other substances in the aorta and coronary arteries and that aging and maturity reduces the response to adenosine. A decreased aortic response also involves a reduction of the optimal transduction signal to the adenosine receptor [68]. During aging it has been reported that voltage and calcium activated potassium channels (MaxiK) reduce their expression, modifying vascular tone and reducing the vasodilation capacity [69].

Aging also increases the coronary artery response to vasoconstrictor factors. The rise in systemic arterial pressure with age can be correlated to elevated endothelin-1 (ET-1) receptor density in the smooth muscle cells [70]. However, the contractile response to ET-1 decreases with age [71]. The change in the sensitivity to endothelin with age is not homogeneous in all arteries; in aortic and renal arteries of old rats sensitivity is reduced, while in the mesenteric artery it is increased [72]. Endothelin levels in the blood vessels decline with age [73].

Studies done in resistance arteries such as the rat tail artery, show that the sensitivity and contents of vasoconstrictor substances such as noradrenaline (NA) fall during aging [74]; however, the response to NA, phenylephrine and high potassium rises with age. When the endothelium is removed, the response to NA is different depending on the vascular bed (aorta or tail artery) [75]. The decline in sensitivity to NA in the rat aortic artery is due to a post receptor mechanism [42], since the β-receptor mechanism does not change during aging [76]. With other mediators, the response does not change in vivo. The myotropic effect of angiotensin II (ATII) [77] and the 5-hydroxytryptamine receptor deteriorate through age (in rats less than 90 days old) [78].

Some studies indicate that there are no changes in the response to NA during aging when endothelin is present in the perfusion system of rat arteries bathed "in vitro" [79]. Responses to ET-1 and NA can change depending on the rat strain [76,77]. The functional change implies an altered response of the vascular smooth muscle [79].

In contrast with reports in rats, rabbit heart frequency does not change with age, but blood pressure rises in a significant way in older animals compared with three month old animals. The vessels of older animals are thicker and less sensitive to NA. The responses to potassium, histamine and isoproterenol do not vary with age [80]. There is a diminution in the adrenergic nerve function that innervates rabbit vessels, which reflects a lower NA release after nervous stimulation and a decrease in NA recapture. These two effects are counterbalanced; there is only a slight decrease in the contractile response to adrenergic nerve stimulation, which is exacerbated when the capture mechanisms are blocked [81].

In the human basilar artery, aging reduces the maximal contraction produced by KCl, NA and 5-hydroxytryptamine. This drop in the contractile response is due to an unspecific structure change in the media cell structure [78].

Vascular intracellular signalling functions differently in the isolated smooth muscle of young and old rats; intracellular second messenger secretion is altered due to age- related changes in the signals sent by the endothelial cells. Traffic of intracellular messengers is altered by the calcium-calmodulin II enzyme [65]. The GMPc concentration falls with age, following the same pattern of nitric oxide synthase expression [56]. Some studies have demonstrated that with age there is an increase in the inositol phosphate levels in response to its agonists [82]. Protein kinase G1 activation is reduced and it has been suggested that this decrease may explain the vascular relaxation in older organisms [67].

Cardiovascular Risk Factors and Aging

Hypertension is an age-dependent disorder [83], and almost half of the elderly human population (more than 65 years old) is hypertensive [84]. Several models of hypertensive rats have been used to examine the influence of hypertension on the developing and aging cardiovascular system. Important alterations have been described which are discussed in the following sections. Insulin resistance is associated with aging and contributes to vascular malfunction. The prevalence of type 2 diabetes increases with age and affects almost 20 % of people over age 65 [85] and there are twice as many hypertensive patients among diabetics compared to non-diabetics. Models of diabetic rats have also been studied to analyze the role of diabetes in altering the aging cardiovascular system. The main alterations induced by hypertension and diabetes on the aging processes in the cardiovascular system are mentioned in Table 4.

Table 4. Cardiovascular risk factors and aging

1. Hypertension renders vessels stronger, more rigid and hyperactive.
2. Vascular responses are affected in a different way in insulin-dependent diabetes and non insulin-dependent diabetes.
3. Diabetes increases the sympathetic arterial constriction.
4. Arterial capacity to compensate rises in contractility are diminished in old diabetic animals.
5. High insulin levels cause a constrictor response in old organisms.

Aging and Hypertension

Changes Related to the Onset of Hypertension

Numerous studies focus on comparing the differences in development and aging patterns between hypertensive and normal rats. The contractile responses of vascular smooth muscle to NA, KCl, 5-hydroxytryptamine, electrostimulation and calcium-free physiological solution are increased during development and maturity in normal rats. Endothelium-dependent relaxation mediated by acetylcholine as well as isoproterenol, which is mediated by the β-receptor, falls during rat maturation [86].

Peripheral resistance in hypertension cannot be accounted for by a general abnormality in the calcium-dependent contractile machinery nor by changes in agonist-induced calcium sensitivity of vascular smooth muscle. There are no differences in the calcium responses of mesenteric, renal and femoral arteries between normal and hypertensive rats, nor among groups of different ages [87]. Calcium permeability induced by potassium potentials is normal in the vascular smooth muscle cells of spontaneously hypertensive rats; nevertheless, the calcium permeability induced by NA is increased [87].

The different response that endothelin 1 evokes in spontaneously hypertensive rats during the onset of hypertension, can be in part related to altered responses of receptors to this mediator and to the onset of the elevation of the arterial pressure, which causes hemodynamic imbalances [88].

In an experimental hypertension model in rats, based on a fructose-rich diet, endothelin expression is increased in blood vessels, while NO levels are not modified [89]. In another rat model of hypertension obtained by administering 30% sucrose in the drinking water for 20 weeks, an increased insulin-dependent endothelin response of the vessels has been found [90].

The 5-hydroxytryptamine and α-2 adrenergic receptors are elevated in the Kyoto Wistar rats compared to those of spontaneously hypertensive rats. This finding suggests the participation of the α adrenergic receptors as well as the 5-hydroxytryptamine receptor in the course and maintenance of hypertension [91].

In a mouse model with high blood pressure, the oxidant and anti-oxidant status in the aorta was explored and an increase in superoxide dismutase activity and a decrease in catalase activity were found to be responsible for the increased release of H_2O_2 in this vessel [83].

Alterations Related to Aging in Hypertensive Rats

Hypertensive rat vessels are stronger, more rigid and hyperactive than those in normal rats; therefore, they are capable of responding in a considerably wider range of tensions despite the high pressure to which the individuals may be exposed. This characteristic of the responses is enhanced when the hypertension is corrected. In contrast, in normal arteries, during aging, there is practically no change in the resistance, nor in contractility or sensitivity to vasoactive substances [65]. In spontaneously hypertensive old rats, the smooth muscle capacity to remove calcium is reduced, compared with that of the Kyoto Wistar rats [92].

During the late stages of aging in spontaneously hypertensive rats (SHR), there is an inhibition of the vascular relaxation pathway involving not only NO production by endothelial cells but also the bio-availability of NO and the smooth muscle response to NO. This inhibition is partially reversed during chronic antioxidant treatment [93].

The strain of the rats alters the aging response to ET-1 and NA, but it is not modified by hypertension or hyperlipidemia [79]. Also there are no differences in the responding capacity to endothelin in isolated arteries of Kyoto Wistar rats of different ages. In contrast, an increase in the response to ET-1 was found with age in spontaneously hypertensive rats (SHR) [94]. This difference seems to be specific to ET-1, since the response capacity to NA did not change. The drop in the capacity of the aortas to respond with age in SHR rats could be due to chronic hypertension and a desensitizing reaction to ET-1. This could be related to chronic hyperactive production of endothelin "in vivo", which can be genetically determined or can be related to the endothelial damage produced by hypertension [88].

The inositol phosphate production stimulated by NA and endothelin dropped with age in SHR rats and the reduction was greater in these rats when compared to the Kyoto Wistar rats [82]. Therefore, the age and the strain modulate inositol phosphate production induced by agonists [82].

Aging and Diabetes

Insulin modifies vascular responses at different levels and there are contradictory reports that point out that it can increase or decrease contractility. Elements of the evidence that insulin acts as a hypotensive agent are: *1)* high insulin levels like those present in insulinoma patients do not cause hypertension [95]; *2)* insulin has vasodilator properties raising α2-adrenergic relaxation through a pertussis toxin-sensitive mechanism, which stimulates the endothelial production of nitric oxide [96,97]; *3)* insulin is also associated with a vasodilation mediated by the β-adrenergic response [98], which raises the type-C natriuretic peptide endothelial secretion [99]; *4)* insulin reduces the intracellular calcium levels, lowering the flux through the voltage and ligand dependent channels and raising calcium ATPase activity [100]; *5)* insulin diminishes the contractile responses; the calcium response of the smooth muscle of the porcine right coronary arteries decreases [101,102], and the vasoconstrictor effects of endothelin in porcine pericardic arteries also diminish [103].

There is evidence that indicates a vasoconstrictor effect of insulin such as: *1)* ET-1 levels are high in patients with diabetes mellitus [104] and during euglycemic clamp experiments with hyperinsulinemia in subjects with non-insulin dependent diabetes mellitus (NIDDM) [105]; *2)* hypertriglyceridemia increases the stimulatory effect of insulin upon endothelin secretion in studies correlating hyperinsulinemia and hypertension [106]; *3)* there is a relationship between high insulin levels and hypertension in many different species [107]; *4)* insulin stimulates endothelin production by endothelial cells from pigs and bovines [108]; *5)* insulin induces an increase in the gene expression of ET-1 [109]; *6)* insulin raises calcium levels by elevating the activity of Na^+-H^+ and Na^+-Ca^{2+} transporters [99].

Severe rises in plasmatic insulin produce sympathetic excitation and vasodilatation in young adult rats. Aging is associated with insulin resistance and alters sympathetic responses. In contrast to the vasodilatation seen in young animals, insulin causes vasoconstriction in healthy elderly animals. The absence of a relaxing action of insulin in old organisms leads to a slight excitation of the sympathetic system, which provokes vasoconstriction. The constrictor response to insulin empowers insulin resistance in aging subjects [110]. Older hyperinsulinemic animals show an exaggerated selective reaction to 5-hydroxytryptamine and some changes in the endothelium-dependent relaxation induced by ADP as well as a deficiency in the adenilate ciclase enzyme in the smooth muscle.

Insulin-dependent diabetes (IDDM) and non insulin-dependent diabetes (NIDDM) affect vascular responses differently. In diabetic rats the response to β-adrenergic stimulation is diminished and this response reduction is not related to an adenylate ciclase malfunction; however, there is a non-selective disorder in the calcium dependent responses [111,112]. Diabetes lowers the aortic tissue sensitivity to niphedipine and alters the excitation-contraction coupling mechanisms of vascular smooth muscle, enhancing calcium entrance after stimulation. These mechanisms could be responsible for the diabetes-dependent vascular complications [113]. Arterial capacity to compensate the rises in contractility is altered in obese rats (insulin-resistant) and this is accentuated by age [114].

Conclusion

In spite of the tremendous progress by researchers studying cultured cells, free radicals, longevity determining genes and other promising paths, aging is still little understood. Adding to the confusion is the fact that age-related changes do not occur uniformly, either among species, cells or individuals who differ in their susceptibility to specific disorders and in exposure to environmental stresses.

Of all the theories proposed to explain aging, oxidative stress appears to be the most experimentally tested and the primary explanation to date for aging in the cardiovascular system in animal models. Aging in the cardiovascular system is characterized by an increase in blood pressure, a reduction in cardiac output and in the response to stress. In blood vessels, aging is related to structural and functional changes in the endothelium, smooth muscle and extracellular matrix. Age-related vascular changes vary among different species and in vessels irrigating various organs. The mechanisms by which hypertension and diabetes alter the aging mechanisms of the cardiovascular system have been studied in different animal models.

Cardiovascular aging is altered by diseases such as hypertension and diabetes but also aging in general makes organisms more susceptible to such ills as heart disease, stroke and cancer. In humans, the increased life span has increased the incidence of such diseases and they in turn modify the aging processes of the organisms. However, even if science could eliminate today's leading killers of older individuals, aging would continue to occur, ensuring that different maladies would take their place. It would also guarantee that one crucial body component or another, such as the cardiovascular system, would eventually experience a catastrophic failure.

We still do not know how far life might be extended, but prolonging survival could have profound social, environmental and economic consequences. The primary goal of biomedical research and efforts to slow aging should not be the mere extension of life, but rather prolonging the duration of healthy life. Systematic investigations into aging are in progress and could one day provide methods to slow our inevitable decline and extend health and longevity.

REFERENCES

[1] Rivard A, Principe N, Andres V. Age-dependent increase in c-fos activity and cyclin A expression in vascular smooth muscle cells. A potential link between aging, smooth muscle cell proliferation and atherosclerosis. *Cardiovasc Res* 2000; 45(4): 1026-1034.

[2] Rose M, Charlesworth B. A test of evolutionary theories of senescence. *Nature* 1980; 287: 141-142.

[3] Rusting RL. Why do we age? *Sci Am* 1992; 267: 87-95.

[4] Harman D. Aging: overview. *Ann N Y Acad Sci* 2001; 928: 1-21.

[5] Lutz PL, Prentice HM, Milton SL. Is turtle longevity linked to enhanced mechanisms for surviving brain anoxia and reoxygenation. *Exp Gerontol* 2003; 38(7):797-800.

[6] Economos AC. Rate of aging, rate of dying and non-Gompertzian mortality- encore... *Gerontology* 1985; 31: 106-111.

[7] Finch CE, Ruvkun G. The genetics of aging. *Annu Rev Genomics Hum Genet* 2001;2:435-462.

[8] Kirkwood TB. Genes that shape the course of ageing. *Trends Endocrinol Metab* 2003; 14: 345-347 .

[9] Kirkwood TB, Rose MR. Evolution of senescence: late survival sacrificed for reproduction. *Philos Trans R Soc Lond B Biol Sci* 1991; 332: 15-24.

[10] Tatar M, Bartke A, Antebi A. The endocrine regulation of aging by insulin-like signals. *Science* 2003; 299(5611): 1346-1351.

[11] Carter CS, Ramsey MM, Ingram RL, Cashion AB, Cefalu WT, Wang ZQ, Sonntag WE. Models of growth hormone and IGF-1 deficiency: applications to studies of aging

processes and life-span determination. *J Gerontol A Biol Sci Med Sci* 2002; 57(5):B177-188.

[12] Bartke A, Chandrashekar V, Dominici F, Turyn D, Kinney B, Steger R, Kopchick JJ. Insulin-like growth factor 1 (IGF-1) and aging: controversies an new insights. *Biogenrontology* 2003; 4(1): 1-8.

[13] Manda K, Bhatia AL. Melatonin-induced reduction in age-related accumulation of oxidative damage in mice. *Biogerontology* 2003; 4(3): 133-139.

[14] Simon AF, Shih C, Mack A, Benzer S. Steroid control of longevity in Drosophila melanogaster. *Science* 2003; 299(5611):1407-1410.

[15] Hayflick H. The cell biology of human aging. *Sci Am* 1980; 242: 42-49.

[16] Harman D. Free-radical theory of aging. Increasing the functional life span. *Ann N Y Acad Sci* 1994; 717: 1-15.

[17] Roth GS, Ingram DK, Lane MA. Caloric restriction in primates and relevance to humans. *Ann N Y Acad Sci* 2001; 928: 305-315.

[18] Cerami A, Vlassara H, Brownlee M. Glucose and aging *Sci Am* 1987 256: 82-89.

[19] Wei YH, Ma YS, Lee HC, Lee CF, Lu CY. Mitochondrial theory of aging matures – roles of mtDNA mutation and oxidative stress in human aging. *Zhonghua Yi Xue Za Zhi* 2001; 64: 257-270.

[20] Melov S, Coskun PE, Wallace DC. Mouse models of mitochondrial disease, oxidative stress, and senescence. *Mutat Res* 1999;434(3):233-242).

[21] Charlesworth B. Evolutionary mechanisms of senescence *Genetica* 1993; 91:11-19.

[22] Rose MR, Graves JL Jr. What evolutionary biology can do for gerontology. *J Gerontol* 1989; 44: B27-.

[23] Dilman VM. Ontogenetic model of ageing and disease formation and mechanisms of natural selection. *J Theor Biol* 1986; 118: 73-81.

[24] Li J, Holbrook NJ. Common mechanisms for declines in oxidative stress tolerance and proliferation with aging. *Free Radic Biol Med* 2003; 35(3): 292-299.

[25] Reaven PD. Napoli C, Merat S, Witztum JL. Lipoprotein modification and atherosclerosis in aging. *Exp Gerontol* 1999; 34(4): 527-537.

[26] Ohkuwa T, Sato Y, Naoi M. Glutathione status and reactive oxygen generation in tissues of young and old exercised rats. *Acta Physiol Scand* 1997;159(3):237-244.

[27] Harris NR, Rumbaut RE. Age-related responses of the micorcirculation to ischemia-reperfusion and inflammation. *Pathophysiology* 2001;8(1):1-10.

[28] Abete P, Napoli C, Santoro G, Ferrara N. et al. Age-related decrease in cardiac tolerance to oxidative stress. *J Mol Cell Cardiol* 1999; 31 (1):227-236.

[29] Boucher F, Tanguy S, Besse S, Tresallet N, Favier A, de Leiris J. Age-dependent changes in myocardial susceptibility to zero flow ischemia and reperfusion in isolated perfused rat hearts: relation to antioxidant status. *Mech Ageing Dev* 1998;103(3):301-316.

[30] Dobson Jr JG, Fray J, Leonard JL, Pratt RE. Molecular mechanisms of reduced {beta}-adrenergic signaling in the aged heart as revealed by genomic profiling. *Physiol Genomics* 2003; 15(2):142-147.

[31] Phaneuf S, Leeuwenburgh C. Cytochrome c release from mitochondria in the aging heart: a possible mechanism for apoptosis with age *Am J Physiol Regul Integr Comp Physiol* 2002;282(2):R423-430.

[32] Pollack M, Leeuwenburgh C. Apoptosis and aging: role of the mitochondria. *J Gerontol A Biol Sci Med Sci* 2001;56(11):B475-482.

[33] Muscari C, Giaccari A, Giordano E, Clo C, Guarnieri C, Caldarera CM. Role of reactive oxygen species in cardiovascular aging. *Mol Cell Biochem* 1996;160-161:159-166.

[34] Kurokawa T, Ozaki N. Sato E, Ishibashi S. Rapid decrease of glycogen concentration in the hearts of senescence-accelerated mice during aging. *Mech Ageing Dev* 1997; 97(3);227-236.

[35] von Zglinicki T, Marzabadi MR, Roomans GM. Water and ion distributions in myocytes cultured under oxidative stress mimic changes found in the process of aging. *Mech Ageig Dev* 199; 58(1):49-60.

[36] Hagen TM, Moreau R, Suh JH, Visioli F. Mitochondrial decay in the aging rat heart: evidence for improvement by dietary supplementation with acetyl-L-carnitine and/or lipoic acid. *Ann N Y Acad Sci* 2002; 959:491-507.

[37] Bai J, Cederbaum AI. Mitochondrial catalase and oxidative injury. *Biol Signals Recept* 2001;10(3-4):189-199.

[38] Feng R, He W, Ochi H. A new murine oxidative stress model associated with senescence. *Mech Ageing Dev* 200; 122(6):547-559.

[39] Nohl H, Staniek K, Gille L Imbalance of oxygen activation and energy metabolism as a consequence or mediator fo aging. *Expl Gerontol* 1997; 32 (4-5):485-500.

[40] Bejma J, Ramires P, Ji LL. Free radical generation and oxidative stress with ageing and exercise: differential effects in the myocardium and liver. *Acta Physiol Scand* 2000; 169(4):343-351.

[41] Matz RL, Schott C, Stoclet JC, Andriantsitohaina R. Age-related endothelial dysfunction with respect to nitric oxide, endothelium-derived hyperpolarizing factor and cyclooxygenase products. *Physiol Res* 2000; 49(1): 11-18

[42] Carvajal A, Velasco A, Martin Arias LH, Maroto M.J. Age-related changes in contractile responses to noradrenaline in isolated blood vessels from rat and rabbit. *Auton Pharmacol* 1995; 15(5): 321-326

[43] van der Loo B, Labugger R, Aebischer CP, Skepper JN, Bachschmid M, Spitzer V, Kilo J, Altwegg L, Ullrich V, Luscher TF. Cardiovascular aging is associated with vitamin. E increase. *Circulation* 2002; 105(14):1635-1638.

[44] Inagami T, Naruse M, Hoover R. Endothelium as an endocrine organ. *Ann Rev Physiol* 1995; 57: 171-189.

[45] Furchgott R.F., Zawadzki J.V. The obligatory role of endothelial cells in the relaxation of arterial smooth muscle by acetylcholine. *Nature* 1980; 288: 373-376.

[46] Ignarro L. J., Byrns R.E., Buga G.M y Wood K.S Endothelium-derived relaxing factor (EDRF) released from artery and vein appears to be nitric oxide (NO) or a closely related radical species. (Abstract). *Fed Proc Am Soc Exp Biol* 1987; 46:644P.

[47] Palmer RMJ, Ferrige AG, Moncada S. Nitric oxide release accounts for the biological activity of endothelium-derived relaxing factor. *Nature* 1987;327:524-526.

[48] Cohen RA, Vanhoutte PM. Endothelium-dependent hyperpolarization. Beyond nitric oxide and cyclic GMP. *Circulation* 1995;92:3337-3349.

[49] Muller-Delp JM, Spier SA, Ramsey MW, Delp MD. Aging impairs endothelium-dependent vasodilation in rat skeletal muslce arterioles. *Am J Physiol* 2002; 283: H1662-H 1672.

[50] Gryglewski RJ, Palmer RM, Moncada S. Superoxide anion is involved in the breakdown of endothelium-derived vascular relaxing factor. *Nature* (Lond.) 1986;320:454-456.

[51] Dreww B, Leeuwenburgh C. Aging and the role of reactive nitrogen species. *Ann NY Acad Sci* 2002; 959:66-81.

[52] Moncada S, Palmer RMJ, Higgs EA. Nitric oxide: physiology, pathophysiology, and pharmacology. *Pharmacol Rev* 1991;43:225-246.

[53] van der Loo B, Labugger R, Skepper JN, Bachschmid M, Kilo J, Powell J.M. et al. Enhanced peroxynitrite formation is assocated with vascular aging. *J Exp Med* 2000; 192: 1731-1743.

[54] Goettsch W, Lattmann T, Amann K, Szibor M, Morawietz H, Munter K, et al. Increased expression of endothelin-1 and inducible nitric oxide synthase isoform II in aging arteries in vivo: implications for atherosclerosis. *Biochem Biophys Res Commun* 2001;280: 908-913.

[55] Matsushita H, Chang E, Glassford AJ, Cooke JP, Chiu CP, Tsao PS. Activity Is Reduced in Senescent Human Endothelial Cells: Preservation by hTERT Immortalization. *Circ Res* 2001; 89(9): 793-798

[56] Barton M, Cosentino F, Brandes RP, Moreau P, Shaw S, Luscher TF. Anatomic heterogeneity of vascular aging: role of nitric oxide and endothelin. *Hypertension* 1997; 30(4): 817-824 .

[57] Challah M, Nadaud S, Philippe M, Battle T, Soubrier F, Corman B,Michel JB. Circulating and cellular markers of endothelial dysfunction with aging in rats. *Am J Physiol* 1997; 273(4 Pt 2):H1941-1948.

[58] Hoffmann J, Haendeler J. Aicher A, Rossig L et al. Aging enhances the sensivity of endothelial cells toward apoptotic stimuli: important role nitric oxide. *Circ Res* 2001; 89 (8): 709-715.

[59] Ruiz-Torres A, Gimeno A, Melon J, Mendez L, Munoz FJ, Macia M. Age-related loss of proliferative activity of human vascular smooth muscle cells in culture. *Mech Ageing Dev* 1999; 110(1-2): 49-55.

[60] Wen YY, Wang SX, Chen MQ. Studies on age-related changes in vascular smooth muscle and their Ca2+ mechanisms. *Clin Exp Pharmacol Physiol* 1999; 26(10): 840-841.

[61] Dinenno FA, Jones PP, Seals DR, Tanaka H. Age-associated arterial wall thickening is related to elevations in sympathetic activity in healthy humans. *Am J Physiol Heart Circ Physiol* 2000; 278(4): H1205-1210.

[62] Johnson CP, Baugh R, Wilson CA, Burns J. Age related changes in the tunica media of the vertebral artery: implications for the assessment of vessels injured by trauma. *J Clin Pathol* 2001; 54(2): 139-145.

[63] Moon SK, Thompson LJ, Madamanchi N, Ballinger S, Papaconstantinou, Horaist C, Runge MS, Patterson C. Aging, oxidative responses, and proliferative capacity in cultured mouse aortic smooth muscle cells. *Am J Physiol Heart Circ Physiol* 2001; 280(6):H2779-2788.

[64] Shaw LM, Ohanian J, Heagerty AM. Calcium sensitivity and agonist-induced calcium sensitization in small arteries of young and adult spontaneously hypertensive rats. *Hypertension* 1997; 30(3 Pt 1): 442-448.

[65] Lundberg MS, Crow MT. Age-related changes in the signaling and function of vascular smooth muscle cells. *Exp Gerontol* 1999; 34(4): 549-57.

[66] Folkow B, Karlstrom G. Age- and pressure-dependent changes of systemic resistance vessels concerning the relationships between geometric design, wall distensibility, vascular reactivity and smooth muscle sensitivity. *Acta Physiol Scand* 1984; 122(1): 17-33.

[67] Lin CS, Liu X, Tu R, Chow S, Lue TF. Age-related decrease of protein kinase G activation in vascular smooth muscle cells. *Biochem Biophys Res Commun* 2001; 287(1): 244-248.

[68] Hinschen AK, Rose'Meyer RB, Headrick JP. Age-related changes in adenosine-meiated relaxation of coronary and aortic smooth muscle. *Am J Physiol Heart Circ Physiol* 2001; 280(5): H2380-2389.

[69] Marijic J, Li Q, Song M, Nishimaru K, Stefani E, Toro L. Decreased expression of voltage- and Ca(2+)-activated K(+) channels in coronary smooth muscle during aging. *Circ Res* 2001; 88(2): 210-216.

[70] Lu MH, Chao CF, Chin YH, Yu KR, Pai L. The correlation of blood pressure, age and endothelin-1binding sites in aortic smooth muscle cells of rats. *Jpn Circ J* 1998; 62(7):532-536.

[71] Pirrelli A, Mitolo-Chieppa D. Endothelin-1-receptor-mediated responses in resistance vessels of young and adult spontaneously hypertensive rats. *J Hypertens* 2000; 18(7): 893-900.

[72] Ishihata A, Katano Y, Morinobu S, Endoh M. Influence of aging on the contractile response to endothelin of rat thoracic aorta. *Eur J Pharmacol* 1991; 200(1): 199-201.

[73] Weinheimer G, Dooley DJ, Cazzonelli M, Osswald H. Aging and endothelin-1 induced vascular contractions. *Experientia* 1990; 46(10): 1008-1009.

[74] Tabernero A, Vila E. Effect of age on noradrenaline response in rat tail artery and aorta: role of endothelium. *J Auton Pharmacol* 1995; 15(5): 327-333.

[75] Fouda AK, Atkinson J. Sensitivity to noradrenaline and electrical stimulation decreases with age in the rat tail artery. *Naunyn Schmiedebergs Arch Pharmacol* 1986; 334(1): 37-39.

[76] Hayashi S, Toda N. Age-related changes in the response of rabbit isolated aortae to vasoactive agents. *Br J Pharmacol* 1978; 64(2): 229-237.

[77] Couture R, Regoli D. Vascular reactivity to angiotensin and noradrenaline in rats. Effect of aging and of uninephrectomy. *Clin Exp Hypertens* 1980; 2(1): 1-24.

[78] Hatake K, Wakabayashi I, Kakishita E, Hishida S. Effect of aging on contractile response to KCl, norepinephrine and 5-hydroxytryptamine in isolated human basilar artery. *Gen Pharmacol* 1992; 23(3): 417-420.

[79] Filippelli A, Palla A, Lampa E, Rossi F. Aging and in vitro vascular responses to endothelin-1 in several rat strains. *Pharmacol Res* 1993; 28(3): 193-202.

[80] Duckles SP. Age-related changes in adrenergic neuronal function of rabbit vascular smooth muscle. *Neurobiol Aging* 1983; 4(2): 151-156.

[81] Owen TL. Effect of age on blood pressure and small vessel reactivity in male rabbits. *Blood Vessels* 1986; 23(6):271-278.

[82] Pasanisi F, Hamilton CA, Wadsworth R, Pryce C, Nixon G, Reid JL. Phosphoinositide metabolism and aging in aorta from SHR and WKY rats: effects of endothelin-1 and noradrenaline. *Clin Exp Hypertens* 1994; 16(1): 119-133.

[83] Uddin M, Yang H, Shi M, Polley-Mandal M, Guo Z. Elevation of oxidative stress in the aorta of genetically hypertensive mice. *Mech Ageing Dev* 2003; 124(7): 811-817.

[84] García-Peña C, Thorogood M, Reyes S, Salmeron-Castro J, Duran C. The prevalence and treatment of hypertension in the elderly population of the Mexican Institute o Social Security. *Salud Publica* 2001; 43(5): 1-6.

[85] Wallace JI. Management of diabetes in the elderly. *Clinical Diabetes* 1999; 17(1): 19-26.

[86] Soltis EE, Newman PS. Ontogeny of vascular smooth muscle responsiveness in the postweaning rat. *Dev Pharmacol Ther* 1992; 18(1-2): 44-54.

[87] Mulvany MJ, Nyborg N. An increased calcium sensitivity of mesenteric resistance vessels in young and adult spontaneously hypertensive rats. *Br J Pharmacol* 1980; 71(2): 585-596.

[88] Cargnelli G, Rossi G, Bova S, Pessina AC. In vitro vascular reactivity to endothelin: a comparison between young and old normotensive and hypertensive rats. *Clin Exp Hypertens* 1990; 12(8): 1437-1451.

[89] Lee DH, Lee JU, Kang DG, Paek YW, Chung DJ, Chung MY. Increased vascular endothelin-1 gene expression with unaltered nitric oxide synthase levels in fructose-induced hypertensive rats. *Metabolism* 2001; 50(1): 74-78.

[90] Nava P, Guarner V, Posadas R, Perez I, Baños G. Insulin-induced endothelin release and vasoactivity in hypertriglyceridemic and hypertensive rats. *Am J Physiol* 1999; 277 (*Heart Circ Physiol* 46): H399-H404.

[91] Agrawal DK, McNeill JH. Effect of diabetes on vascular smooth muscle function in normotensive and spontaneously hypertensive rat mesenteric artery. *Can J Physiol Pharmacol* 1987; 65(11): 2274-2280.

[92] Wuorela H, Arvola P, Kahonen M, Vapaatalo H, Porsti I. Arterial smooth muscle responses in adult and moderately aged spontaneously hypertensive rats. *Pharmacol Toxicol* 1994; 74(3): 167-173.

[93] Payne JA, Reckelhoff JF, Khalil RA. Role of oxidative stress in age-related reduction of NO-cGMP-mediated vascular relaxation in SHR. *Am J Physiol Regul Integr Comp Physiol* 2003; 285(3): R542-551.

[94] Montagnani M, Vulpis V, Nazzaro P, Potenza MA, Rinaldi R, Nacci C, De Salvia MA, Siro Brigiani G, Pirrelli A, Mitolo-Chieppa D.J Endothelin-1-receptor-mediated responses in resistance vessels of young and adult spontaneously hypertensive rats. *Hypertension* 2000; 18(7):893-900.

[95] Sawicki PT, Heinemann L, Starke A, Berger M. Hyperinsulinaemia is not linked with blood pressure elevation in patients with insulinoma. *Diabetologia* 1992; 35: 649-652.

[96] Lembo G, Iaccarino G, Vecchione C, Barbato E, Morisco C, Monti F, Parrella L, Trimarco B. Insulin enhances endothelial α_2-adrenergic vasorelaxation by a pertussis toxin mechanism. *Hypertension* 1997; 30: 1128-1134.

[97] Gros R, Borkowski KR, Feldman RD. Human insulin-mediated enhancement of vascular β-adrenergic responsiveness. *Hypertension* 1994; 23: 551-555.

[98] Igaki T, Itoh H, Suga S, Komatsu Y, Ogawa Y, Doi, K, Yoshimasa T, Nakao K. Insulin suppresses endothelial secretion of C-type natriuretic peptide, a novel endothelium-derived relaxing peptide. *Diabetes* 1996; 45 Suppl 3: S62-S64.

[99] Levy J, Zemel MB, Sowers JR. Role of cellular calcium metabolism in abnormal glucose metabolism and diabetic hypertension. *Am J Med* 1989; 87 (suppl 6A): 7S-16S.

[100] Kahn AM, Husid A, Odebunmi T, Allen JC, Seidel CL, Song T. Insulin inhibits vascular smooth muscle contraction at a site distal to calcium concentration. *Am J Physiol* 1998; 274: E885-E892.

[101] Shimizu S, Bowman PS, Thorne G 3rd, Paul RJ. Effects of hypoxia on isometric force, intracellular Ca (2+), pH and energetics in porcine coronary artery. *Circ Res* 2000; 86: 862-870.

[102] Dick GM, Sturek M. Effects of physiological insulin concentration on the endothelin sensitive Ca2+ store in porcine coronary artery smooth muscle. *Diabetes* 1996; 45: 876-880.

[103] Hasdai D, Holmes DR Jr, Richardson DM, Izhar U, Lerman A. Insulin and IGF-1 attenuate the coronary vasoconstrictor effects of endothelin but not of sarafotoxin 6c. *Cardiovasc Res* 1998; 39: 644-650.

[104] Takahashi K, Ghatei MA, Lam HC, Halloran DJO, Bloom SR. Elevated plasma endothelin in patients with diabetes mellitus. *Diabetologia* 1990; 33: 306-310.

[105] Ferri C, Carlomagno A, Coassin S, Baldoncini R, Cassone Faldetta MR, Laurenti O, Properzi G, Santucci A, De Mattia G. Circulating endothelin-1 levels increase during euglycemic hyperinsulinemic clamp in lean NIDDM men. *Diabetes Care* 1995; 18: 226-233.

[106] Piatti PM, Monti LD, Conti M, Baruffaldi K, Galli L, Phan CV, Guazzini B, Pontiroli AE, Pozza G. Hypertriglyceridemia and hyperinsulinemia are potent inducers of endothelin-1 release in humans. *Diabetes* 1996; 45: 316-321.

[107] Hall JE, Brands MW, Hildebrandt DA, Mizelle HL. Obesity-associated hypertension; hyperinsulinemia and renal mechanisms. *Hypertension* 1992; 19: I-45-55.

[108] Hu RM, Levin ER, Pedram A. Insulin stimulates production and secretion of endothelin from bovine endothelial cells. *Diabetes* 1993; 42: 351-358.

[109] Oliver FJ, de la Rubia G, Feener EP, Lee ME, Loeken MR, Shiba T, Quertermous T, King GL. Stimulation of endothelin-1 gene expression by insulin in endothelial cells. *J Biol Chem* 1991; 266: 23251-23256.

[110] Hausberg M, Hoffman RP, Somers VK, Sinkey CA, Mark AL, Anderson EA. Contrasting autonomic and hemodynamic effects of insulin in healthy elderly versus young subjects. *Hypertension* 1997; 29(3): 700-705.

[111] Feletou M, Moreau N, Boulanger M, Duhault J. Effect of aging and drug-induced weight reduction on rat vascular reactivity. *J Cardiovasc Pharmacol* 1993; 21(1): 120-127.

[112] Feletou M, Moreau N, Duhault J. Vascular responsiveness in young, diabetic, and aging hyperinsulinemic rats. *Life Sci* 1994; 54(23): 1801-1813.

[113] Mahmoudian M, Behnaz F, Rezaei E. Diabetes-induced changes in the contractility of the aorta and pA2 of nifedipine in the rat. *Acta Diabetol* 1996; 33(2): 114-117.

[114] O'Brien SF, Russell JC, Davidge ST. Vascular wall dysfunction in JCR:LA-cp rats: effects of age and insulin resistance. *Am J Physiol* 1999; 277(5 Pt1): C987-993.

In: Hypertension: New Research
Editor: Elwood F. Benhagen, pp. 69-103 ISBN: 1-59454-204-X

Chapter III

Recent Progress in Idiopathic Portal Hypertension with an Emphasis on Intrahepatic Vascular, Portal Tract and Parenchymal Alterations

Yasuni Nakanuma, Seiko Sawada, Kazuto Kozaka, Yoh Zen, Makoto Hashizume, and Yasunori Sato

Department of Human Pathology, Kanazawa University Graduate School of Medicine, Kanazawa, and
Department of Emergency Medicine, Kyushu University Graduate School of Medicine, Fukuoka, Japan

Abstract

Idiopathic portal hypertension (IPH) is characterized by a long-standing presinusoidal portal hypertension of unknown etiology and by the definite absence of cirrosis, and obliteration of intrahepatic small portal veins and dense portal fibrosis may be related to its pathogenesis. While the etiologies of IPH remains only speculative, some unidentified agent(s) may affect the intrahepatic small vasculatures or portal tracts, or may play a role in the increased portal venous blood flow. Portal fibrosis may be explainable by imbalanced synthesis and degradation of collagen and elastic fiber involving connective tissue growth factor and matrix metalloproteinase-9. During the long clinical course of IPH, several pathological changes may develop secondarily, including subcapsular parenchymal atrophy, atrophy of the liver, focal and mild intralobular fibrosis, and portal venous phlebosclerosis and thrombosis. Subcapsular parenchymal and hepatic atrophy may result from hepatocellular dropout via apoptosis or necrosis due to chronic portal venous blood insufficiency. Portal venous thromboemboli of the larger intrahepatic portal veins may be responsible for segmental or zonal hepatic parenchymal collapse. Increased expression of heme oxygenase-1 and endothelin-1 in the hepatic lobules of IPH livers may be related to the altered sinusoidal hemodynamics. Focal and mild intralobular pericellular fibrosis and thin fibrous septa may be due to activation of hepatic stellate cells. However, liver cirrhosis does not occur eventually. Taken together, a new staging or categorization of IPH with a combination of hepatic parenchymal atrophy and portal venous thrombosis was proposed: non-atrophic liver without subcapsular parenchymal atrophy (stage I), non-atrophic liver with subcapsular parenchymal atrophy (stage II), atrophic liver with subcapsular parenchymal atrophy (stage III), and portal venous occlusive thrombosis (stage IV). IPH livers are likely to progress from stage I to stage III, and stage IV develop rarely in stage I, and more frequently in stage III than in stage II, and means a poor prognosis. This staging is applicable to clinical cases without consideration of histologic sampling errors. Nodular parenchymal hyperplastic changes are also frequently found in IPH liver, resembling nodular regenerative hyperplasia, and partial nodular transformation, or even focal nodular hyperplasia, probably due to heterogeneity of intravascular lesion in the liver. These histopathologic feastuers of IPH livers may be shared in IPH and its equivalents characterized by long-standing presinusoidal portal venous high pressure with reduced portal venous inflow into the hepatic parenchyma, though the etiopathogenesis of such disease complex may be different in the several districts in the world.

Key words: idiopathic portal hypertension, portal venous insufficiency, portal vein thromboembolism, nodular hyperplasia of hepatocytes, hepatic parenchymal atrophy

INTRODUCTION

Portal hypertension with patent portal and hepatic veins and with massive splenomegaly in the absence of a known cause of liver diseases including cirrhosis is occasionally experienced in the East and also the West [1-5]. Clincially, portal hypertension is usually silent for a variable but relatively longer period in such diseases, and they are often discovered due to late complications such as hemorrhage from gastroesophageal varices and severe anemia. Idiopathic portal hypertension (IPH) belongs to such disease and is characterized by intrahepatic portal venous block at small portal veins and dense portal fibrosis [6, 7]. Similar diseases or equivalents of IPH have been also reported in other geographic districts in the world [1, 4, 5, 8], while their etiopathogenesis may be different. So far, the early or acute or primary lesions causally related to intrahepatic portal venous block or related to etiopathogenesis have not been identified in IPH and also its counterparts.

In this review, we first describe the clinical features of IPH and its stagings, and then the pathology of the IPH liver and its pathophysiology and also refer to its related diseases. The recent progress in the etiopathogenesis of IPH is also reviewed. This review is based on more than 100 liver specimens from cases fulfilling the criteria for IPH obtained from the file of hepatobiliary diseases in our laboratory and affiliated hospitals.

For better understanding of the pathology and pathophysiology of IPH, the anatomy of intrahepatic portal tracts including portal veins are briefly described [9, 10]. The large intrahepatic portal tracts are characterized by the presence of intrahepatic large bile ducts (segmental and area bile ducts and their 1st to 3rd branches), and the small portal tracts by the presence of interlobular bile ducts with an external diamater less than 100 μm. The medium-sized portal tracts are between them. The portal veins in the large portal tracts, medium-sized portal tracts, and small portal tracts are called intrahepatic large portal veins, intrahepatic medium-sized portal veins, and the intrahepatic small portal veins, respectively. In addition to the main portal vein branch in individual portal tracts, the microvasculature near the limiting plate and those within portal tracts, particularly around bile ducts, were classifiable as "inlet venules" and "peribiliary capillary plexus (PBP)", respectively.

Clinical Findings

Main Clinical Features, Diagnosis and Prognosis

IPH is clinically characterized by presinuosoidal portal hypertension (varices and portosystemic collateral vessels), massive splenomegaly, decreased levels of one or more blood elements (hypersplenism), and relatively mild abnormalities in liver function tests [11]. The ratio of female to male in patients with IPH was about 3:1, and the age of patients with IPH range between 6 and 67 years old (mean, 40 years) [12]. There are no laboratory findings characteristic to IPH. A similar disorder called noncirrhotic portal fibrosis (NCPF) in India, and hepatoportal sclerosis or portal obliterative vasculopathy in the United States and idiopathic trophical splenomegaly in the tropical countries seems to be the counterpart of IPH in Japan [1, 2, 4, 5, 8, 13, 14]. While new cases of IPH are rapidly declining recently in Japan suggesting a role of infection in its etiopathogenesis indirectly [15], NCPF is still a common cause of portal hypertension in India and it represents 20-25% of the cases that bleed due to esophageal varices [16, 17]. However, it remains unclear whether the etiology of IPH of Japan is identical to that of NCPF. As for the sex and age distribution, IPH affects preferentially middle to old aged women in Japan, while NCPF in India usually affects young men [7,11,17-19], suggesting the clinciopathologic heterogeneity of this disease group in the world.

To make a diagnosis of IPH, histopathological study is necessary. For pathologists, the most important task is to exclude liver cirrhosis, particularly macronodular liver cirrhosis. Liver biopsy specimens, particularly needle biopsies, show nonspecific and non-diagnositc changes. That is, dense portal fibroelastosis with subintimal thickening or luminal obliteration of small portal vein branches, and a striking peri-ductal fibrosis, support a diagnosis of IPH [1,15]. When portal hypertension occurs in association with a radiologically patent portal vein and an apparently normal liver histology, IPH is always one possibility.

The disease is relatively benign if variceal bleeding is controlled or prevented, and does not progress to cirrhosis. However, a certain number of IPH cases with hepatic failure have been reported [20-22]. Ichimura et al. [22] followed 171 patients with IPH, and reported that 20 patients died; 6 from bleeding of the gastro-intestinal tract, 5 from hepatic insufficiency and 9 from other causes. Superimposition of occlusive thrombosis of the intrahepatic large portal veins and/or portal vein trunk means a poor prognosis. In fact, IPH patients frequently die of portal venous thrombosis, and a number of autopsy cases of IPH are found to be complicated by fresh occlusive portal venous thrombosis in the sclerotic portal veins.

New Staging System of IPH by Imaging Modalities and Gross Findings

IPH shows a long clinical course, and it seems therefore plausible that the secondary changes due to peripheral portal venous insufficiency develop and progress in their degree and extent gradually. Radiological finding of central hypertrophy and peripheral atrophy of

IPH [23] may reflect subcapsular atrophy of liver and even hepatic atrophy. Superimposition of occlusive thrombosis of the intrahepatic large portal veins and/or portal vein trunk could belong to such secondary changes. These experiences suggest that the combination of these progressive or sedondary changes are applicable for the categorization or staging of IPH. So far, there has been no staging system or categorization of IPH livers available in the literature.

The staging of IPH is preferably applicable clinically to the patients by the imaging modalities. While the liver histology is necessary for the diagnosis of IPH, this is not preferred for the staging or categorization of IPH, because the histologic changes of IPH are known to be very heterogeneous and sampling errors are unavoidable [2,4,14,15]. Recently, we proposed a new staging system for IPH [24]. That is, we adopted three main, grossly recognizable morphologic factors in the new staging; the presence or absence of peripheral parenchymal atrophy, the size or weight of the liver, and obstructive portal vein thrombosis of the intrahepatic large portal veins and/or portal vein trunk. All of these factors are recognizable grossly by a combination of several imaging modalities and/or portography. Magnetic resonance imaging (MRI) in IPH patients gives an information on the subcapsular atrophy [25], and liver volume is also able to be calculated by computed tomography (CT) [26]. Portal venous thrombotic occlusion is also evaluable radiologically.

By using the ratio of the distance between the hepatic capsule and marker branch of the intrahepatic portal vein near the capsule to that between the hepatic capsule and marker branch of inthrahepatic portal vein hear the hepatic hilus as an index of subcapsular atrophy index, and the liver volume calculable by CT as a liver atrophy index [26], a promising result on the staging system is now being accumulated (Koaka et al, in submission). The parenchymal nodular changes of the liver are not recommended for the staging of IPH livers, because they are not always present and the correlation between the nodular formation and the progression of IPH remains to be clarified.

IPH livers could be grouped into four groups (Stage I, II, III, and IV). ***Stage I*** is characterized by the absence of subcapsular parenchymal atrophy. The liver is usually not atrophic and even swollen, and the surface is smooth. ***Stage II*** shows presence of subcapsular parenchymal atrophy in non-atrophic liver as a whole. The surface is uneven or waving and even nodular. The cut surface shows distinct subcapsular atrophy. ***Stage III*** is defined by the presence of subcapsular parenchymal atrophy in the atrophic liver. The surface is uneven or waving, and even vaguely nodular. The cut surface shows distinct subcapsular atrophy. Occasionally, there is collapse involving areas or segments of the liver. Presence of obstructive thrombosis of intrahepatic large portal veins or portal vein trunk characterizes ***Stage IV.*** This occurs at all stages, but is rare at stage 1, and more frequent at stage III than at stage II.

From standpoint of peripheral portal venous insufficiency and hepatic atrophy, stage I is early IPH, while stages II is more or less advanced stage and stage III is more. In stage I, II and III livers, the intrahepatic large portal veins and extrahepatic portal veins are patent while they show venous wall thickening and even calcification in this order, suggesting repeated organization of portal venous thrombosis. As for stages I, II, and III, the histopathological changes may progress in this order. We would like to strongly encourage the clinicians to use this staging system for the long-term follow up of IPH patients and for the evaluation of the prognosis of IPH patients. This stading system seems to be applicable to counterparts of IPH and related diseases, too.

PATHOLOGY AND PATHOPHYSIOLOGY OF IPH

There have been many studies on the liver pathology of IPH, and representative pathologic features of IPH livers are well established [14,15,27]. It is generally thought that the liver has already reached pathologically to the end-stage of IPH, when a diagnosis of IPH is made clincially. The followings are the representative pathologic changes of IPH.

Grossly, the liver is atrophic as a whole or deformed variably (***Figure 1A***). Nodular parenchymal areas with alternating atrophic areas are also seen (***Figure 1B***). Fibrotic portal tracts are spaced unevenly and often positioned closely together, especially at the subcapsular regions [7,28]. Such gross remodeling is also a characteristic feature of the equivalents of IPH [1,4]. Histopathologically, dense portal fibrosis with stenosis or obliteration of intrahepatic small portal veins (***Figure 2A,2B***), phlebosclerosis of intrahepatic portal veins, and sinusoidal dilatation and dilated aberrant blood vessels in the parenchyma are frequently seen (***Figure 3A, 3B, 3C).*** While the IPH liver has no cirrhosis and appears normal histologically, particularly to the pathologists without interest in liver pathology, reticulin or elastica van Gieson (EVG) stains show that the normal lobular architecture, particularly mutual position of portal tracts and central veins, is profoundly distorted and hepatocellular cords is disorganized, suggesting that the intrahepatic hemodynamics are significantly disturbed (***Figure 3A***). While a majority of these lesions are secondary to long-standing presinusoidal portal hypertension and peripheral portal venous insufficiency, there could be some hepatic and portal changes related to the primary or initiating factor(s), particularly in the biopsy livers.

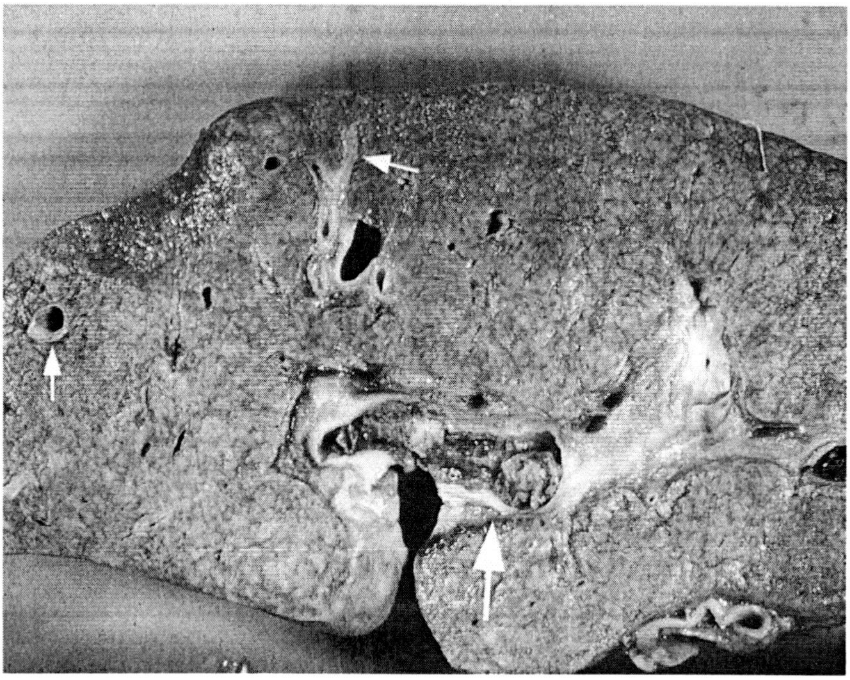

Figure 1-A: Cut surface of autopsy liver of idiopathic portal hypertension. The liver is atrophic, and portal tracts and hepatic veins (small arrows) are unusually approximated to the hepatic capsule. Dilated intrahepatic large portal vein (large arrow) is occluded by fresh thrombi. Hepatic parenchyma appears fine nodule, reflecting nodular regenerative hyerplasia.

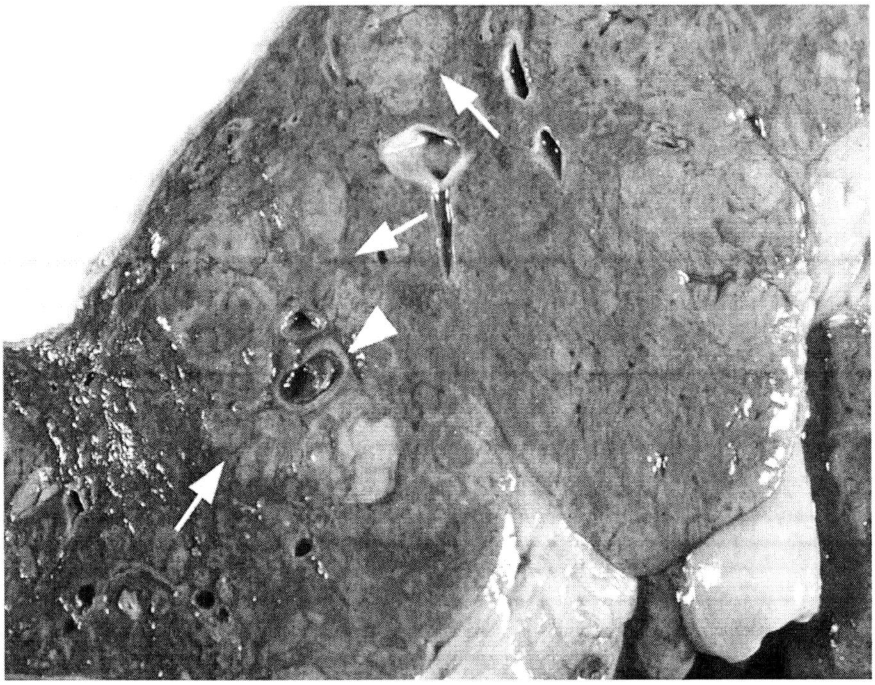

Figure 1-B: Cut surface of autopsy liver of idiopathic portal hyperetnsion. The hepatic parenchyma shows nodular hyperplasia (arrows) around the intrahepatic portal tract containing fresh thrombi (arrow head). The remaining hepatic parenchyma are also diffusely nodular.

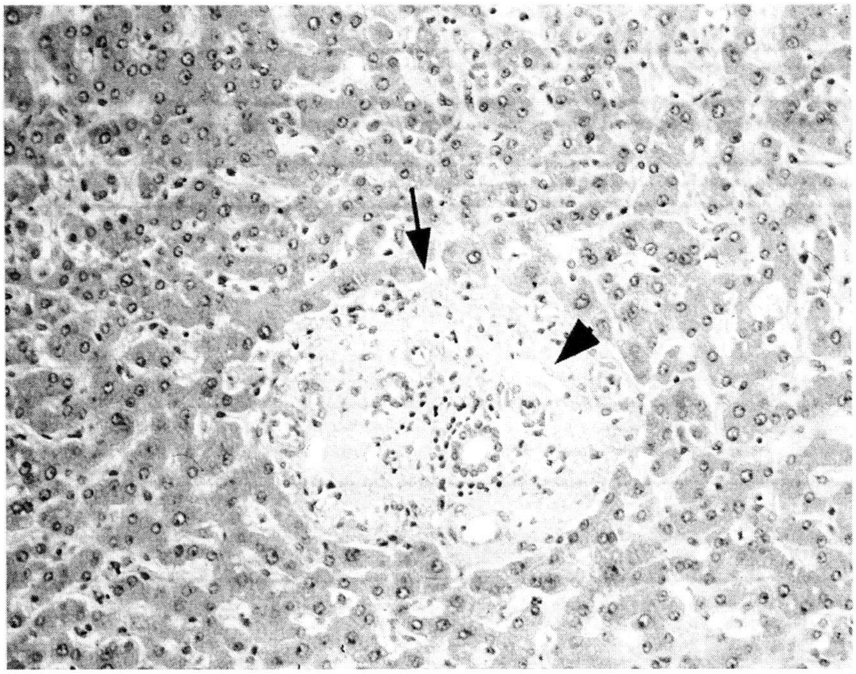

Figure 2-A: Small portal tract (arrow) in idiopathic portal hypertension is densely sclerotic, and hepatic artery and bile ducts are identifiable. But, portal vein is very stenotic (arrow head). There is a scanty lymphoid cells in this portal tract. HE.

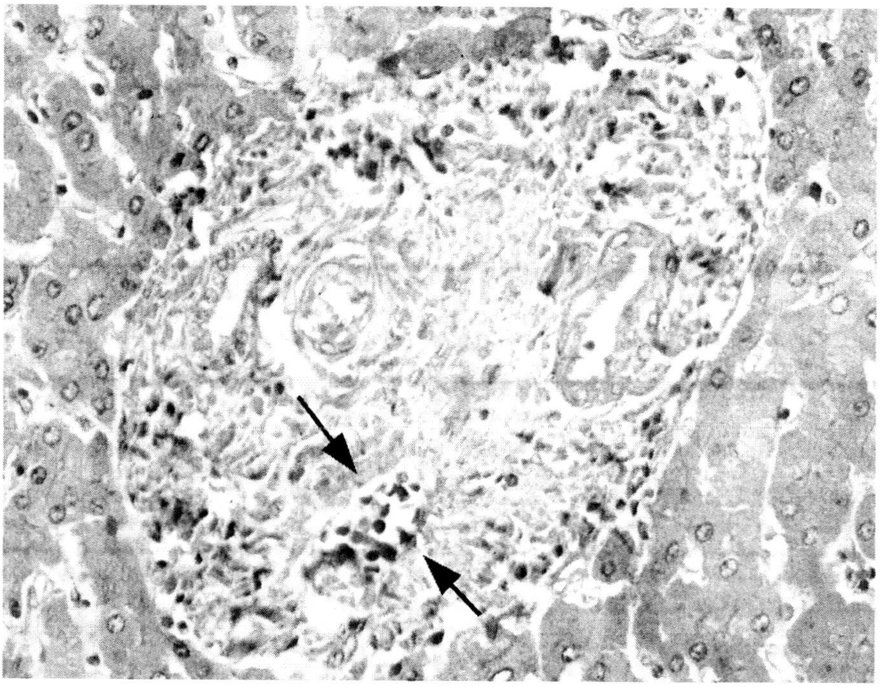

Figure 2-B: Small portal tract in idiopathic portal hypertension, is densely fibrotic, and portal vein is stenotic and also muscular hyperplasia is seen around this portal vein (arrows). Azan-Mallory stain.

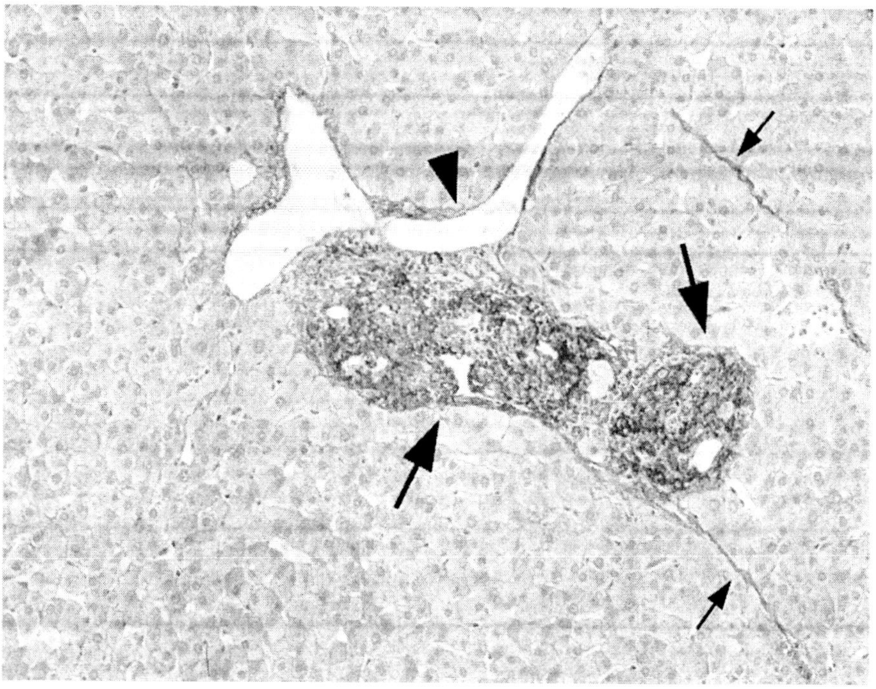

Figure 3-A: The lobular pattern is severely distorted. Two densely elastotic portal tracts (large arrows) are approximated to each other, and there is dilated aberrant vessels adjacent to these portal tracts (arrow head). There are thin fibrous septa in the parenchyma (small arrows), and central vein is unusually located. Idiopathic portal hypertension. Elastica van Gieson staining.

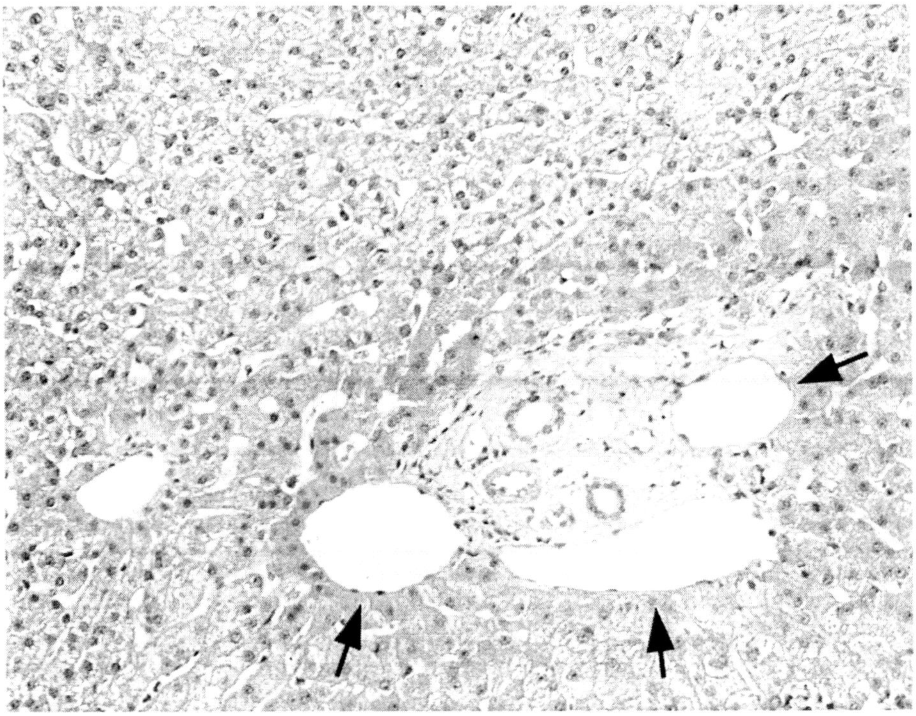

Figure 3-B: There are several dilated aberrant vessels (arrows) around fibrotic portal tract (periportal angiomatosis). Original portal vein in this portal tract is unclear. Idiopathic portal hypertension. HE.

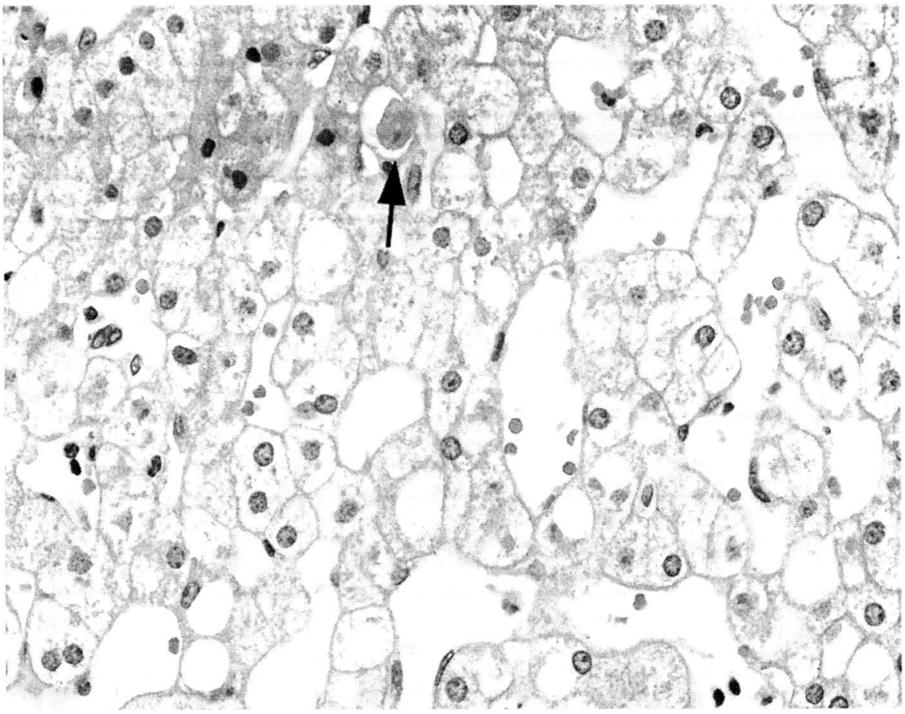

Figure 3-C: Hepatic parenchyma shows sinusoidal dilatatiaon, hepatocellular atrophy and one acidophilic body (arrow) in idiopathic portal hypertension. HE.

Recent studies on IPH and its counterparts suggested that current definitions and criteria and nomenclature for these diseases are confused [4]. For example, while active regenerative changes or hepatocellular nodular hyperplasia are originally said to be characteristically absent in IPH [14,15], there have been many studies in the IPH livers on the occurrence of hepatic parenchymal nodular lesions clearly different from regenerative nodules of liver cirrhosis (***Figure 1B, 4A, 4B***). Portal venous thromboembolic lesions, particularly occlusive thromboemboli, are a kind of exclusive lesion in IPH, though they are also known to develop not infrequently in IPH, particularly frequently found in autopsy livers of IPH, and they may even participate and contribute to the development and progression of hepatic parenchymal and intrahepatic portal venous lesions. The most important issue is that a majority of these findings found in IPH and its counterparts are nonspecific, and meticulous examination can detect similar lesions in the livers unrelated to IPH or in those without portal hypertension [29]. Primary and acute vascular lesions often remain still to be clarified, and the pathognomonic lesions or markers of IPH are still lacking. Histologic heterogeneity is a fundamental character of IPH and this is also a big problem in the evaluation of the liver pathology of IPH. Thus, a consensus on the diagnostic criteria of IPH and its related diseases should be discussed in near future.

Pathology and Pathophysiology of Intrahepatic Vasculatures and Blood Flow of IPH

Altered hemodynamics of IPH include sustained intrahepatic presinusoidal portal hypertension, marked splenomegaly, and increased intrahepatic portal venous resistance in the absence of cirrhosis. Portal venous blood flow into the liver is increased and the portal vein trunk and intrahepatic large portal veins are usually dilated, while hepatic arterial flow into the liver is decreased, and arterio-portal venous (A-P) shunts is negligible [6,7,11,14,30]. Marked splenomegaly with increased portal venous blood inflow does not seem to be explainable simply by chronic congestion [15], and its mechanisms remain an enigma. By contrast, in liver cirrhosis, portal venous blood flow into the liver is almost normal while intrahepatic vascular resistance at the postsinusoidal level is markedly increased [30]. In addition, hepatic arterial blood flow into the liver is increased, and there are many A-P shunts in the liver. Extrahepatic portal-systemic shunts are present in both IPH and liver cirrhosis, and the development of such spontaneous shunts tends to protect IPH patients from variceal bleeding [16].

Portal Venous System

The portograms in IPH frequently show dilatation of the portal veins at the hepatic hilus and of intrahepatic large portal veins, irregular and often obtuse-angled divisions of the peripheral branches, occasional abrupt interruptions, and an avascular area beneath the liver surface are frequently seen [31]. Non-opacification of some of the large intrahepatic portal branches and a paucity of medium-sized portal branches, could be seen as a late and secondary complication of portal venous thromboembolism [31].

Grossly visible intrahepatic large portal veins and extrahepatic portal veins are open or even dilated in IPH livers, though they show constantly phlebosclerosis and intimal thickening to various degrees, probably due to the organization of repeated mural and possibly occlusive portal venous thromboembolism and sustained portal hypertension. Portal venous blood stasis may be responsible for the thrombosis. However, the theory that IPH represents an undiagnosed intrahepatic portal vein thrombosis has not been demonstrated. Thrombotic processes of the portal venous system eventually occur, particularly after splenectomy [24] (***Figure 1A, 1B***).

Obliteration or luminal narrowing of intrahepatic small portal veins (***Figure 2A, 2B***) is a rather constant histologic finding [15,32,33], and this is also shown by morphometrical studies [33,34]. For example,the number of small portal vein branches are reduced in IPH, and the ratio of portal venous luminal area to portal tract area of IPH is significantly reduced compared with alcoholic fibrosis/cirrhosis and more normal liver. It seems conceivable that small portal venous obliteration or stenosis is responsible for susptained presinusoidal portal hypertension. However, it is also possible that such lesions may be an adaptive response of small portal veins against increased portal venous inflow into the liver or high portal venous pressure [27,35].

Phlebosclerosis of intrahepatic portal veins, particularly medium-sized and large ones, is a frequent and also constant lesion which is easily recognizable at wedge biopsy or autopsy. This lesion is usually associated with intima thickening and medial muscular hypertrophy (arterialization) [1]. These lesions are probably an adaptive response against high pressure of intrahepatic portal vein and increased inflow of portal blood into the liver because similar lesions are reproducible in experimental anastomosis of the hepatic artery and portal veins in animals. Simlar lesions also occur mildly in cirrhosis with long-standing portal hypertension [36].

In addition to the main portal vein branches, inlet venules and PBP are also affected in IPH. That is, inlet venules are reduced in number, particularly in the portal tracts with portal venous obliteration, and PBP is not increased in IPH compared to normal livers. Instead, PBP and inlet venules are increased and dilated in extrahepatic portal obstruction (EHO), chronic active hepatitis, extrahepatic portal venous obstruciton and alcoholic cirrhosis [9]. The alterations of the inlet venules may reflect an abnormal microcirculation in the small portal tracts, and the reduction of inlet venules plays an important role in the development of portal venous high pressure and is responsible for reduced portal venous inflow into the hepatic sinusoids of IPH. PBP is known to provide the sites for intrahepatic A-P shunts [37], and no increase or dilatation of PBP in smaller portal tracts of IPH livers may be compatible with negligible A-P shunts in IPH, when compared to liver cirrhosis. However, PBP in larger portal tracts are variably increased.

Hepatic Arterial and Lymphatic Changes in Portal Tracts

A decrease of the portal venous inflow into the liver is known to be always and immediately associated with a compensatory increase of hepatic arterial flow in man and also in experimental animals [38, 39]. In IPH livers, small-sized hepatic arterial branches are not increased in number or in the luminal area in spite of decreased lumen of the small portal veins, reflecting the decreased arterial blood flow in the liver [34]. This is supported by our morphometrical study. That is, the ratio of hepatic arterial luminal area to portal tract area inalcoholic cirrhosis is significantly higher than that in normal liver; however, that for IPH was similar to normal in spite of decreased peripheral portal venous inflow [34]. In alcoholic cirrhosis, the number of mast cells and macrophages known to be the source of angiogenic substances is significantly increased in the portal tract compared with normal liver, while in IPH livers they are not increased. In alcoholic cirrhosis, an increase of hepatic arterial lumen with a reduction in portal venous lumen may be explainable by an increase of angiogenesis-related cells in portal tracts [34]. However, such compensatory arterial changes and increase of mast cells and macrophages are not evident in IPH, and this compensatory failure may be a feature of IPH.

As for hepatic lymph vessels or lymph flow in IPH, Oikawa et al [33] reported that the number of lymphatics was higher in IPH samples than in control samples, suggesting that increased lymph flow may in turn reduce the high portal vein pressure in IPH. The ratio of the total area of these branches to that of the portal tract, was lower in IPH samples than in the control samples. These morphometric changes in IPH may be associated with a reduction in portal blood flow and increased lymph flow, and the latter may in turn reduce the high portal vein pressure in IPH.

Hepatic Sinusoids

Hepatic lobular patterns are variably disturbed in IPH. That is, atrophic or hyperplastic hepatic lobules, distorted hepatocellular cord patterns, unusual spacing of portal tracts and central veins, sinusoidal dilatation or compression, and aberrant blood vessels are recognizable in a variable combination or distribution (***Figure 4A, 4B***). The presence of these lesions suggests ongoing disturbed hemodynamics in hepatic sinusoids. Altered expression of vasoactive molecules demonstrated in the hepatic lobules, may relate to such disturbed hemodynamics, directly or indirectly.

Aberrant blood vessels and sinusoidal dilatation in the hepatic parenchyma: Aberrant blood vessels, which are defined as dilated blood vessels in the hepatic parenchyma, are encountered in IPH livers (***Figure 3A, 3B***). They are also called as shunt vessels and multiple central veins [24,35,40]. Aberrant blood vessels are known to show the same immunoreactivity as portal veins for collagen type IV, laminin, and factor VIII. Some are immediately adjacent to the peripheral portal tract, and they are called periportal angiomatosis, probably herniation of portal vein branches or inlet venules into the adjoining parenchyma. They also tend to develop in extrahepatic portal obstruction (EHO) (***Figure 5***) [14,35,41]. They are concluded to arise from the spared inlet venules, which might have been used as intrahepatic shunts draining portal blood flow blocked by occluded or obliterated portal vein branches and inlet venules [35]. Increased portal pressure would be expected to enhance the development of aberrant vessels.

Sinusoidal dilatation with or without congestion is not infrequent in IPH (***Figure 3C, 4A, 4B***), probably reflecting altered sinusoidal hemodynamics. In some cases, the sinusoidal dilatation is topologically associated with aberrant blood vessels in the hepatic parenchyma. In others, the sinusoidal dilatation is related to fibrous core (probably obliterated central veins) or then fibrous septa, suggesting their heterogeneous pathogenesis [42]. Sinusoidal dilatation may also occur by obstruction of portal vein branches [5].

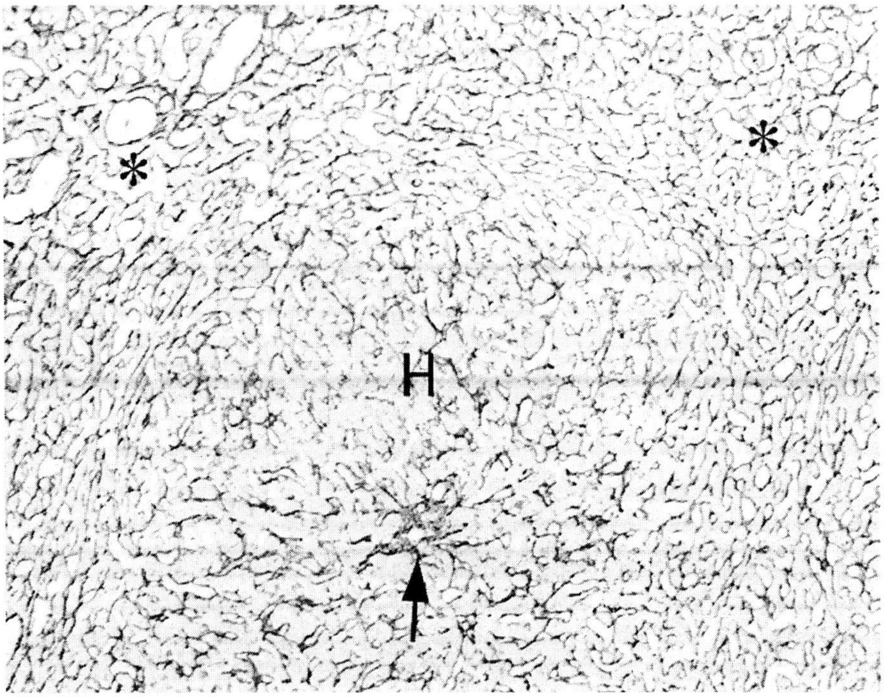

Figure 4-A: Hepatic parenchyma around the portal tract (arrow) shows hyperplastic changes (H), while the surrounding parenchyma is atrophic, and sinusoidal dilatation and mild pericellular fibrosis (*). Idiopathic portal hypertension. Gomori's reticulin stain.

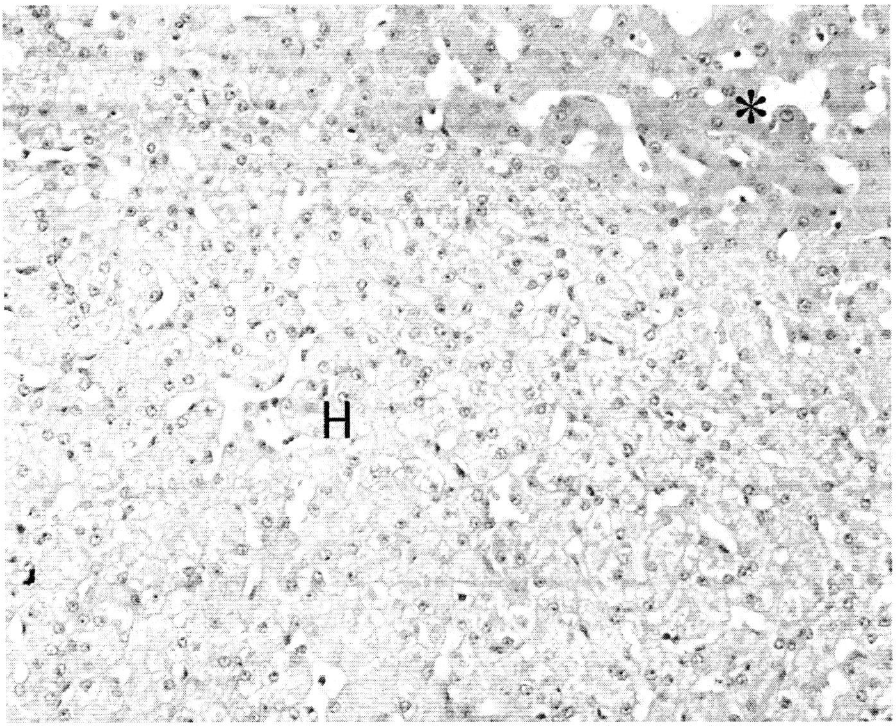

Figure 4-B: Hepatic parenchyma shows hyperplastic change (H) and also atrophic changes (*). The latter shows sinusoidal dilatation. Idiopathic portal hypertension. HE.

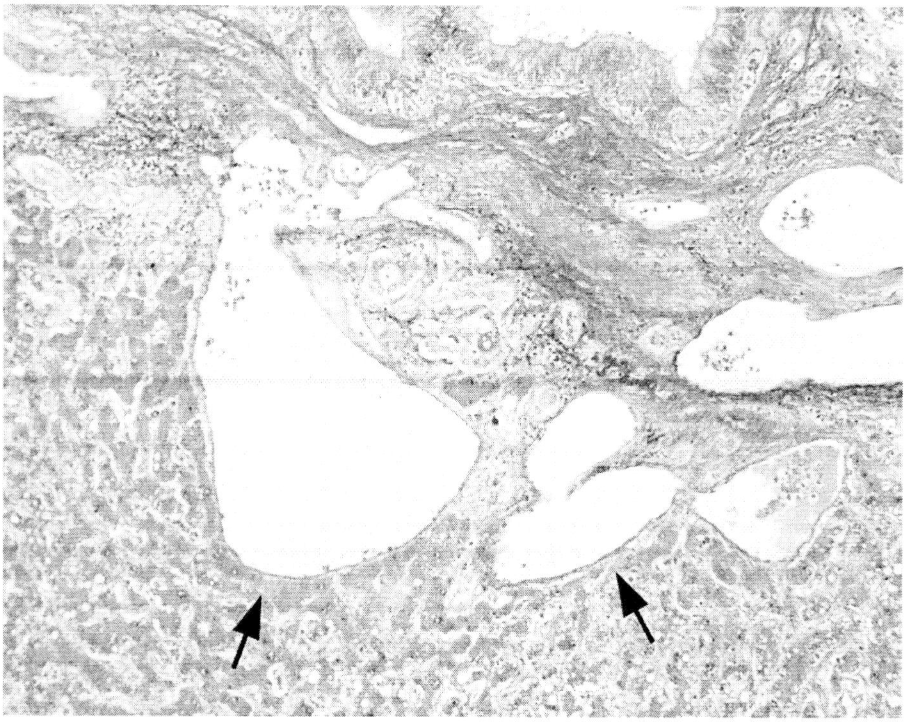

Figure 5: Dilated aberrant vessels (arrows) adjacent to the portal tract reflects shunt vessels in extrahepatic portal venous obstruction. Elastica van Gieson stain.

Expression and participation of vasoactive molecules: Recently, there have been several studies on the pathophysiological roles of vasoactive molecues such as heme oxygenase (HO)-1 and endothelin (ET)-1 in IPH and cirrhosis, particularly in the sinusoidal hemodynamics. The former is known as the stress-inducible and cabon monoxide (CO)-producing enzyme [43,44], and CO is known to serve as an ednogeneous regulator necessary for maintining microvascular blood flow. CO is also involved in controlling the hepatic vasculat tone in a variety of experimental models.

That is, Makino et al [43] reported that HO-1 is expressed in a majority of Kupffer cells and also observed in hepatocytes in cirrhosis, while such expression is negligible in normal livers. Total HO-1 activities become significantly greater in cirrhotic liver than those from normal individuals. IPH livers display a significant decrease in HO-1 expression in Kupffer cells, and its hepatocellular expression is not detectable [43]. Marked difference in HO-1 expression in the hepatic sinusoids may reflect the different local hemodynamics between cirrhosis and IPH. These results suggest that Kupffer cells could alter their expression of HO-1 in response to local hemodynamic changes in hepaptic parenchyma in liver cirrhosis. In IPH, the sinusoidal blood flow into the hepatic lobules is reduced by the block at the level of small portal veins, so that up-regulation of HO-1 and increased production of CO is not necessary or not important in the regulation of sinusoidal hemodynamics, compared to cirrhosis. Wall shear stress arising in the sinusoids related to the blood flow may explain the difference in HO-1 expression between cirrhosis and IPH.

ET-1 is known to mediate increased resistance to hepatic sinusoidal blood flow. Kamath et al [45] and Ohara et al [46] reported that ET-1 is localized at periportal hepatocytes and perisinusoidal cells in the hepatic parencnyma of IPH and cirrhosis, and that their expression is up-regulated in liver cirrhosis and also to a lesser degree in IPH, when compared to normal livers. The expressions of ET-1, ET-A receptors, ET-B receptors, and inducible NOS (iNOS) are also detected in patients with cirrhosis, and to a mild degree in IPH. The peripheral venous plasma concentration of ET-1 is also increased in liver cirrhosis and to a mild degree in IPH. These data suggest that ET-1 and its receptors are involved significantly in response to increased blood flow into the sinusoid in cirrhosis. Relatively increased expression of ET-1 and its receptors may also reflect altered sinusoidal blood flow in IPH.

Hepatic Venous Outflow

In IPH livers, frequent hepatic vein-to-hepatic vein anastomoses, narrower angles between large veins and their tributaries, smooth and wavy middle-sized to large branches (giving a general "weeping willow" appearance), homogeneous sinusoidal filling, and minimal to no filling of the portal venous system on wedged retrograde portography are frequently and characteristically found in IPH livers by imagings [47]. By contrast, such findings are rare in liver cirrhosis. Histopathologically, hepatic vein tributaries show eccentric or concentric fibrosis with luminal narrowing as seen in liver cirrhosis [14, 48], and they may reflect reduced blood flow in the hepatic venous lumen. However, fresh thromboemboli are not seen in hepatic venous systems of IPH.

Infrequently, the unusual of prolapse of hepatocytes into portal tracts and also into the subendothelial space of hepatic veins are seen in IPH (***Figure 6***), and this could be related to the abnormal intrahepatic blood flow or to intrahepatic vasculopathy [49].

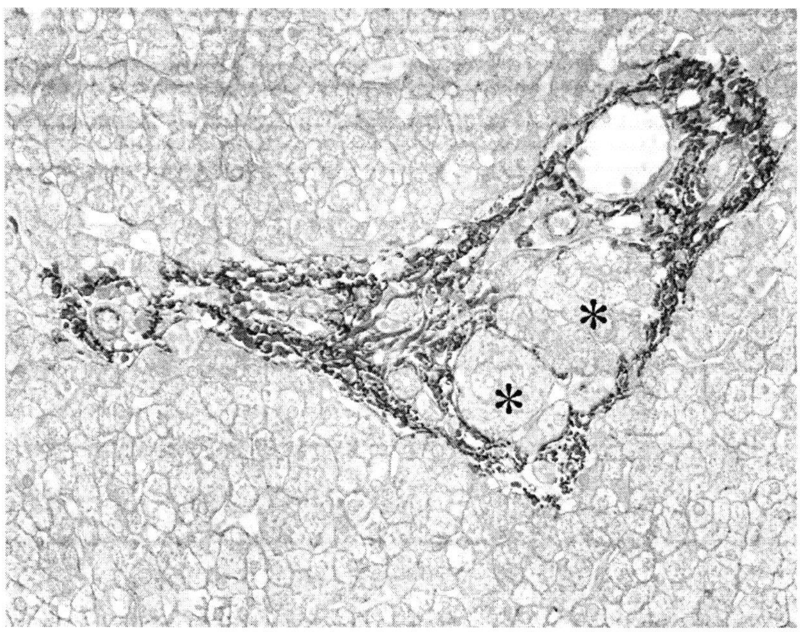

Figure 6. There is clear and unusual growth of hepatocytes (*) in the portal tract. This is not a neopalstic feature but is related to intralobular circulation disturbance in idiopathic portal hypertension. Elastica van Gieson stain.

Dense Portal Fibrosis

Portal tracts are always affected in IPH, and portal dense fibrosis (sclerosis) and periductal fibrosis are frequently seen in IPH livers (***Figure 2A, 2B, 7A, 7B***). However, the degree and characters of these changes differ depending upon the anatomical levels of the portal tracts and their distribution is also heterogeneous in the liver [1,3,5,24]. Because portal vein branches are frequently stenotic or obliterated in such sclerotic portal tracts, the fibrogenetic processes involving the portal tract is causally related to such occlusive vascular lesions. Otherwise, both of these changes may develop secondarily against increased intrahepatic portal blood flow into or high pressure in IPH livers as an adaptation response of liver.

Dense fibroelastosis of portal tracts: Small and medium-sized portal tracts show fibroelastosis with their variable enlargement, and they are usually round and occasionally show spike-like fibrous septa into the hepatic parenchyma. Intrahepatic large portal tracts also shows a variable fibrosis. Extensive elastosis of small portal tracts are frequently seen in IPH (***Figure 7A, 7B***), and some appear as rudimentary, although such changes are also occasionally seen in normal atrophic livers of very old persons. These changes may be the result of ischemic portal changes. Interestingly, portal vein branches and even interlobular bile ducts are frequently missing in such elastic portal tracts of IPH. Portal tract inflammation characterized by infiltration of a few lymphoid cells is occasionally encountered, especially in wedge biopsied liver specimens.

Disordered synthesis and degradation of fibrosis and extracellular matrix (ECM) in small and medium-sized portal tracts may be responsible for the generation of such dense portal fibroelastosis. Matrix metalloproteinase (MMP)-9 is known to play an important role in the degradation of elastin and also collagen [50]. Immunohistochemically, MMP-9 positive mononuclear cells are fewer in their number in the fibrotic portal tract of IPH liver, when compared with alcoholic cirrhosis [42].

Connective tissue growth factor (CTGF), a cystein-rich peptide with heparin-binding molecules, can enhance fibroblastic proliferation and chemotaxis, and stimulates the synthesis of ECM for fibroblasts (51~53). It is known that the serum level of CTGF is increased in patients with progressive systemic sclerosis (PSS), and pulmonary fibrosis [54]. In addition, it appears that production of CTGF is involved in the development or maintenance rather than the initiation of fibrosis in PSS.CTGF is also one of the strongest fibrogenetic factors of the liver [51]. In the group with chronic hepatitis, an increase of CTGF immunostaining is associated with a higher score of fibrosis, CTGF is strongly expressed during liver fibrogenesis, and hepatic stellate cells seem to be the major cellular source of CTGF in the liver [51]. In IPH, the exact molecular mechanism of the fibrogenesis in portal fibrosis remains speculative. Recently, Shiomi et al [52] reported by using Atlas cDNA expression Arrays that CTGF gene was over-expressed in IPH liver tissues. Our recent study disclosed that CTGF is expressed in periductal mononuclear cells. Shiomi et al. [52] also showed the expression of CTGF in interstitial cells around the intraheaptic portal vein in IPH. CTGF is also expressed on ECM of portal tracts in IPH and also in alcoholic cirrhosis [42]. These data suggest that CTGF can bind to heparin sulfate proteoglycan (HSPG), which exists in the fibrotic portal tracts [51], and may contribute to portal fibrosis. As HSPG is frequently seen in the portal tract of alcoholic cirrhosis and IPH, CTGF may bind and be stored in ECM of portal tracts and work continuously as fibrogenetic factor (unpublished observation).

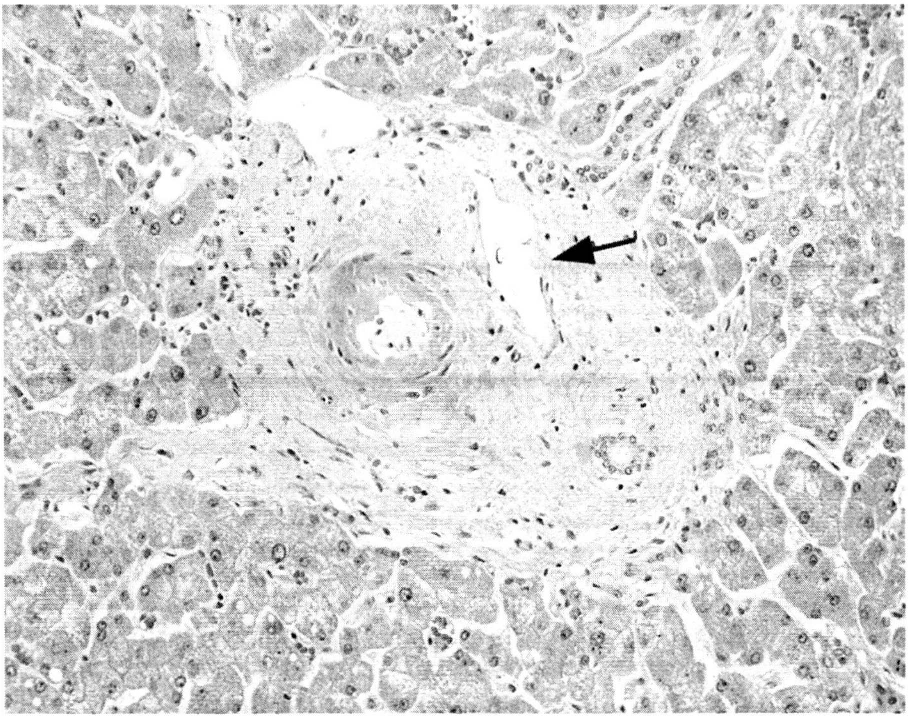

Figure 7A: Small portal tract of IPH liver shows fibrous enlargement with stenotic portal vein branch (arrow) and scanty inflammatory cell infiltration. Idiopathic portal hypertension. HE.

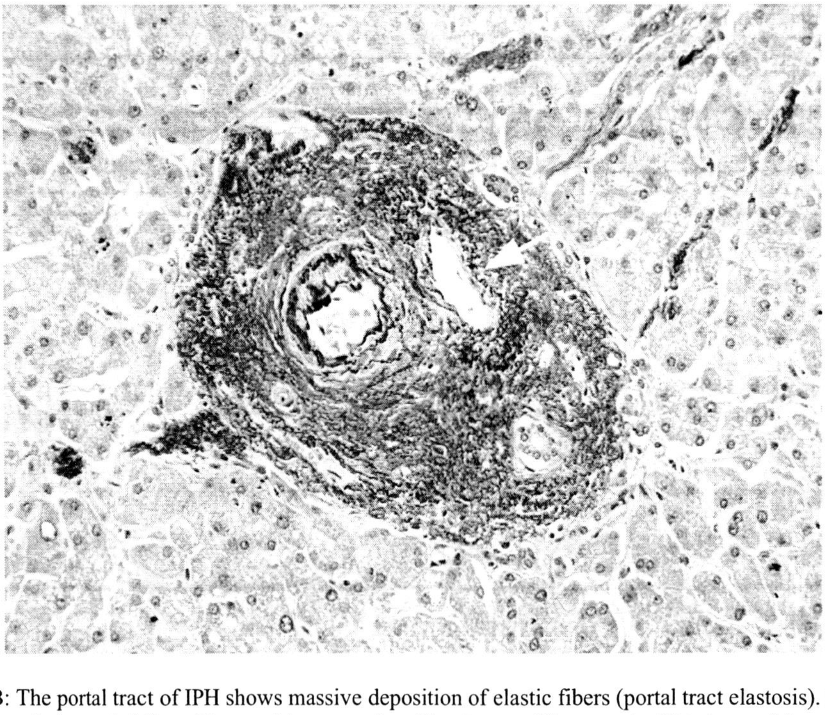

Figure 7B: The portal tract of IPH shows massive deposition of elastic fibers (portal tract elastosis). Portal vein is stenotic (arrow). Idiopathic portal hypertension. Elastica van Gieson stain. This is a serial section of Figure 5-A

Recently, it was shown that the patients of PSS showed increased serum level of CTGF [53, 54]. Shiomi et al [52] also found that serum level of CTGF was significantly higher in IPH and chronic fibrosing liver diseases than controls, and CTGF level was extraordinary high in some IPH patients.

There have been several case reports including our recent two cases presenting with both diffuse PSS and IPH [55], raising a possibility that CTGF is an important factor in the portal tract lesions of IPH as speculated in the skin lesions of PSS. Dense fibrosis is found in both the dermis and intrahepatic portal tract of these cases. In addition, small vascular and endothelial damages are commonly observed to various degrees in these fibrotic areas of both organs. The activation of fibroblasts and vascular endothelial damages by CTGF and other cytokines may be involved in the dermal lesions in PSS and also operative in the portal tract lesions in IPH.

Taken together, increased CTGF expression and decreased MMP-9 expression in the portal tracts of IPH may cause disturbance of elastin and collagen sysntehsis and degreadtion, thus inducing excessive elastin and collagen deposition in small portal tracts [42]. However, the factors for inducing or regulating these pro-fibrotic molecules and enviroment within portal tracts of IPH, remain only speculative.

Periductal fibrosis*:** Periductal fibrosis is also frequently seen at the level of interlobular bile ducts and septal bile ducts of IPH (Figure 8***). Such bile ducts are easily found in wedge biopsy or autopsy lviers, though usually not encountered in needle liver biopsies. This fibrotic pattern is not lamellar, thus different from onion-skin like periductal fibrosis of primary sclerosing cholangitis. This may be due to an insufficiency of blood flow in PBP, because these periductal fibrotic changes of IPH resemble the adverse effects of transcatheter arterial embolization (TAE) or chemoembolization therapy known to affect PBP [56]. It is possible that portal venous vascular compression by portal fibrosis or arterial hypoperfusion leads to the ischemic enviroment of portal tracts including the bile ducts and then these ductal changes in IPH. CTGF expressing mononuclear cells around the bile ducts may be also involved. Loss of bile ducts is also known as a rare complication of IPH as seen in TAE or chemoembolization therapy [57].

Hepatic Parenchymal Changes of IPH Livers

Recent pathologic and hemodynamic studies disclosed that portal hypertension in IPH may develop in a close association with a specific injury to the intrahepatic small portal veins or portal structures. In this sense, the hepatic parenchyma could be spared from the pathologic changes in IPH. However, in IPH livers, there are various types of hepatic parenchymal changes described below.

That is, distortion of hepatic lobular architecture, isolated aberrant vessels with a random distribution in the hepatic parenchyma and mild and focal intralobular fibrosis are frequently seen in a variable combination and distribution in IPH livers. In addition, hepatocellular atrophy with sinusoidal dilatation, hepatic parenchymal collapse and hepatocellular nodular hyperplasia are also not uncommon [2,58,59]. While these parenchymal changes are probably secondary to the obliteration of small portal veins with decreased afferent irrigation in the parenchyma and portal tract sclerosis, these changes characterize and even modify the histopathology of the IPH liver.

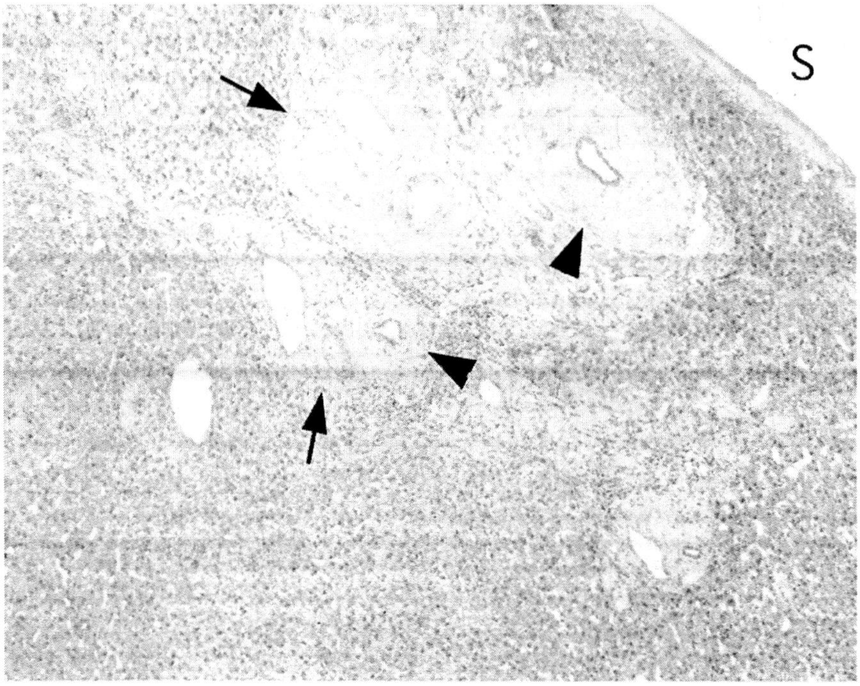

Figure 8A: Portal tracts (arrows) show unusual approximation to the hepatic surface (S) and also to each other, suggesting the atrophy of the hepatic parenchyma (subcapsular atrophy). The interlobular bile duct shows dense periductal fibrosis (arrow heads). Idiopathic portal hypertension. HE.

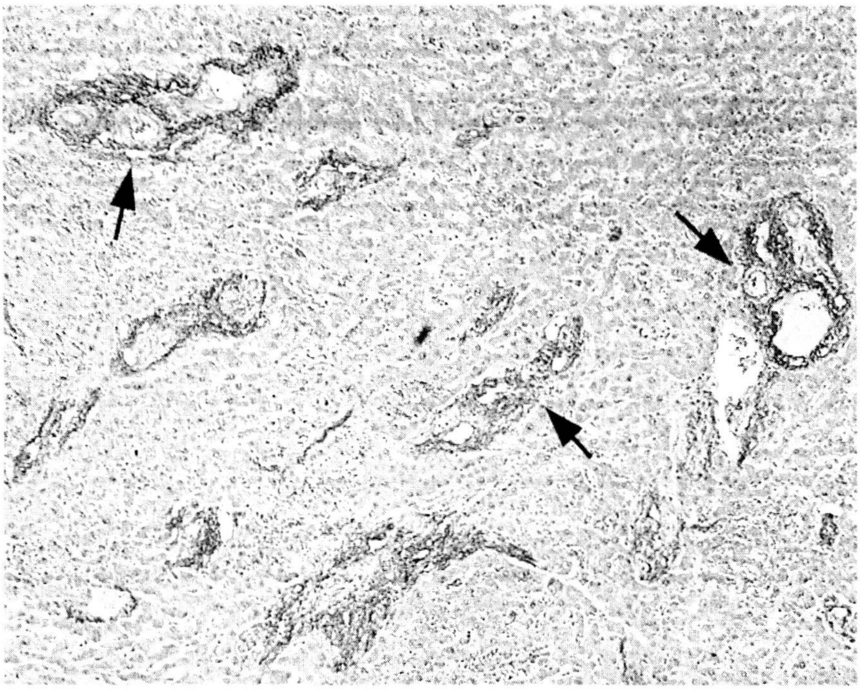

Figure 8B: Several portal tracts (arrows) showing elastosis and fibrosis, and central veins are unusually approximated. Sizes of hepatic lobules are markedly reduced. Idiopathic portal hypertension. Elastica van Gieson stain.

Hepatic Parenchymal Atrophy and Collapse (Extinction)

Hepatic parenchymal atrophy of IPH is recognizable by the following three parameters. First, the weight of the liver is reduced in more than one half of IPH cases, though there is a wide variation. IPH livers at autopsy are always atrophic and some are markedly. Second, hepatic parenchymal atrophy is preferentially recognizable grossly at the hepatic periphery or subcapsular regions (subcapsular hepatic atrophy or subcapsular scarring with the collapse of the underlying parenchyma) (***Figure 1A, 8A***). There is unusual approximation of portal tracts and hepatic vein tributaries close to the hepatic capsule or to each other due to lobular atrophy (***Figure 8B***). In these areas, hepatic parenchyma is variably lost or collapsed. Waving of hepatic surface or nodular surface reflects such atrophy. The liver with nodular surface appearing as liver cirrhosis, is an extreme feature of subcapsular hepatic atrophy with slender fibrous septa formation. In the deeper areas of these cases, however, such fibrosis and nodularity are minimal or absent. Third, the atrophy of hepatic parenchyma is recognizable by reduced size of hepatic lobules [14,59]. This is type of atrophy is accentuated in the perivenular areas and also between hyperplastic hepatocellular nodules, and hepatocytes are more or less atrophic or small.

Pathogenesis of hepatic parenchymal atrophy: In human livers, atrophy of hepatocytes or hepatic lobules is found in the cases of portal vein obliteration [20,59]. In fact, Wanless et al.[59,60] reported that apoptosis of hepatocytes could be a transient response to acute ischemia and that atrophy and nodular hyperplasia of hepatocytes are chronic response to ischemia, and that vascular obstruction or ischemia and irregular intrahepatic irrigation are an important cause of apoptosis and atrophy and hyperplasia found in chronic liver disease including IPH.

Our recent study disclosed that the livers of IPH showed frequently the hepatic parenchymal changes such as sinusoidal dilatation with hepatocellular atrophy and hyperplasia [42]. Disordered intrahepatic hemodynamics, particularly continuous portal venous insufficiency due to obliteration of small portal veins and dense fibroelastosis of small portal tracts, may be responsible for the development of these hepatic parenchymal alterations [14,42]. Sinusoidal dilatation usually associated with hepatocellular atrophy is preferentially seen in perivenular areas and also between hyperplastic hepatocytic nodules, and the hepatocytes are more or less atrophic or small. In these areas, pericellular fibrosis and thin fibrous septa were also frequently seen (see below).

These continuous parenchymal ischemic conditions may lead to the uneven dropout of hepatocytes from the hepatic lobules followed by the atrophy of hepatic lobules and subcapsular atrophy and then decreased weight of the liver. Hepatocellular apoptosis and focal necrosis were infrequently and focally found or occasionally clustered in the hepatic parenchyma in IPH livers (***Figure 3C***). They are more or less frequent in the areas with sinusoidal dilatation. Hepatocellular apoptosis is a process of ischemic hepatic parenchymal atrophy or dropout [59]. Two types of eosinophilic hepatocellular changes are presumed to be apoptotic in origin; round acidophilic bodies and stellate-shaped acidophilic bodies. Either of these apoptotic changes is usually found focally in the hepatic parenchyma in IPH. Focal necrosis characterized by the dropout of hepatocytes and lymphoid cell infiltration is only occasionally associated with pigmented macrophages scattered in the hepatic parenchyma. The significance of this lesion remains only speculative. However, there were no interface hepatitis, zonal necrosis or lymph follicle formation in the portal tracts as seen in viral or autoimmune chronic active hepatitis.

Hepatic parenchymal collapse (extinction): In addition to the above-mentioned continuous peripheral portal venous insufficiency, portal venous thromboembolism is also known to superimpose not infrequently in IPH livers. Some of such thrombi may resolve and disappear and also responsible for the irregular intimal thickening and phlebosclerosis of the intrahepatic large portal vein and also portal vein trunk, but some may cause portal venous occlusion which lead to hepatic parenchymal collapse or extinction to a variable exent [60]. Occasionally, the hepatic segment or area are totally collapsed due to thrombotic occlusion of the intrahepatic large portal vein(s) [1,4,14].

Hepatic Parenchymal Fibrosis

So far, two types of intralobular fibrosis are identifiable in IPH livers (***Figure 9A,9B***): pericellular fibrosis and slender fibrous septa. These changes are more or less mild and focal, when compared to other fibrotic progressive liver diseases such as alcoholic hepatitis or chronic viral hepatitis. While intralobular fibrosis in other liver diseases with progressive hepatic fibrosis is probably due to activated hepatic stellate cells (HSC) or Ito cells [21,61], the pathogenesis of such intralobular fibrosis in IPH livers remains unexplored, so far.

Our recent study [42] showed that pericellular fibrosis around the hepatocytes was focally seen in the perivenular areas, particularly between hyperplastic hepatocellular nodules. In these areas, hepatocytes are more or less atrophic and the sinusoids are more or less dilated. This type of fibrosis may link eventually to the neighboring central veins. Intralobular fibrous slender septa is seen in more than 50% of IPH cases, and this septa and pericellular fibrosis merge sometimes. These findings suggest that microcirculatory changes are related to the development of mild and focal pericellular fibrosis or thin fibrous septa. Interestingly, in these areas, α-smooth muscle actin (α-SMA) positive, activated HSC (myofibroblasts) are increased or accumulated. These activated HSC are known to produce actively ECM proteins including collagen, laminin and fibronectin responsible for sinusoidal capillization and also secrete profibrotic molecules such as transforming growth factor (TGF)-β for hepatic fibrosis of chronic progressive liver diseases such as alcoholic fibrosis and chronic viral hepatitis [61-65]. It seems likely that these activated HSC seem to be increased in the parenchymal areas showing these intralobular fibrosis. In this situation, these activated HSC may be a key cell in the parenchymal fibrosis in IPH. Ischemic state in the hepatic lobules due to decreased portal venous inflow may activate HSC and then contribute to the development and progression of mild fibrosis in IPH.

Taken together, these findings suggest that such parenchymal changes related to portal venous insufficient blood flow into the hepatic lobules may contribute to the development and progression of intralobular fibrosis and parenchymal atrophy mainly via hepatocellular atoptosis in IPH.

Incomplete septal cirrhosis (ISC) which is also associated with presinusoidal long-standing portal hypertension, shows more fibrotic changes but not sufficient to be diagnosed as evident cirrhosis [2,24,40]. In ISC, slender septal fibrosis containing elastin is an extension of portal fibrosis and perivenular fibrosis, and this fibrosis demarcates the parenchyma into inconspicuous nodules (***Figure 9B***). These livers also show abnormal spacing between the portal tracts and central veins, and small hypoplastic portal tracts are found within the parenchyma. While this may belong to one spectrum of IPH or its equivalent, and could be a late manifestation of IPH [2,20,21], the exact differentiation from macronodular cirrhosis is difficult occasionally in biopsy specimens.

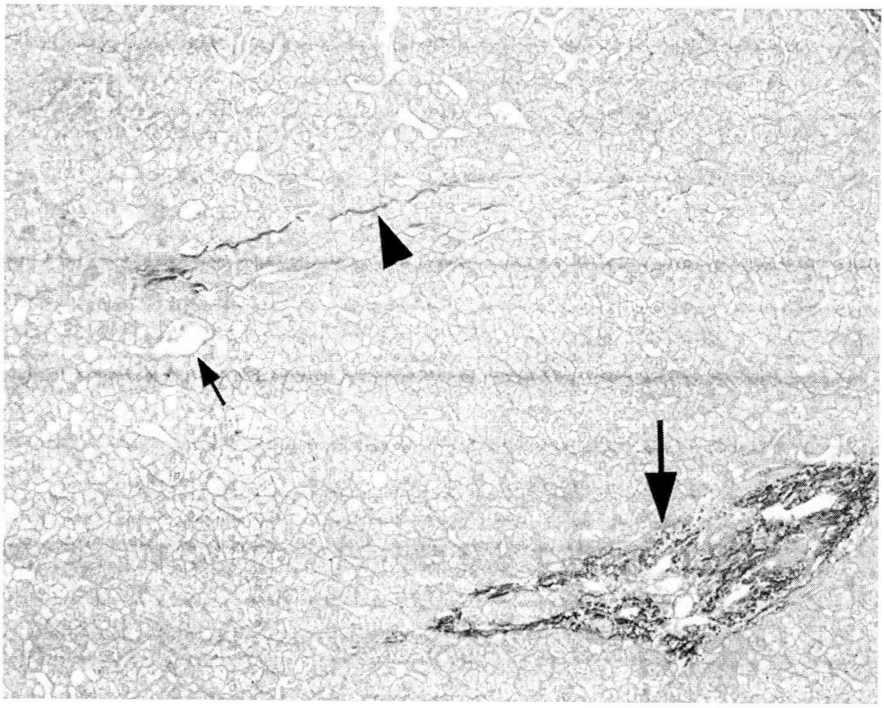

Figure 9A. There is thin fibrous septa (arrow head) in the parenchyma. There is sinusoidal dilatation, too. Hepatic lobular pattern is distorted. Large arrow, portal tract; small arrow, central vein. Idiopathic portal hypertension. Elastica van Gieson stain.

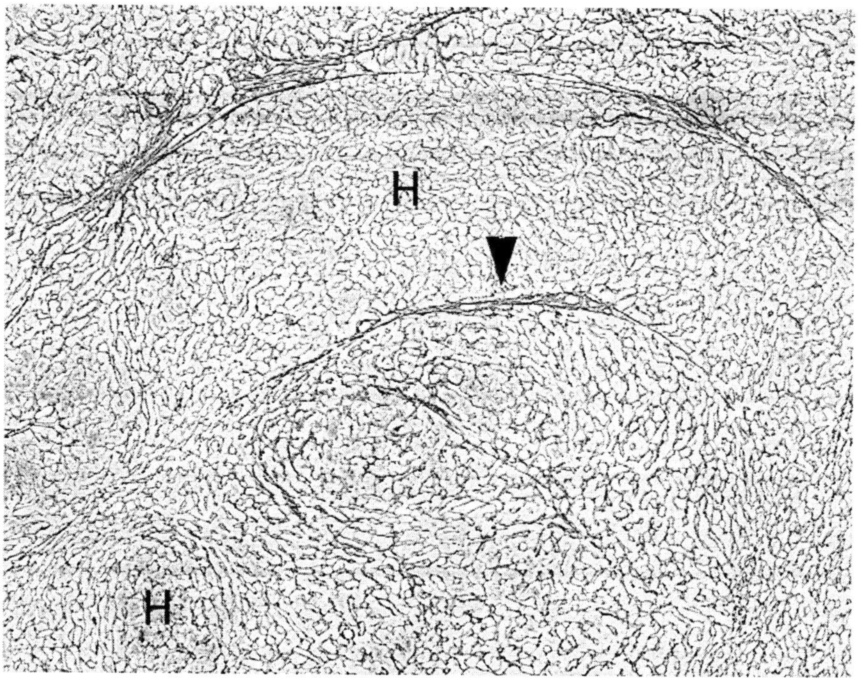

Figure 9B. Hepatic lobular pattern is distorted. There are thin fibrous septa (arrow heads), and hepatic parenchyma seems nodular. Idiopathic portal hypertension. Gomori's reticulin stain.

Nodular Hepatocellular Hyperplasia

It is well known that grossly visible and microscopically identifiable nodular hyperplastic hepatocellular lesions are encountered occasionally in the livers of portal venous hypoplasia or agenesis, and also in those of EHO and Budd-Chiari syndrome [3-5]. Among these lesions, focal nodular hyperplasia, nodular regenerative hyperplasia, partial nodular transformation, and non-cirrhotic macroregenerative nodules, and hepatocellular adenoma-like hyperplastic nodules have been reported, and they are speculated to occur secondarily due to abnormal intrahepatic irrigation [66-68].

Earlier studies on IPH insisted that active hepatocellular regenerative changes or nodule formation are characteristically absent in IPH, and therefore, IPH is different from macronodular cirrhosis with thin septa and portal hypertension, though there have been many studies on the hyperplastic change in IPH livers in recent years [11,14]. However, IPH livers with these nodular changes are clearly different from liver cirrhosis. In fact, nodular regeneration is found in one third or more of IPH cases (***Figure 1B, 4A, 4B, 9B***) [2,58], and both of atrophy and nodular hyperplasia of the hepatic parenchyma are regarded as a chronic response to long-standing ischemia in IPH and other vascular diseases [59]. However, it remains unclear why hepatocellular hyperplasia is predominant in some cases and absent in others. In this context, the hepatic morphology of IPH could be regarded as an abnormal remodelling of the liver associated with the frequent development of hepatocellular hyperplastic nodules and frequent obliteration of intrahepatic small portal veins [5]. It should be noted that there have been, however, no reports on the occurrence of HCC in the IPH liver with such nodular hyperplastic lesions, and therefore, these nodular hyperplastic changes are not related to the neoplastic processes of the liver.

Nodular regenerative hyperplasia (NRH): NRH is characterized by non-cirrhotic regenerative nodules in the liver and occurs in portal hypertensive cases and also in cases without portal hypertension [2,5,69]. Generally, these nodulations involve the whole liver. NRH with presinusoidal portal hypertension could be IPH itself, because nodular regenerative hyperplasia of variable degree and extent is found in a considerable number of IPH cases. Distinguishing NRH with portal hypertension from IPH with variable parenchymal nodular hyperplasia is difficult, and such cases may form a spectrum with respect to nodular hyperplasia in non-cirrhotic portal hypertension and both features appear to relate to obliteration of small portal veins [2,5,69]. This is supported by an animal model affecting small inrahepatic portal veins, presenting with NRH and portal hypertension [70].

Partial nodular transformation (PNT): This lesion is characterized by grossly visible parenchymal nodulations and buldgings, mainly involving the hepatic hilar and perihilar regions [71]. It is known to occur frequently in acute and subacute portal venous thromboembolism [72]. This lesion is also encountered in IPH livers, particularly those with fresh occlusive thromboemboli of portal veins or portal vein trunk and those with extensive subcapsular dropout or extinction. At present, it remains undetermined if this lesion is an exaggerated compensatory reaction of the hepatic parenchyma to several stimuli or a single disease entity. Similar gross lesions may occur as a compensatory hypertrophy of the liver in partial biliary occlusion such as biliary atresia and infantile bile duct paucity syndrome including Allagille syndrome [73].

Focal nodular hyperplasia (FNH) and FNH-like lesions: The nodular changes similar to FNH of the liver as seen in liver cirrhosis have also been reported in IPH [4]. In IPH livers, these lesions are focal or occasionally multiple in distribution, and their morphologies are incomplete or immature when compared to FNH without non-cirrhotic portal hypertension. Portal vein thromboemboli could be an initiating event for the development of FNH like nodules in IPH livers.

At present, it seems conceivable that such nodular parenchymal changes are one of the constitutional components of IPH or it's equivalents. Intrahepatic vascular lesions with deficient and irregular afferent irrigation disturbance may be responsible for the development and maintenace of portal hypertension and also for the nodular hepatocellular hyperplasia in IPH [4].

Pathologic Spectrum of IPH and Its Equivalents

Because IPH liver shows the above-mentioned nodular and fibrotic lesions and small portal venous obliterative lesions and large portal venous thrombotic lesions in a variable combination, subclassification of IPH based on the above-changes has been proposed. That is, in some cases of IPH, nodular regenerative changes of hepatocytes are predominant in the absence of parenchymal fibrotic changes, and such cases can be called NRH. In other cases, however, subcapsular fibrosis and slender fibrosis in the parenchyma is clear and can be called as ISC [2,4]. PNT or FNH lesions are also encountered clearly in several cases of IPH. Several cases showed typical features of IPH without fibrotic or nodular hyperplastic changes. Some cases showed more than one features. Ibarrola and Colina reported that it was frequently difficult to apply the nomenclature system proposed so far to non-cirrhotic hypertension cases of unknown cause experienced in the West, while some cases were typical of IPH or NRH or ISC. Further discussion on the nomenclature on this disease group should be done in near future.

Correlation to Equivalents and Related Diseases of IPH

Equivalent Diseases of IPH with Different Names

There have been reported several kinds of diseases similar to or counterparts of IPH but with different names such as hepatoportal sclerosis, NCPF, non-cirrhotic intrahepatic portal hypertension, and benign intrahepatic portal hypertension [1,8]. They share clinical and laboratory features and also pathological features such as portal venous and portal tract abnormalities and also parenchymal atrophy and nodular parenchymal hyperplasia [14]. In fact, several pathologists examined the autopsy livers of both IPH and NCPF, and they concluded that their pathological features were very similar or identical to each other [14]. However, it remains unclear whether their etiopathogenesis is the same or may differ according to different districts in the world or even in the same district.

Similar but Different Diseases

There are similar diseases to IPH, but are thought different from IPH at present. The followings are examples.

Myeloproliferative disorders

In myeloproliferative disorders such as myelofibrosis or polycythemia vera, non-cirrhotic portal hypertension can develop. In such cases, thrombosis of portal veins and hepatic veins is a common cause of portal hypertension [74]. However, in a few cases with portal hypertension, increased portal blood flow from marked splenomegaly associated with extramedullary hematopoiesis could be a factor in portal hypertension. NRH with widespread obliteration of portal vein radicals (obliterative portal venopathy) are known to occur in hematological disease including polycythemia vera, agnogenic myeloid metaplasia, primary thrombocythemia, rheumatoid arthritis with thrombocytosis, multiple myeloma, and erythrocytosis associated with polycystic renal disease. The following pathogenesis of NRH is proposed: Thrombi, perhaps largely composed of platelet aggregates formed in the portal venous circulation or spleen, embolize to the liver and results in obliterative vascular lesions. Atrophy and regenerative nodule formation occur in response to the interruption of the portal blood supply [13].

Presinusoidal portal hypertension related to medical treatments and intoxication

There is an association between a long-standing presinusoidal portal hypertension resembling IPH and the use of chemotherapeutic agents, particularly thioguanine [75,76]. Chronic arsenic intoxication is also known to be associated with such a syndrome [76]. Mild sclerosis of some small portal triads and perisinusoidal fibrosis are the only abnormality seen. A peculiar pattern of progressive portal-tract fibrosis, and inconspicuous intralobular and conspicuous capsular fibrosis accompanied by splenomegaly was also observed in five workers with vinyl chloride polymerization [77].

Furthermore, a similar syndrome occurs following renal transplantation [78]. These patients had been treated with azathioprine and prednisolone for several years. In these patients, the spleen might have played an important role in the development of this syndrome. Microscopic examination of liver biopsies taken at the operation revealed lymphoplasmacytic infiltration with bile duct hyperplasia but no evidence of periportal fibrosis except for very mild perisinusoidal fibrosis.

Extrahepatic portal venous obstruction (EHO) in adults

Adult EHO cases with the clinicopathological features similar to those IPH have been occasionally reported [79]. Such cases might have started as IPH originally, and portal venous thrombosis and portal venous obstruction might have occurred secondarily in their long clinical course (stage IV). These EHO cases should be differentiated from EBO without features of IPH. Thrombotic processes of the portal venous system tend to occur, particularly after splenectomy [20]. In the latter, the liver histology failes to show obliteration of small portal veins and dense portal fibroelastosis [15].

In addition, there are also patients with spontaneous portal-systemic shunt and hepatic encephalopathy without splenomegaly in whom the liver histology resembles IPH but with normal portal pressure [80]. Such cases could be also a variant of IPH in which portal blood flow into the shunt and thereby clinically detectable portal hypertension and splenomegaly do not occur.

Etiopathogenesis of IPH

The primary factor(s) involved in the development of long-standing presinusoidal portal hypertension of IPH and its equivalents remain unclear. As for the genetic factors, the family clustering is not evident in IPH, and the phenotype frequencies of the specificities of HLA-A and -B loci in patients with IPH did not differ from those in healthy controls [12].

The following factors are now proposed for the etiologic factors of IPH.

Infectious Etiology

The number of IPH patients is rapidly decreasing in Japan in recent years, perhaps due to the improvements of the environment or public health, suggesting that infection(s) or infection-related immunopathological assaults might have been operative in the development of IPH. Particularly, systemic or intrabdominal infection might have been participated in this disease [81]. Several experimental approaches have been made to obtain clues as to the etiopathogenesis of IPH, and Okuda et al successfully produced a hepatic lesion and hemodynamics similar to that in IPH by repeated injection of aggregated killed non-pathogenic Escherichia coli (E.coli) directly into the portal vein [82,83]. In the treated dogs, portal pressure was elevated and middle-to-small-sized portal branches were decreased in number as studied by portography. The histology of the liver showed dense fibrosis in the portal tract and aberrant vasculatures around the portal area. Bile duct damages were also seen.These changes closely mimic those seen in human IPH. It is possible that gut-derived antigens such as bacteria absorbed from the intestine to the portal venous system plays an etiologic role in the development of IPH. Furthemore, tabbits were given killed nonpathogenic E.coli intraportally or intravenously. The animals to which a mixture of killed E. coli and rabbit antiserum (aggregated E. coli) was given intraportally developed remarkable histologic changes in the liver. The early inflammatory reactions in the portal area and parenchyma were followed by rapid disappearance of inflammation and development of portal fibrosis with bile duct proliferation. This procedure also produced splenomegaly, and in some animals marked portal hypertension. These histologic changes resemble portal fibrosis seen in IPH and, less closely, pericholangitis associated with inflammatory bowel disease in humans. As for chronic infection of HBV or HCV, IPH is not causally related to such viruses [12].

Immunological Factors

As to the primary cause(s) of IPH, many studies have suggested that it might be an immune-mediated disease. That is, certain immunologic abnormalities seem to play an etiologic role in the portal venous obliteration and also relate to the massive splenomegaly. Clinically, a number of immunological abnormalities such as hypergammaglobulinemia and antinuclear antibodies with high titer occur in IPH patients. LE cell phenomena were also positive in some patients [84,85]. In addition, the association of IPH with systemic lupus erythematosus (SLE), chronic thyroiditis, mixed connective tissue disease, and PSS has been occasionally reported [86-89]. Usually, IPH and other autoimmune or collagen vascular disease develop simultaneously [90]. The presence of anticardiolipin antibody, indicated by positivity for lupus anticoagulant, was suggestive of the presence of a common immunological mechanism in the etiology of IPH and SLE. Raynaud's phenomenon associated with positive anti-RNP antibody is also associated with IPH.

As for the histological findings suggestive of immunopathologic processes, edematous and fibrous thickening of the intima with chronic inflammatory cell infiltration in the intima of portal vein branches is occasionally observed. This lesion may be a kind of nonsuppuraive phlebitis [27,88]. Although this lesion is focal, it is rather characteristic of IPH and may be a primary lesion of IPH according to Ohbu [27]. It is exclusively found in IPH livers. HLA-DR antigen which is involved in immune recognition and other immunologic reactions, is strongly expressed on the microvasculature of portal tracts more frequently in IPH and this expression may be a factor initiating immunologic assault on portal microvessels in IPH [32,88,90]. Increased level of interferon (IFN)-γ in portal venous blood derived from the massive spleen may be responsible for this HLA-DR expression [91].

While in autopsy livers of IPH, there are no or only scanty lymphoid cells in the liver tissue, there are occasionally a lymphoid cells in portal tracts of wedge biopsy specimens, particularly at early stages [6]. Recently, we have recently experienced one case of early IPH in which hepatic changes recognizable histologically are lymphoid cell infiltration of the portal tract and of subendothelial regions of portal vein branches, suggesting an altered immunophenomenon of this disease at early stage [92]. While such lymphoid cells have been neglected so far, they may have some pathogenetic significance in the development of portal and vascular lesions in IPH.

As for the adhesion molecules which are important in the interaction between lymphocytes and accessory and target cells, the serum level of soluble VCAM-1 is found to be increased [91]. The level of soluble ICAM-1 of IPH patients was slightly high but not different from that in patients with other diseases. VCAM-1 is expressed in the sinusoidal lining cells and portal venous endothelial cells in several IPH patients. Increased expression of VCAM-1 may reflect an immunopathological phenomenon in the occurrence of IPH.

Because cytokines and the balance of T helper (h) 1 and Th2 CD4+ T cells have been reported to be important for regulating the immune response. The mean value of soluble TNF receptor-II was significantly higher in IPH patients than that of control subjects and fatty liver patients. The ratios of Th1 and Th2 in both peripheral and spleen lymphocytes of IPH patients were significantly increased compared with the ratios found in peripheral lymphocytes of control subjects. The increase in the ratios was due to a decrease in the percentage of Th2 CD4+ T cells, suggesting that the imbalance of Th1 and Th2 CD4+ T cells and TNF may be associated with the pathogenesis of IPH [93]. The autologous mixed lymphocyte reaction (AMLR) reflecting immune control mechanisms showed that the AMLRs both in the spleen and peripheral blood were significantly suppressed in IPH patients compared to those of normal healthy subjects [94]. By allogeneic MLR, there was a tendency that the disturbance of non-T cells was more intensive than that of T cells. The depressed cause of AMLR in patients with IPH was suggested mainly to disturbance of the antigen-presenting ability of non-T cells. However, the exact role of such disturbed immune control to the pathogenesis of IPH remains only spceculative.

Thrombosis and Clotting Abnormalities

Mural and even occlusive thromboembolism of hilar and intrahepatic large portal veins is known to occur secondary in IPH (***Figure 1A, 1B***), and this may aggravate the liver pathology of IPH. The calculated incidence of portal vein thrombosis was angiographically

0.573% of all cirrhotic patients without splenectomy in the past [7], though the incidence of portal vein thrombosis unrelated to splenectomy was angiographically 2.86% in IPH. Hypercoagulable states such as polycythemia rubra vera, oral contraceptives, pregnancy, and deficiencies in natural anticoagulants such as protein C and factor V Leiden mutation produce a favorable medium for thrombus generation in the portal vein [94-98]. However, in IPH such deficiency or mutation of these factors have not been reported.

Wanless reported that when thrombosis in the extrahepatic portal veins extends to the intrahepatic small portal veins, the liver histology become mimicking IPH and a diagnosis of IPH may be done [99]. However, direct evidence for portal venous thrombosis as a primary factor of IPH is still lacking in IPH patients experienced in Japan [11].

IPH Related to Toxic or Chemical Environmental Factors

Presinusoidal portal hypertension resembling IPH is known to develop in patients treated with chemotherapeutic agents and during arsenic intoxication and vinly chloride polymerization [76,77]. The histologic and clinical hemodynamic similarity of these cases to IPH suggests that IPH at times results from unknown toxic, possible environmental, chemicals and drugs. So far, no definite or concrete materials have been shown to be responsible for the development of IPH.

PERSPECTIVES

The recent progress in the study of IPH with respect to pathology and pathophysiology was reviewed. The liver pathology of IPH is characterized by occlusive changes of the intrahepatic small portal veins, portal dense fibrosis, and irregularly distributed parenchymal atrophy and mild and focal lobular and slender septal fibrosis in the parenchyma, particularly in the subcapsular region. Atrophic changes and focal and slight fibrotic changes in the hepatic lobules are probably secondary to reduced portal venous inflow into the parenchyma. These alterations are associated with altered expression of several vasomodularing molecules such as HO-1 and endothelin-1 and activation of HSC. The fibrogenesis and elastosis of portal tracts in IPH may be related to up-regulation of CTGF and down-regulation of MMP-9, though the causes for activation of these molecules remain unclear. Furthermore, there were several kinds of hepatocellular nodular lesions, probably due to heterogeneous and dys-synchronous affection of the intrahepatic vasculatures in IPH livers. Portal venous thrmoboembolism could also not infrequently superimpose and be responsible for variable collapse of hepatic parenchyma and also for phlebosclerosis. Taking the gross findings reflecting secondary changes into the consideration, a new staging system of IPH was proposed (stage I, II, III and IV). Stage I is characterized by no atrophy of the liver and patent portal vein, and Stage IV by occluding portal venous thromboemboli.

Almost all cases of IPH are found to have massive splenomegaly with anemia or pancytopenia except for spontaneous P-V shunts, and massive splenomegaly contributes to the increased portal venous blood flow into the liver. Furthermore, from such massive spleens, several kinds of biologically active subustacnes such as INF-γmay inflow into the liver. IFN-γ in portal venous blood is known to be increased [91]. Such situations regarding massive splenomegaly may contribute to the progression of IPH and the develoment of IPH liver pathology. splenomegaly in IPH was presumed to be caused by proliferation of sinus endothelial cells, and by the increased splenic blood flow in the irregularly widened interendothelial slits of the sinuses [100]. However, the studies on the participation of massive spleen in the pathogenesis of IPH, particularly the causal relationship, remains limited.

The most important issues of the pathobiology of IPH to be addressed and clarified in the near future are 1). What are the primary or acute lesions in the liver?. 2). Are the dense portal fibrosis and obliteration of small portal tracts a primary lesion for the development of portal hypertension or secondary adaptive lesion to increased blood flow into the liver and/or high pressure of portal vein ? 3). Is the causal relation of massive splenomegaly to the liver pathology and sustained portal hypertension in IPH ? and 4). What are the etiologies in IPH and its equivalents ?

Acknowledgements

This study was supported by the Japanese Study Group of Intrahepatic Hemodynamic Alterations (Chairman: Prof. Makoto Hashizume, Professor of Emergency Medicine, Kyushu University Graduate School of Medicine, Fukuoka, Japan).

References

[1] Aikat BK, Bhusnurmath SR, Chhuttani PN, Mitra SK, Dutta DV. The pathology of noncirrhotic portal fibrosis: a review of 32 autopsy cases. *Hum Pathol* 1979;10:405-418

[2] Nakanuma Y, Hoso M, Sasaki M, Terada T, Katayanagi K, Nonomura A, Kurumaya H, Harada A, Obata H. Histopathology of the liver in non-cirrhotic portal hypertension of unknown aetiology. *Histopathology* 1996;28:195-204.

[3] Hillaire S, Bonte E, Denninger MH, Casadevall N, Cadranel JF, Lebrec D, Valla D, Degott C. Idiopathic non-cirrhotic intrahepatic portal hypertension in the West: a re-evaluation in 28 patients. *Gut*. 2002;51:275-280.

[4] Ibarrola C, Colina F. Clinicopathological features of nine cases of non-cirrhotic portal hypertension: current definitions and criteria are inadequate. *Histopathology*. 2003;42:251-264.

[5] Roskams T, Baptista A, Bianchi L, Burt A, Callea F, Denk H, De Groote J, Desmet V, Hubscher S, Ishak K, MacSween R, Portmann B, Poulson H, Scheuer P, Terracciano L, Thaler H. Histopathology of portal hypertension: a practical guideline. *Histopathology*. 2003;42:2-13.

[6] Ohnishi K, Saito M, Sato S, Terabayashi H, Iida S, Nomura F, Nakano M, Okuda K. Portal hemodynamics in idiopathic portal hypertension (Banti's syndrome). Comparison with chronic persistent hepatitis and normal subjects. *Gastroenterology* 1987;92:751-758.

[7] Okuda K, Ohnishi K, Kimura K, Matsutani S, Sumida M, Goto N, Musha H, Takashi M, Suzuki N, Shinagawa T, et al. Incidence of portal vein thrombosis in liver cirrhosis. An angiographic study in 708 patients. *Gastroenterology* 1985;89:279-286.

[8] Mikkelson WP, Edmondson HA, Peters RL, Redeker AG, Reynolds TB. Extra- and intrahepatic portal hypertension without cirrhosis (hepatoportal sclerosis). *Ann Surg* 1965;162:602-620

[9] Terada T, Hoso M, Nakanuma Y. Microvasculature in the small portal tracts in idiopathic portal hypertension. A morphological comparison with other hepatic diseases. *Virchows Arch A Pathol Anat Histopathol.* 1989;415:61-67.

[10] Nakanuma Y, Hoso M, Sanzen T, Sasaki M. Microstructure and development of the normal and pathologic biliary tract in humans, including blood supply. *Microsc Res Tech.* 1997;38:552-570.

[11] Okuda K, Kono K, Ohnishi K, Kimura K, Omata M, Koen H, Nakajima Y, Musha H, Hirashima T, Takashi M, et al. Clinical study of eighty-six cases of idiopathic portal hypertension and comparison with cirrhosis with splenomegaly. *Gastroenterology* 1984;86:600-610.

[12] Satoh H, Iwasaki Y, Ohkubo A, Beppu T, Futagawa S, Sugiura M, Juji T. Human leukocyte antigen (HLA) in patients with idiopathic portal hypertension (IPH). Tohoku *J Exp Med.* 1980;131:393-397.

[13] Wanless IR, Godwin TA, Allen F, Feder A. Nodular regenerative hyperplasia of the liver in hematologic disorders: a possible response to obliterative portal venopathy. A morphometric study of nine cases with an hypothesis on the pathogenesis. *Medicine* (Baltimore) 1980;59:367-379.

[14] Okuda K, Nakashima T, Okudaira M, Kage M, Aida Y, Omata M, Sugiura M, Kameda H, Inokuchi K, Bhusnurmath SR, Aikat BA. Liver pathology of idiopathic portal hypertension. Comparison with non-cirrhotic portal fibrosis of India. The Japan idiopathic portal hypertension study. *Liver* 1982;2:176-192.

[15] Okudaira M, Ohbu M, Okuda K. Idiopathic portal hypertension and its pathology. *Semin Liver Dis*. 2002;22:59-72.

[16] Dhiman RK, Chawla Y, Vasishta RK, Kakkar N, Dilawari JB, Trehan MS, Puri P, Mitra SK, Suri S. Non-cirrhotic portal fibrosis (idiopathic portal hypertension): experience with 151 patients and a review of the literature. *J Gastroenterol Hepatol.* 2002;17:6-16.

[17] Sarin SK, Aggarwal SR. Idiopathic portal hypertension. Digestion. 1998;59:420-423.

[18] Nakak NC, Ramalingaswami V. Obliterative portal venopathy of the liver associated with so-called idiopathic portal hypertension or tropical splenomegaly. *Arch Pathol* 1969;87:359-369

[19] Vakili C, Farahvash MJ, Bynum TE. "Endemic" idiopathic portal hypertension: report on 32 patients with non-cirrhotic portal fibrosis. *World J Surg* 1992;16:118-124.

[20] Bernard PH, Le Bail B, Cransac M, Barcina MG, Carles J, Balabaud C, Bioulac-Sage P. Progression from idiopathic portal hypertension to incomplete septal cirrhosis with liver failure requiring liver transplantation. *J Hepatol* 1995;22:495-499.

[21] Bioulac-Sage P, Le Bail B, Bernard PH, Balabaud C. Hepatoportal sclerosis. *Semin Liver Dis* 1995;15:329-339

[22] Ichimura S, Sasaki R, Takemura Y, Iwata H, Obata H, Okuda H, Imai F. The prognosis of idiopathic portal hypertension in Japan. *Intern Med* 1993;32:441-444.

[23] Matsui O, Takashima T, Kadoya M, Kitagawa K. Computed tomography during arterial portography in idiopathic portal hypertension. *Radiat Med* 1984;2:189-193.

[24] Nakanuma Y, Tsuneyama K, Ohbu M, Katayanagi K. Pathology and pathogenesis of idiopathic portal hypertension with an emphasis on the liver. *Pathol Res Pract.* 2001;197:65-76.

[25] Arai K, Matsui O, Kadoya M, Yoshikawa J, Gabata T, Takashima T, Kobayashi K, Unoura M. MR imaging in idiopathic portal hypertension. *J Comput Assist Tomogr* 1991;15:405-408.

[26] Urata K, Kawasaki S, Matsunami H, Hashikura Y, Ikegami T, Ishizone S, Momose Y, Komiyama A, Makuuchi M. Calculation of child and adult standard liver volume for liver transplantation. *Hepatology*. 1995;21:1317-1321.

[27] Ohbu M, Okudaira M. *Subintimal edematous and cellular lesions of intrahpeatic portal veins in portal hypertension.* Report of intrahepatic hemodynamic alterations of Japanese Health and Welfare Minister, 1996,pp.32-37.

[28] Ludwig J, Hashimoto E, Obata H, Baldus WP. Idiopathic portal hypertension; a histopathological study of 26 Japanese cases. *Histopathology* 1993;22:227-34.

[29] Nakanuma Y, Hoso M. *Specificity of liver lesions of idiopathic portal hypertension. Annual report on idiopathic portal hypertension organized by Japanese Welfare Ministry* (Chairman, Prof. Shunji Futagawa), 1995, pp.50-52 (in Japanese).

[30] Ohnishi K, Chin N, Tanaka H, Iida S, Sato S, Terabayashi H, Nomura F. Differences in portal hemodynamics in cirrhosis and idiopathic portal hypertension. *Am J Gastroenterol* 1989;84:409-412.

[31] Futagawa S, Fukazawa M, Horisawa M, Musha H, Ito T, Sugiura M, Kameda H, Okuda K. Portographic liver changes in idiopathic noncirrhotic portal hypertension. AJR *Am J Roentgenol* 1980;134:917-923.

[32] Terada T, Nakanuma Y, Hoso M, Obata H. Expression of HLA-DR antigen on hepatic vascular endothelial cells in idiopathic portal hypertension. *Clin Exp Immunol* 1991;84:303-307.

[33] Oikawa H, Masuda T, Sato S, Yashima A, Suzuki K, Sato S, Satodate R. Changes in lymph vessels and portal veins in the portal tract of patients with idiopathic portal hypertension: a morphometric study. *Hepatology* 1998;27:1607-1610.

[34] Tsuneyama K, Ohba K, Zen Y, Sato Y, Niwa H, Minato H, Nakanuma Y. A comparative histological and morphometric study of vascular changes in idiopathic portal hypertension and alcoholic fibrosis/cirrhosis. *Histopathology*. 2003;43:55-61.

[35] Ohbu M, Okudaira M, Watanabe K, Kaneko S, Takai T. Histopathological study of intrahepatic aberrant vessels in cases of noncirrhotic portal hypertension. *Hepatology* 1994;20:302-308.

[36] Siderys H, Judd D, Herendeen T. The experimental production of elevated portal pressure by increasing portal vein flow. *Surg Gynecol Obstet* 196;120:514-516.

[37] Koda W, Harada K, Tsuneyama K, Kono N, Sasaki M, Matsui O, Nakanuma Y. Evidence of the participation of peribiliary mast cells in regulation of the peribiliary vascular plexus along the intrahepatic biliary tree. *Lab Invest*. 2000;80:1007-1017.

[38] Itai Y, Moss AA, Goldberg HI. Transient hepatic attenuation difference of lobar or segmental distribution detected by dynamic computed tomography. *Radiology*. 1982;144:835-839.

[39] Nagino M, Nimura Y, Kamiya J, Kanai M, Hayakawa N, Yamamoto H. Immediate increase in arterial blood flow in embolized hepatic segments after portal vein embolization: CT demonstration. *AJR Am J Roentgenol*. 1998;171:1037-1039.

[40] Sciot R, Staessen D, Van Damme B, Van Steenbergen W, Fevery J, De Groote J, Desmet VJ. Incomplete septal cirrhosis: histopathological aspects. *Histopathology.* 1988;13:593-603.

[41] Terada T, Takegoshi T, Doishita K, Nakanuma Y. Histological study of intrahepatic cavernous transformation in a patient with primary myelofibrosis and portal venous thrombosis. *Virchows Arch A Pathol Anat Histopathol.* 1988;412:339-345.

[42] Tsuneyama K, Kouda W, Nakanuma Y. Portal and parenchymal alterations of the liver in idiopathic portal hypertension: a histological and immunochemical study. *Pathol Res Pract.* 2002;198:597-603.

[43] Makino N, Suematsu M, Sugiura Y, Morikawa H, Shiomi S, Goda N, Sano T, Nimura Y, Sugimachi K, Ishimura Y.Altered expression of heme oxygenase-1 in the livers of patients with portal hypertensive diseases. *Hepatology.* 2001;33:32-42.

[44] Kyokane T, Norimizu S, Taniai H, Yamaguchi T, Takeoka S, Tsuchida E, Naito M, Nimura Y, Ishimura Y, Suematsu M. Carbon monoxide from heme catabolism protects against hepatobiliary dysfunction in endotoxin-treated rat liver. *Gastroenterology.* 2001;120:1227-1240.

[45] Kamath PS, Carpenter HA, Lloyd RV, McKusick MA, Steers JL, Nagorney DM, Miller VM. Hepatic localization of endothelin-1 in patients with idiopathic portal hypertension and cirrhosis of the liver. *Liver Transpl.* 2000;6:596-602.

[46] Ohara N, Futagawa S, Watanabe S, Fukasawa M, Takamori S. Clinical investigation of endothelin-1 and nitric oxide in patients with portal hypertension focusing on plasma levels and immunohistological staining of liver tissues. *Hepatol Res.* 2001;21:40-54.

[47] Futagawa S, Fukazawa M, Musha H, Isomatsu T, Koyama K, Ito T, Horisawa M, Nakayama S, Sugiura M, Kameda H, Okuda K. Hepatic venography in noncirrhotic idiopathic portal hypertension. Comparison with cirrhosis of the liver. *Radiology* 1981;141:303-309.

[48] Nakanuma Y, Ohta G, Doishita K. Quantitation and serial section observations of focal venocclusive lesions of hepatic veins in liver cirrhosis. *Virchows Arch A Pathol Anat Histopathol.* 1985;405:429-438.

[49] Sasaki M, Nakanuma Y, Watanabe K. Hepatocellular prolapse of hepatic portal tracts and subendothelial space of central veins in idiopathic portal hypertension. *Histopathology.* 1995;27:67-70.

[50] Palombo D, Maione M, Cifiello BI, Udini M, Maggio D, Lupo M. Matrix metalloproteinases. Their role in degenerative chronic diseases of abdominal aorta. *J Cardiovasc Surg* (Torino). 1999;40:257-260.

[51] Paradis V, Dargere D, Vidaud M, De Gouville AC, Huet S, Martinez V, Gauthier JM, Ba N, Sobesky R, Ratziu V, Bedossa P. Expression of connective tissue growth factor in experimental rat and human liver fibrosis. *Hepatology* 1999;30:968-976.

[52] Morikawa H, Hishiguchi S, Shiomi S, Kaneda K, Takigawa M. Expression of connective tissue growth factor in patients with IPH. Kupffer *Cell Foundation,* 2001;8:229-230.

[53] Holmes A, Abraham DJ, Chen Y, Denton C, Shi-wen X, Black CM, Leask A. Constitutive connective tissue growth factor expression in scleroderma fibroblasts is dependent on Sp1. *J Biol Chem.* 2003;278:41728-41733.

[54] Sato S, Nagaoka T, Hasegawa M, Tamatani T, Nakanishi T, Takigawa M, Takehara K. Serum levels of connective tissue growth factor are elevated in patients with systemic

sclerosis: association with extent of skin sclerosis and severity of pulmonary fibrosis. *J Rheumatol* 2000;27:149-154.

[55] Tsuneyama K, Harada K, Katayanagi K, Watanabe K, Kurumaya H, Minato H, Nakanuma Y. Overlap of idiopathic portal hypertension and scleroderma: report of two autopsy cases and a review of literature. *J Gastroenterol Hepatol*. 2002;17:217-223.

[56] Kobayashi S, Nakanuma Y, Matsui O. Histopathology of portal tracts in livers after transcatheter arterial chemo-embolization therapy for hepatocellular carcinoma. *J Gastroenterol Hepatol* 1994;9:45-54.

[57] Nakanuma Y, Ohta G, Takeshita H, Yamazaki Y, Doishita K, Shimizu M. Florid duct lesions and extensive bile duct loss of the intrahepatic biliary tree in chronic liver diseases other than primary biliary cirrhosis. *Acta Pathol Jpn* 1983;33:1095-1104.

[58] Arakawa M, Kage M, Fukuta K. *Nodular lesion and portal hypertension*. Report of intrahepatic hemodynamic alterations of Japanese Health and Welfare Minister, 1988;pp.44-47.

[59] Shimamatsu K, Wanless IR. Role of ischemia in causing apoptosis, atrophy, and nodular hyperplasia in human liver. *Hepatology* 1997;26:343-350.

[60] Wanless IR, Wong F, Blendis LM, Greig P, Heathcote EJ, Levy G. Hepatic and portal vein thrombosis in cirrhosis: possible role in development of parenchymal extinction and portal hypertension. *Hepatology*. 1995;21:1238-1247.

[61] Fridman SL, Rockey DC, McGuire RF, Maher JJ, Boyles JK, Yamasaki G. Isolated hepatic lipocytes and Kupffer cells from normal human liver: morphological and functional characteristics in primary culture. *Hepatology* 1992;15:234-243.

[62] Greenwel P, Schwarz M, Peyrol S, Grimaud JA, Rojkind M. Characterization of fat-storing cell lines derived from normal and Ccl4 cirrhosis livers: difference in the production of interleukin 6. *Lab Invest* 1991;65:644-653

[63] Ramadori G. The stellate cell (Ito cell, fat-storing cell, lipocyte, perisinusoid cell) of the liver: new insight into pathophysiology of an intriguing cell. *Virchow Archiv [B]* 1991;61:147-151.

[64] Schmitt-Graff A, Kruger S, Bochard F, Gabbiani G, Denk H. Modulation of alpha smooth muscle actin and desmin expression in perisinusoidal cells of normal and diseased human livers. *Am J Pathol* 1991;138:1233-1242.

[65] Yamaoka K, Nouchi T, Marumo F, Sato C.α-smooth-muscle actin expression in normal and fibrotic human livers. *Digestive Diseases and Science* 1993;38:1473-1479.

[66] Kondo F. Benign nodular hepatocellular lesions caused by abnormal hepatic circulation: etiological analysis and introduction of a new concept. *J Gastroenterol Hepatol*. 2001;16:1319-1328.

[67] Kondo F, Nagao T, Sato T, Tomizawa M, Kondo Y, Matsuzaki O, Wada K, Wakatsuki S, Nagao K, Tsubouchi H, Kobayashi H, Yasumi K, Tsukayama C, Suzuki M. Etiological analysis of focal nodular hyperplasia of the liver, with emphasis on similar abnormal vasculatures to nodular regenerative hyperplasia and idiopathic portal hypertension. *Pathol Res Pract*. 1998;194:487-495.

[68] Nakanuma Y, Wada M, Haratake J, Ohta G. Nodular hyperplasia with a central telangiectatic fibrosis in the liver of non-cirrhotic portal fibrosis (idiopathic portal hypertension). *Acta Pathol Jpn*. 1982;32:1093-1101.

[69] Stromeyer FW, Ishak KG. Nodular transformation (nodular "regenerative" hyperplasia) of the liver. A clinicopathologic study of 30 cases. *Hum Pathol*. 1981;12:60-71.

[70] McEntee MF, Wright KN, Wanless I, DeVovo R, Schneider JF, Shull R. Noncirrhotic portal hypertension and nodular regenerative hyperplasia of the liver in dogs with mucopolysaccharidosis type I. *Hepatology*. 1998;28:385-390.

[71] Sherlock S, Feldman CA, Moran B, Scheuer PJ. Partial nodular transformation of the liver with portal hypertension. *Am J Med.* 1966;40:195-203.

[72] Terayama N, Terada T, Hoso M, Nakanuma Y. Partial nodular transformation of the liver with portal vein thrombosis. A report of two autopsy cases. *J Clin Gastroenterol.* 1995;20:71-76.

[73] Teradaki S, Terada M, Nakanuma Y. Allagille syndrome and hepatic compensatory hyperplasia. In: *Biopsy Diagnosis of hepatic nodules with respect to dignostic procedures*. Ed by Yasuni Nakanuma, O.Matsui. Bukodo Tokyo, Japan, 1st ed., pp.148-149 (in Japanese).

[74] Wanless IR, Peterson P, Das A, Boitnott JK, Moore GW, Bernier V. Hepatic vascular disease and portal hypertension in polycythemia vera and agnogenic myeloid metaplasia: a clinicopathological study of 145 patients examined at autopsy. *Hepatology* 1990;12:1166-1174.

[75] Shepherd P, Harrison DJ. Idiopathic portal hypertension associated with cytotoxic drugs. *J Clin Pathol* 1990;43:206-210.

[76] Huet PM, Guillaume E, Cote J, Legare A, Lavoie P, Viallet A. Noncirrhotic presinusoidal portal hypertension associated with chronic arsenical intoxication. *Gastroenterology* 1975;68:1270-1277.

[77] Thomas LB, Popper H, Berk PD, Selikoff I, Falk H. Vinyl-chloride-induced liver disease. From idiopathic portal hypertension (Banti's syndrome) to Angiosarcomas. *N Engl J Med* 1975;292:17-22.

[78] Yoshimura N, Oka T, Ohmori Y, Yasumura T, Kohnosu H, Kobashi T. Idiopathic portal hypertension in renal transplant recipients: report of two cases. *Surg Today* 1994;24:1111-1114

[79] Onitsuka A, Yano Y, Yamada N, Tanabe H, Hino A, Ozeki Y, Hayashi M, Horiya Y, Goto *A. Case report of idiopathic portal hypertension with Cruveilhier-Baumgarten syndrome and portal thrombosis.* Nippon Shokakibyo Gakkai Zasshi 1984;81:1485-1488.

[80] Sugimura T, Tsuji Y, Ibayashi H, Sakai H, Nawata H. Portal-systemic shunting in a patient with normal portal vain pressures and histological evidence of idiopathic portal hypertension. *J Gastroenterol Hepatol* 1996;11:301-304.

[81] Boyer JL, Hales MR, Klatskin G. "Idiopathic" portal hypertension due to occlusion of intrahepatic portal veins by organized thrombi. A study based on postmortem vinylite-injection corrosion and dissection of the intrahepatic vasculature in 4 cases. *Medicine* (Baltimore). 1974;53:77-91.

[82] Kono K, Ohnishi K, Omata M, Saito M, Nakayama T, Hatano H, Nakajima Y, Sugita S, Okuda K. Experimental portal fibrosis produced by intraportal injection of killed nonpathogenic Escherichia coli in rabbits. *Gastroenterology* 1988;94:787-796.

[83] Sugita S, Ohnishi K, Iida S, Nomura F, Okuda K. Histological changes in the liver and portal hypertension subsequent to repeated intraportal injections of killed E. coli in the dog. *Liver* 1988;8:1-9.

[84] Inagaki H, Nonami T, Kawagoe T, Miwa T, Hosono J, Kurokawa T, Harada A, Nakao A, Takagi H, Suzuki H, Sakamoto J. Idiopathic portal hypertension associated with systemic lupus erythematosus. *J Gastroenterol* 2000;35:235-239.

[85] Mori K, Ishimura E, Goto H, Shoji S, Seki S, Yamashita T, Wakasa K, Nishizawa Y, Morii H. Idiopathic portal hypertension associated with high serum titer of autoantibodies and liver dysfunction. *J Gastroenterol* 1996;31:123-128.

[86] Nakanuma Y, Nonomura A, Hayashi M, Doishita K, Takayanagi N, Uchida T, Obata Y, Noma K, Ikoma J, Yoshikawa K, et al. Pathology of the liver in "idiopathic portal hypertension" associated with autoimmune disease. The Ministry of Health and Welfare Disorders of Portal Circulation Research Committee. *Acta Pathol Jpn* 1989;39:586-592.

[87] Nayyar AK, Sharma BK, Sarin SK, Malhotra P, Broor SL, Sachdev G. Characterization of peripheral blood lymphocytes in patients with non-cirrhotic portal fibrosis: a comparison with cirrhotics and healthy controls. *J Gastroenterol Hepatol* 1990;5:554-559.

[88] Terada T, Nakanuma Y, Obata H. HLA-DR expression on the microvasculature of portal tracts in idiopathic portal hypertension. Immunohistochemical characteristics and relation to portal phlebosclerosis. *Arch Pathol Lab Med* 1991;115:993-997.

[89] Saito K, Nakanuma Y, Takegoshi K, Ohta G, Obata Y, Okuda K, Kameda H. Non-specific immunological abnormalities and association of autoimmune diseases in idiopathic portal hypertension. A study by questionnaire. *Hepatogastroenterology* 1993;40:163-166.

[90] Sekiguchi Y, Amano K, Takano Y, Saito K, Itoh I, Tsuzaka K, Abe T, Takeuchi T. Portal and pulmonary hypertension in a patient with MCTD. *Ryumachi* 1999;39:657-663 (in Japanese).

[91] Yamaguchi N, Tokushige K, Haruta I, Yamauchi K, Hayashi N. Analysis of adhesion molecules in patients with idiopathic portal hypertension. *J Gastroenterol Hepatol 1*999;14:364-369.

[92] Nakanuma Y, Kouda W, Nakano T, Uneno K, Tachibana S, Araki I. A case report of early idiopathic portal hypertension. *Pathol Res Pract.* 2001;197:759-763; discussion 765-767.

[93] Tokushige K, Yamauchi K, Komatsu T, Takasaki K, Hayashi N. Predominant T helper 1 cells in patients with idiopathic portal hypertension. *J Gastroenterol Hepatol.* 2000;15:1312-1317.

[94] Yamaue H, Tanimura H, Iwahashi M, Tsunoda T, Tani M, Tamai M, Inoue M. Impairment of autologous mixed lymphocyte reaction in the spleen and peripheral blood lymphocytes of patients with idiopathic portal hypertension. *Gastroenterol Jpn.* 1990;25:193-198.

[95] Egesel T, Buyukasik Y, Dundar SV, Gurgey A, Kirazli S, Bayraktar Y. The role of natural anticoagulant deficiencies and factor V Leiden in the development of idiopathic portal vein thrombosis. *J Clin Gastroenterol* 2000;30:66-71.

[96] Orozco H, Guraieb E, Takahashi T, Garcia-Tsao G, Hurtado R, Anaya R, Ruiz-Arguelles G, Hernandez-Ortiz J, Casillas MA, Guevara L. Deficiency of protein C in patients with portal vein thrombosis. *Hepatology* 1988;8:1110-1111.

[97] Wanless IR. Vascular disorders. In: MacSween RNM, Anthony PP, Scheuer PJ, Burt AD, Portmann BC (Eds) *Pathology of the liver*, 3rd ed., Churchill Livingstone Inc, Edinburgh, 1994;pp.535-562.

[98] Cohen J, Edelman RR, Chopra S. Portal vein thrombosis: a review. *Am J Med.* 1992;92:173-182.

[99] Wanless IR. Pathology of non-cirrhotic portal hypertension. In Okuda K, Benhamou JP eds. *Portal hypertension; clinical and physiological aspects.* Tokyo:Springer-Verlag, 1991, pp.393-399.

[100] Maesawa C, Sakuma T, Sato T, Masuda T, Muro-oka G, Satodate R. Structural characteristic of splenic sinuses in idiopathic portal hypertension. *Pathol Int.* 1995;45:642-648.

In: Hypertension: New Research
Editor: Elwood F. Benhagen, pp. 105-139
ISBN: 1-59454-204-X

Chapter IV

CONTRIBUTION OF HEPATIC STELLATE CELLS TO THE REGULATION OF INTRAHEPATIC MICROCIRCULATION AND THE PATHOPHYSIOLOGY OF PORTAL HYPERTENSION

***H. Reynaert*[1,*], *N. Uyama*[2] *and A. Geerts*[2]**
[1]Department of Gastroenterology-Hepatology, University Hospital AZ-VUB
[2]Laboratory for Molecular Liver Cell Biology,
Vrije Universiteit Brussel (VUB), Brussels, Belgium
Grant support: Scientific Fund W. Gepts, AZ-VUB

ABSTRACT

For many years it has been accepted that hepatic stellate cells play a key role in the pathogenesis of hepatic fibrosis. Accumulating evidence from *in vitro* and *in vivo* studies suggests that these cells are also implicated in the regulation of intrahepatic blood flow in normal liver, and in the pathogenesis of intrahepatic portal hypertension.

The liver is a well perfused organ with dual blood supply by the hepatic artery and the portal vein. The intrahepatic vasculature is made up by a number of discrete components, but the liver sinusoid is the principal site of blood flow regulation in the normal liver. The anatomical location of hepatic stellate cells, which embrace the liver sinusoids, provides a favorable arrangement for perisinusoidal constriction, and control of sinusoidal vascular tone and blood flow.

Portal hypertension is a major complication of cirrhosis. It is responsible for most of the lethal complications, and is caused by both increased portal blood flow and augmented vascular resistance. In turn, the increased vascular resistance results from

* Correspondence: H. Reynaert, M.D. Department of Gastroenterology-Hepatology University Hospital, Vrije Universiteit Brussel (AZ-VUB) Laarbeeklaan 101 B-1090 Brussels Belgium Tel: + 32 2 477 68 11 Fax: +32 2 477 68 10 E-mail: Hendrik.Reynaert@az.vub.ac.be

anatomical abnormalities and functional vascular alterations which are caused by an imbalance of local concentrations of vasoconstrictors and vasodilators. In chronic liver disease, hepatic stellate cells are activated and transdifferentiate to a myofibroblast-like phenotype. These activated cells have, among many other properties, enhanced contractile properties. Although the contractile apparatus and signaling pathways of contraction and relaxation of hepatic stellate cells are not as well studied as those of skeletal or smooth muscle cells, recent studies have shed light on some aspects of hepatic stellate cell contractility. Activated hepatic stellate cells respond with increased contractility to a number of vasoactive substances, including endothelin-1. In this way they contribute to the increased intrahepatic vascular resistance, characteristic of portal hypertension. On the other hand, several substances which relax activated hepatic stellate cells, and could potentially decrease portal pressure, have been identified. Since hepatic stellate cells contribute to the pathogenesis of both intrahepatic vascular resistance and hepatic fibrogenesis, they are currently regarded as therapeutic targets to prevent and treat different complications of chronic liver disease.

INTRODUCTION

Portal hypertension is responsible for several potentially lethal complications of cirrhosis, including the development of esophago-gastric varices, ascites, hepato-renal syndrome, hepato-pulmonary syndrome and porto-systemic encephalopathy. Over the last decades, our knowledge of the pathophysiology of portal hypertension has greatly increased, which now provides a rational approach to new treatment options.

As in any vascular system, portal venous pressure is proportional to blood flow and vascular resistance. According to Ohm's law, the change in portal pressure along a vessel equals the product of the portal blood flow and the resistance to flow ($\Delta P = Q \times R$).[1] In normal liver, the intrahepatic resistance changes with variations in portal blood flow, thereby keeping portal pressure within normal limits. In cirrhosis however, both intrahepatic vascular resistance and portal blood flow are increased. These two events disturb the equilibrium in the system and trigger portal hypertension. The initial event in the pathophysiology of portal hypertension is augmented vascular resistance to portal blood flow. Increased blood flow in the portal vein, caused by the hyperdynamic circulation in the splanchnic and systemic blood vessels, occurs at a more advanced stage of portal hypertension and contributes to its persistence and aggravation.

Increased intrahepatic vascular resistance is primarily caused by anatomical changes such as fibrotic scar tissue and regenerative nodules compressing portal and central venules. Furthermore, swelling of hepatocytes and capillarization of hepatic sinusoids (loss of endothelial fenestrations and collagen deposition in the space of Disse) add to the increased vascular resistance. Although architectural changes are most important, it has become clear in recent years that also a dynamic component contributes significantly to the increased hepatic vascular tone which can be reduced by 20 to 30% with pharmacological agents.[2, 3] The dynamic part of hepatic resistance is caused by active contraction of septal and/or portal myofibroblasts, activated hepatic stellate cells (HSCs) and portal venules. At present it is assumed that an imbalance between endogenous vasoconstrictors such as endothelin-1, angiotensin II, α-adrenergic stimuli and others, and vasodilators including nitric oxide (NO) and carbon monoxide (CO), is responsible for the augmented intrahepatic vascular tone.

Several ultrastructural and physiological features of HSCs are similar to pericytes in other organs, suggesting that HSCs may function as liver-specific pericytes. In fact, both the anatomical location of HSCs and the capacity to contract or relax in response to various vasoactive mediators suggest that these cells may play a role in modulating intrahepatic vascular resistance and blood flow at the sinusoidal level.[4-6] Several investigators have shown that activated HSCs contract in response to various agents of which endothelin-1 is the strongest, and that some agents, e.g. NO, promote relaxation of HSCs. Moreover, HSCs play a key role in the development of hepatic fibrosis, the main cause of portal hypertension.[7]

HEPATIC STELLATE CELLS

In a normal human liver, HSCs represent 5 to 8 % of all cells and approximately 13% of the volume of sinusoidal cells. Stellate cells are located in the perisinusoidal space of Disse beneath the endothelial barrier. They have long cytoplasmic processes which run parallel to the sinusoidal endothelial wall. Second order branches sprout out from the processes, embrace the sinusoid and penetrate between hepatocytes reaching neighboring sinusoids (Figure 1).[8] Hepatic stellate cells are in close contact with nerve endings, some of which contain neuropeptides such as substance P, neuropeptide Y, somatostatin and calcitonin gene-related peptide.[8, 9] The exact meaning of this remains to be elucidated, but it is speculated that HSCs could be involved in neurotransmission, via neuropeptides.

In normal liver, HSCs are implicated in several important functions. Hepatic stellate cells play a key role in the intrahepatic uptake, storage and release of vitamin A. Approximately 90% of the total body vitamin A is stored in the liver, and about three quarters of this amount is accumulated in HSCs.[10] Synthesis and degradation of extracellular matrix components is another hallmark of HSCs in the normal liver. Quiescent stellate cells express mainly collagen type III, collagen type IV, and laminin, but only minimal amounts of fibrillary collagen type I. Synthesis of connective tissue is in equilibrium with its degradation by metalloproteinases produced by HSCs. A third characteristic of quiescent HSCs is the secretion of several growth factors including hepatocyte growth factor, vascular endothelial growth factor, endothelin-1, insulin-like growth factor II, transforming growth factor-β, nerve growth factor, neurotrophin, etc. Finally, quiescent HSCs are involved in the regulation of intrahepatic blood flow in the normal liver (see below).

After acute or chronic liver injury of any origin, HSCs are activated and undergo a process of transdifferentiation leading to a myofibroblastic phenotype with proliferative, fibrogenic and contractile properties.[7] The activation process is characterized by two sequential events: initiation which occurs early in the process, followed by perpetuation. Initiation refers to early changes in gene expression and phenotype that render the cells responsive to cytokines and other paracrine stimuli from injured neighboring cells including hepatocytes, Kupffer cells and platelets. Perpetuation on the other hand results from the effects of the stimuli on maintaining the activated phenotype. Whereas initiation is largely due to paracrine stimuli, perpetuation is due to both paracrine and autocrine loops. Morphologically, activated cells are characterized by loss of vitamin A droplets and *de novo* expression of α-smooth muscle actin (Figure 2). Functionally, activated HSCs are characterized by increased proliferation, motility, contractility, and synthesis of extracellular matrix components. These functions are under the control of several growth factors, cytokines, products of oxidative stress and composition of extracellular matrix. Proliferation and migration are mainly regulated by platelet derived growth factor, basic fibroblast growth factor, and insulin-like growth factor. Endothelin-1, thrombin, angiotensin-II and vasopressin have a profound contractile effect and may promote proliferation of HSCs.

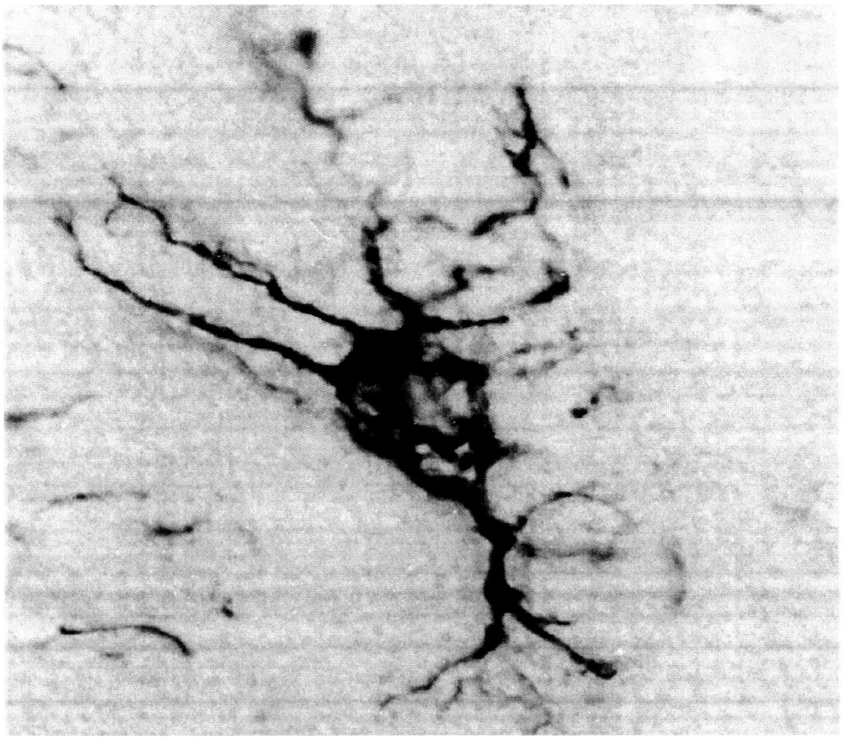

Figure 1: Hepatic stellate cells have long cytoplasmic processes which run parallel to the sinusoidal endothelial wall, embrace the sinusoid and penetrate between hepatocytes. High power light micrograph of a glial fibrillary acidic protein (GFAP) positive cell (original magnification x2740).

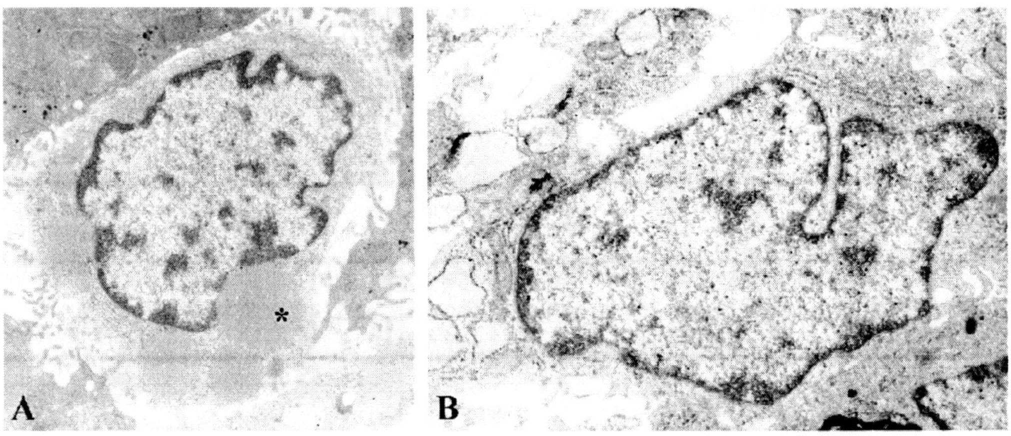

Figure 2: High magnification electron micrograph of HSCs. Quiescent hepatic stellate cells (A) are laden with lipid droplets (*) whereas the activated cells (B) are characterized by loss of vitamin A droplets (x6100).

Transforming growth factor-β is the principal factor involved in extracellular matrix accumulation. Tumor necrosis factor-α and interleukin-1 have pro-inflammatory effects whereas interleukin-10 and interferon-γ have anti-inflammatory effects.[11] Of all these substances, platelet derived growth factor (secreted by sinusoidal endothelial cells, Kupffer cells, platelets, monocytes and HSCs) and transforming growth factor-β (released by hepatocytes, sinusoidal endothelial cells, Kupffer cells, platelets, monocytes) are the most important profibrogenic growth factors for HSCs.[11] In acute or self-limited liver damage, all of these changes are transient, whereas in the case of persistent liver injury they lead to chronic inflammation and accumulation of extracellular matrix. As a consequence, the delicate balance between fibrogenesis and fibrolysis is disturbed resulting in liver fibrosis and ultimately cirrhosis. The dramatic progress in understanding the pathogenesis of liver fibrosis has directed the approach of development of antifibrotic drugs towards targeting HSCs. Numerous drugs aiming at inhibiting the accumulation of activated HSCs at the sites of liver injury and preventing the deposition of extracellular matrix are currently under investigation in *in vitro* and *in vivo* experimental models of liver fibrosis, but their efficacy and safety in humans are as yet unknown.[12] Hepatic fibrosis is probably the most important and certainly the most intensively studied aspect of chronic liver disease in which activated HSCs are implicated, but certainly not the one and only. Several observations suggested that, although tumor cells are most important, activated HSCs may play a crucial role in the progression of hepatocellular carcinoma and liver metastasis. Indeed, in addition to carcinoma cells, a stromal compartment, including extracellular matrix, blood vessels and myofibroblasts, is present in liver tumors. The role of HSCs/myofibroblasts in hepatocellular carcinoma is not completely elucidated, but most observations suggest that they could facilitate tumor progression, probably by secretion of HGF.[13, 14] Finally, activated HSCs are involved in the pathogenesis of portal hypertension. The contribution of HSCs to the increased intrahepatic vascular resistance and the possible mechanisms by which HSCs mediate their effects are discussed below.

Blood Flow Regulation in Normal Liver

The liver is a richly perfused organ receiving approximately 25% of cardiac output. About 75% of hepatic blood flow (rich in nutrients but poorly oxygenated) is contributed by the portal vein. The remainder of blood supply (oxygen rich) is provided by the hepatic artery. The intrahepatic vasculature is composed of portal venules, hepatic arterioles, lymphatics, hepatic sinusoids and central venules. Most blood enters the sinusoids from portal venules through inlet sphincters. Branches of hepatic arterioles terminate in sinusoids near their origin from portal venules (arterio-sinus twigs). Furthermore, intersinusoidal sinusoids connect neighboring sinusoids, and finally, sinusoids receive blood from arterio-portal anastomoses via portal venules. Sinusoids drain their blood in central venules through outlet sphincters.[15, 16] The hepatic sinusoid which is the principal site of blood flow regulation, is the narrowest vascular structure within the liver: the highest vascular resistance occurs in the sinusoids.[17] Moreover, it is the vital site for transvascular exchange between blood and hepatocytes. The sinusoidal surface of the hepatocytes is separated from the blood by fenestrated sinusoidal endothelial cells lining the sinusoid, Kupffer cells (liver macrophages) protruding into the lumen of the sinusoid, Pit cells (liver specific natural killer cells) and HSCs also referred to as Ito cells, lipocytes, fat storing cells or hepatic perisinusoidal cells.[8] From the above it is clear that there are several potential sites for sinusoidal blood flow regulation: (i) portal venules, (ii) hepatic arterioles, (iii) central venules and (iv) sinusoids, with inlet sphincters, outlet sphincters, and sinusoidal cells of which HSCs and sinusoidal endothelial cells have contractile properties.

Several data indicate that HSCs play a role in blood flow regulation in normal liver. The first direct evidence was provided by *in vivo* microscopy in normal rat liver.[18-21] Infusion of endothelin-1 in the portal vein caused a marked decrease in sinusoidal diameter and an increase in sinusoidal pressure gradient and resistance. Endothelin-1 was found to induce significant sinusoidal constriction at the sites of HSCs, but not at the sites of Kupffer cells or sinusoidal endothelial cells. Co-administration of L-NAME and an endothelin receptor B (ET_B) agonist resulted in significant bulging of HSCs into the sinusoidal lumen and reorganization of fat droplets in the cell body in a way consistent with shape changes accompanying cell contraction.[22] Recently, some evidence was obtained that locally produced CO might control sinusoidal blood flow in normal liver. Carbon monoxide is, like NO, a gaseous molecule with multiple vascular functions including vascular cell relaxation. Similar to NO, CO plays a role in microvascular blood flow regulation in the liver.[23] Reduction of endogenously produced CO by zinc protoporphyrin IX, a competitive inhibitor of heme oxygenase (HO), elicited a marked increase in hepatic vascular resistance. Morphometric analysis confirmed that sinusoidal contraction co-localized with HSCs.[24] Moreover, HbO_2, a CO-trapping substance that can pass through the sinusoidal fenestrations into the space of Disse, elicited a sinusoidal constriction whereas liposome-encapsulated Hb, which cannot enter the space of Disse, had no effect on sinusoidal tone.[25] These findings suggest that HSCs may be the target cells of CO, at least in a normal liver.

Even though these observations are suggestive, they do not prove that HSCs modulate hepatic blood flow. Indeed, it has been shown that endothelin-1 induced presinusoidal sphincter constriction resulting in decreased sinusoidal blood flow without stellate cell contraction.[26] This raises the question whether sinusoidal diameter narrowing is not due to passive recoil of sinusoids secondary to decreased sinusoidal blood flow. In fact, experimental clamping of the portal vein has been shown to result in passive recoil of sinusoids and portal venules.[27] Discrepant results are probably related to different doses of endothelin-1 and a different morphological method of assessing vessel diameter after tissue fixation of isolated perfused livers. Endothelin-1 probably has sinusoidal as well as extrasinusoidal sites of action, but the sinusoidal sites appeared to be sensitive to lower, more physiological concentrations of endothelin-1.[20]

In vitro experiments are also controversial. It has been demonstrated that HSCs, cultured for 24 hours, relaxed in response to interleukin-1[28] and contracted in response to substance P and endothelin-1.[29, 30] A higher concentration of endothelin-1 was required to obtain a significant increase in intracellular Ca^{2+} ($[Ca^{2+}]_i$) and contraction of quiescent HSCs than of activated HSCs.[30] However, these observations could not be confirmed by other investigators.[31, 32] Possible explanations for discrepant findings include damaging of receptors by isolation of cells and differences in the set-up of contraction experiments. Indeed, although quiescent HSCs may not possess the necessary machinery required for forceful contraction, weaker contractions might occur. To show collagen lattice contraction, a more forceful contraction of cells is required than the force needed to demonstrate contraction of isolated cells by phase contrast microscopy. Arguments against contraction of HSCs in normal liver include: (i) HSCs in normal liver do not have a stellate shape, but rather a spider-like shape which is less likely to be contraction-ready, (ii) effective contraction is limited by spatial constraint in the space of Disse and contraction would be possible only by cells with a powerful contractile machinery, (iii) the presence of lipid droplets prevents microfilament assembly into a long span.[33] Taken together, although some arguments are against, most evidence suggests that HSCs are involved in the regulation of sinusoidal tone and blood flow in normal liver.

Cytoskeleton and Contractile Apparatus of Hepatic Stellate Cells

The cytoskeleton of a cell consists of four different types of cytoskeletal filaments: microfilaments or actin filaments, contractile filaments containing myosin, intermediate filaments, and microtubules. Cytoskeletal filaments are organized in networks in which the filaments are loosely packed and are not aligned, or in bundles in which the filaments are packed in parallel arrays. The two major functions of the cytoskeleton are (i) structural support for the cytoplasma and nuclear membrane, and (ii) action as a dynamic component of cell movement and cell contraction.

Microtubules are not involved in cell contraction and/or movement, and will therefore not be discussed in this review. Likewise, intermediate filaments are mainly involved in cell structure and play but an indirect role in cell contraction. However, since the activation of HSCs is characterized by manifest changes in intermediate filament expression, we will briefly discuss the different intermediate filaments in quiescent and activated HSCs. Intermediate filaments are classified into 6 groups.[34, 35] Class I and II represent acidic and basic keratins. Desmin, vimentin and glial fibrillary acidic protein (GFAP) constitute class III proteins whereas neurofilaments and lamins represent class IV and V respectively. Class VI protein nestin is another member of the intermediate filaments. Although intermediate filament proteins form morphologically indistinguishable filaments, they are differentially expressed in a cell type specific way. Thus, keratins are expressed by epithelial cells, desmin by muscle cells, GFAP by astroglial cells, neurofilaments by neurons, and vimentin by glial and mesenchymal cells. Based on the characteristic expression pattern of different intermediate filament proteins, it is likely that each of them has distinct properties serving the specific needs of different cell types. It has been suggested that different intermediate filaments have different affinities for intracellular structures or different mechanical properties that make intermediate filaments of a particular composition well suited for one cell type, but poorly suited for another. Expression of type III intermediate filaments in HSCs varies according to the species and the state of activation.[10] For instance, desmin is abundant in rodent HSCs, whereas it is absent in quiescent human stellate cells and positive in a minority of activated human HSCs. Of particular interest is the fact that rodent HSCs express desmin, vimentin, and GFAP, and thus intermediate filaments of mesenchymal, muscle and neural cells, which raises the question of the embryonic origin of HSCs.

Actin filaments are most important structures responsible for cell contraction and movement. In humans, six actin genes encoding for 6 actin isoforms have been identified: 3 α-actins (which are mainly present in muscle cells), a β-actin and two γ-actins (present in non-muscle cells). G-actin monomers aggregate into oligomers of 3 to 5 monomers, which in turn elongate into long F-actin filaments.[36] The formation of long actin filaments is a dynamic process of assembly, elongation, dissociation, branching and stabilization which is regulated by multiple proteins, including actin related protein 2/3, profilin, cofilin, and gelsolin. By changing actin polymerization, actin generates forces on the cell membrane which results in cell shape changes and cell movement. Interaction of myosin and actin results in cell contraction. Myosins, actin-based molecular motors, are ubiquitously expressed as multiple isoforms in all eukaryotic cells. In general, myosin is composed of heavy chains and several light chain subunits. Myosin heavy chain is typically constructed of three functional subdomains: the motor domain which interacts with actin and binds ATP, the neck domain which binds myosin or calmodulin light chains, and the tail domain which serves to anchor and position the motor domain.

Recently, based on the comparisons of primary structure of motor domains of myosin heavy chain genes, the human myosin family was divided into 12 classes [37] (table 1). To date, myosin I, II and V have been well characterized, while the functions and biochemical properties of other myosins remain largely unknown. Myosin I, which is a single headed, nonfilamentous member of the myosin family, can bind calmodulin light chain in the neck region. Its tail domain has membrane-binding properties. Eight different isoforms of myosin I have been reported in mammalian cells.[37] Although the molecular details of myosin I function in the cell are not known, it is thought to be a key player for cortical membrane tension, endocytosis and endocytic trafficking, signal transduction, and membrane ruffling.[38-41]

Myosin V, a dimeric, nonfilamentous member of the myosin family, can bind calmodulin light chain in the neck region. Similar to myosin I, myosin V has membrane-binding properties in its tail domain. Three types of myosin V isoforms have been described in mammalian cells: myosin Va, Vb and Vc. Myosin V is thought to play a role in transport a variety of intracellular cargo along actin.[42, 43] Myosin II is the most characterized member of the myosin family. Myosin II is two-headed and can form filaments. It is composed of two heavy chains, two non-phosphorylatable alkali (essential) light chains, and two phosphorylatable regulatory light chains. Myosin II heavy chain can bind myosin light chains, but not calmodulin light chain, in the neck region. Myosin II has, at least, 13 kinds of heavy chain genes including 6 skeletal, 3 cardiac, 1 smooth muscle and 3 non-muscle myosin heavy chain genes (Table 1). Myosin II light chain also has 5 alkali light chain genes and 5 regulatory light chain genes (table 2). As for the function, myosin II can interact with actin and is responsible for the development, migration and contraction of cells. Both the alkali and regulatory light chains are thought to regulate myosin activity. The exact mechanism by which the interaction between myosin and actin causes contraction is beyond the scope of this review. In short, the myosin head of a heavy chain binds an actin subunit and "walks" to the next actin subunit using the energy liberated by hydrolysis of one ATP molecule. Somewhat similar contractile mechanisms are found in non-muscle cells.

Table 1. List of human myosin heavy chain genes

Symbol	Chromosome	RNA Ref seq Number	Name	Comments
CLASS I				
MYO1A	12q13-q15	NM_005379	myosin IA	brush border myosin-I
MYO1B	2q12-q34	XM_290989	myosin IB	
MYO1C	17p13	NM_033375	myosin IC	
MYO1D	17q11-q12	XM_050041	myosin ID	
MYO1E	15q21-q22	NM_004998	myosin IE	
MYO1F	19p13.3-p13.2	NM_012335	myosin IF	
MYO1G	7p13-p11.2	XM_291223	myosin IG	
CLASS II				
MYH1	17p13.1	NM_005963	myosin, heavy polypeptide 1, skeletal muscle, adult,	myosin heavy chain IIx/d
MYH2	17p13.1	NM_017534	myosin, heavy polypeptide 2, skeletal muscle, adult	myosin heavy chain IIa
MYH3	17p13.1	NM_002470	myosin, heavy polypeptide 3, skeletal muscle, embryonic	myosin heavy chain II embryonic
MYH4	17p13.1	NM_017533	myosin, heavy polypeptide 4, skeletal muscle	myosin heavy chain IIb
MYH6	14q12	NM_002471	myosin, heavy polypeptide 6, cardiac muscle, alpha	
MYH7	14q12	NM_000257	myosin, heavy polypeptide 7, cardiac muscle, beta	Associated with familial hypertrophic cardiomyopathy
MYH7B	20q11.23	XM_371398	myosin, heavy polypeptide 7B, cardiac muscle, beta	
MYH8	17p13.1	NM_002472	myosin, heavy polypeptide 8, skeletal muscle, perinatal	myosin heavy chain perinatal
MYH9	22q13.1	NM_002473	myosin, heavy polypeptide 9, non-muscle	nonmuscle myosin heavy chain IIA
MYH10	17p13	NM_005964	myosin, heavy polypeptide 10, non-muscle	nonmuscle myosin heavy chain IIB
MYH11	16p13.13-p13.12	NM_002474	myosin, heavy polypeptide 11, smooth muscle isoform SM1	
		NM_022844	myosin, heavy polypeptide 11, smooth muscle isoform SM2	
MYH13	17p13	NM_003802	myosin, heavy polypeptide 13, skeletal muscle	extraocular muscle myosin heavy chain
MYH14	19q13.33	NM_024729	myosin, heavy polypeptide 14	nonmuscle myosin heavy chain IIC

Table 1. Continued

Symbol	Chromosome	RNA Ref seq Number	Name	Comments
CLASS III				
MYO3A	10p11.1	NM_017433	myosin IIIA	Associated with hearing loss in humans. Expression of this gene is highly restricted, with the strongest expression in retina and cochlea.
MYO3B	2	NM_138995	myosin IIIB	
CLASS V				
MYO5A	15q21	NM_000259	myosin VA (heavy polypeptide 12, myoxin)	Expressed in melanoma cells and neurons. Associated with melanosome transport, Griscelli syndrome
MYO5B	18q21	XM_371116	myosin VB	Associated with plasma membrane recycling
MYO5C	15q21	NM_018728	myosin VC	
CLASS VI				
MYO6	6q13	NM_004999	myosin VI	Associated with intracellular vesicle and organelle transport, inherited deafness
CLASS VII				
MYO7A	11q13.5	NM_000260	myosin VIIA	Associated with Usher syndrome 1B (characterized by profound congenital deafness, vestibular areflexia, and progressive retinitis pigmentosa.)
MYO7B	2q21.1	XM_291001	myosin VIIB	
CLASS IX				
MYO9A	15q22-q23	NM_006901	myosin IXA	
MYO9B	19p13.1	NM_004145	myosin IXB	

Table 1. Continued

Symbol	Chromosome	RNA Ref seq Number	Name	Comments
CLASS X				
MYO 10	5p15.1-p14.3	NM_012334	myosin X	
CLASS XV				
MYO 15	17p11.2	NM_016239	myosin XV	Associated with profound, congenital, neurosensory, nonsyndromal deafness
CLASS XVI				
MYR8	13q33.3	XM_028522	myosin heavy chain Myr 8	
CLASS XVIII				
MYO18A	17q11.2	NM_078471	myosin XVIIIA isoform a	
		NM_203318	myosin XVIIIA isoform b	
MYO18B	22q11.2-q12.1	NM_032608	myosin XVIIIB	
not numbered				
X	17q	x	Gen Bank Accession No (AC023133)	DNA sequence

Information on the expression of myosins by HSCs is scarce and the relationship between mutations of these myosin genes and functions of HSCs remains unknown. HSCs have been shown to express alpha smooth muscle myosin heavy chain (MYH 11) and three sarcomeric myosin heavy chains including perinatal skeletal myosin heavy chain (MYH 8), adult skeletal fast IIa (MYH 2) and IId (MYH 1) myosin heavy chains.[44] In addition, expression of skeletal myosin heavy chain by HSCs was up-regulated when contraction was induced by ET-1.[45] Traditionally, sarcomeric myosins have been thought to be restricted to striated muscle cells. Thus, HSCs might be equipped with skeletal myosins which participate in HSCs contraction. Although the mechanisms by which myosin II proteins are involved in the contraction of HSCs have not been clarified, it has been assumed that, in analogy to other myofibroblast-like cells, myosin II is a key player for contraction of activated HSCs. Activation of myosin II is regulated by Ca^{2+}-dependent and independent mechanisms (Figure 3). Intracellular Ca^{2+}, whether released from endoplasmatic reticulum by inositol 1,4,5-trisphosphate (IP_3) or by Ca^{2+} influx, binds to calmodulin. The Ca^{2+}-calmodulin complex then binds the enzyme myosin light chain kinase which becomes activated and phosphorylates myosin regulatory light chain. In turn, phosphorylated myosin light chain activates contraction. It has been assumed that Ca^{2+} signaling pathways play an important role in mediating the contractile force generated by HSCs in a similar manner to that shown in smooth muscle.[46] A second mechanism of contraction is Ca^{2+}-independent: Rho-kinase, a small GTPase, regulates myosin light chain phosphorylation by inhibiting myosin phosphatase and also by direct phosphorylation of myosin light chain.[47-49] When myosin phosphatase is inactive, myosin light chain phosphorylation, and thus myosin activity and contractility increases. Both Ca^{2+}-dependent and Ca^{2+}-independent mechanisms are important in HSC contractility and migration.[50, 51]

Table 2. List of human myosin light chain genes

Symbol	Chromosome	RNA Ref seq Number	Name	Comments
MLC1SA	12q13.13	NM_002475	myosin alkali light chain 1 slow a	Expressed in both slow-twitch skeletal muscle and in nonmuscle tissue.
MRCL3	18p11.31	NM_006471	myosin regulatory light chain	regulatory, non-sarcomeric
MYL1	2q33-q34	NM_079420	fast skeletal myosin alkali light chain 1 isoform 1f	
		NM_079422	fast skeletal myosin alkali light chain 1 isoform 3f	
MYL2	12q23-q24.3	NM_000432	myosin, light polypeptide 2, regulatory, cardiac, slow	Associated with mid-left ventricular chamber type hypertrophic cardiomyopathy.
MYL3	3p21.3-p21.2	NM_000258	myosin, light polypeptide 3, alkali; ventricular, skeletal, slow	
MYL4	17q21-qter	NM_002476	myosin, light polypeptide 4, alkali; atrial, embryonic	Expressed in embryonic muscle and adult atria
MYL5	4p16.3	NM_002477	myosin, light polypeptide 5, regulatory	Expressed in fetal muscle and in adult retina, cerebellum, and basal ganglia.
MYL6	12q13.13	NM_021019	myosin, light polypeptide 6, alkali, smooth muscle and non-muscle isoform 1	Expressed in smooth muscle and non-muscle tissues.
		NM_079423	smooth muscle and non-muscle myosin alkali light chain isoform 2	
		NM_079425	smooth muscle and non-muscle myosin alkali light chain isoform 3	
		NM_079424	smooth muscle and non-muscle myosin alkali light chain isoform 4	
MYL7	7p21-p11.2	NM_021223	myosin, light polypeptide 7, regulatory	myosin light chain 2a
MYL9	20q11.23	NM_006097	myosin regulatory light polypeptide 9 isoform a	
		NM_181526	myosin regulatory light polypeptide 9 isoform b	

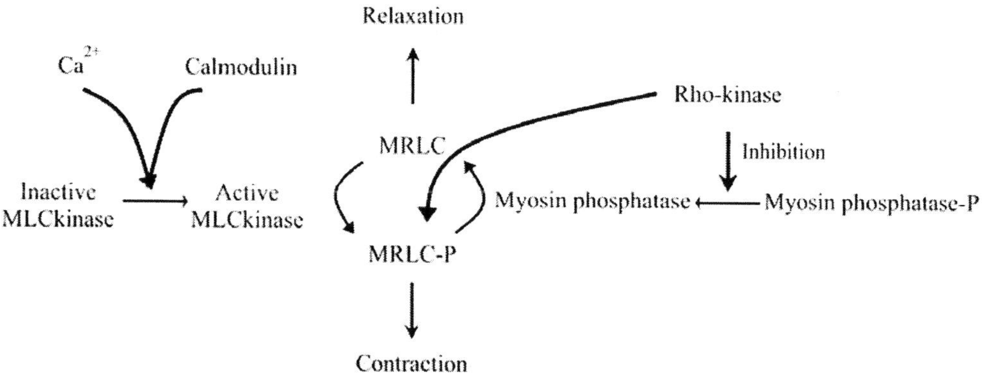

Figure 3: Contraction is regulated via two mechanisms: a Ca^{2+}-dependent and a Ca^{2+}-independent mechanism. Activation of myosin light chain kinase (MLC kinase) by the calmodulin-Ca^{2+}-complex results in phosphorylation of myosin regulatory light chain (MRLC) and contraction. Rho-kinase directly phosphorylates MRLC and inhibits dephosphorylation of MRLC by inhibiting the activation of myosin phosphatase.

Myosin II and actin form contractile bundles, also called stress fibers, which terminate at focal adhesions. The focal adhesions are attached to the extracellular matrix via cell surface receptors, termed integrins. Integrins are heterodimeric transmembrane proteins that consist of an α and a β subunit. Different integrins have been demonstrated in activated HSCs, especially $\alpha_1\beta_1$ and $\alpha_2\beta_1$.[52] Signal transduction of integrins is, among others, mediated via focal adhesion kinase, which is also part of the focal adhesion complex.[53, 54] Extracellular signals are transmitted via integrins and other membrane receptors for growth factors and cytokines through different Rho-GTPases Cdc42, Rac and Rho.[55, 56] This will result in the formation of filopodia (via Cdc42), lamellipodia (via Rac), focal adhesions and stress fibers (via Rho) and increased actin turnover.[55] Thus, intregrins are the principal functional and structural connection between the cell and the extracellular matrix leading to well coordinated cell movements.[55] Cell motility is extremely important in wound healing and tumor progression, two phenomena in which HSCs play a crucial role.

Intracellular Signaling of HSC Contractility (Figure 4)

Recent years have seen considerable progress towards understanding the signaling mechanisms regulating contraction and relaxation in non-muscle cells. Whereas contraction of smooth muscle cells is governed primarily by Ca^{2+} signaling, and Rho signaling plays a secondary role, contractility of non-muscle cells is principally mediated by Rho signaling. It is not known as yet which of both mechanisms plays a greater role in HSC contractility. However, it has been speculated that, as HSCs are activated and exhibit smooth muscle like features, Ca^{2+} signaling becomes more important.[50]

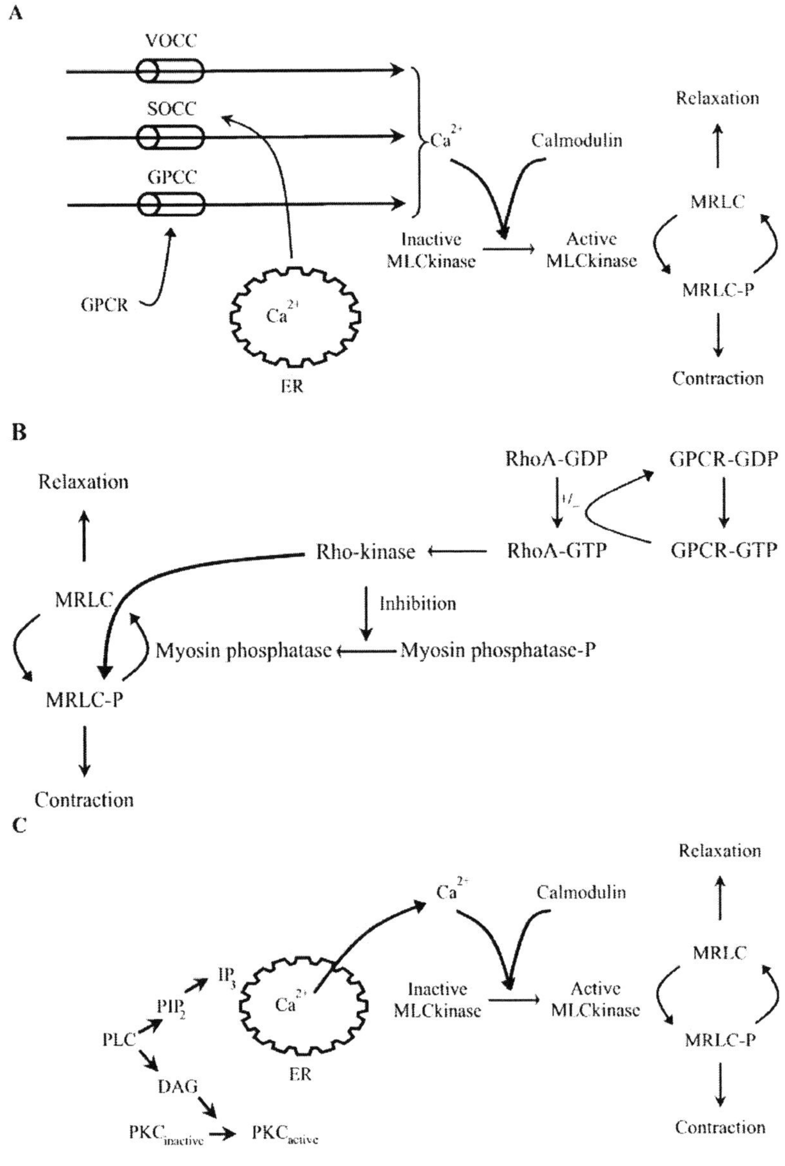

Figure 4: Contraction pathways in activated hepatic stellate cells
A. Calcium channels. Activation of calcium channels via depolaristation (Voltage Operated Calcium Channels or VOCC), via depletion of calcium in intracellular calcium stores (Store Operated Calcium Channels or SOCC), or via G-protein coupled receptors (GPCR) will result in increased intracellular calcium. Calcium then binds calmodulin and the Ca^{2+}-calmodulin complex binds the enzyme myosin light chain kinase (MLCK) which becomes activated and phosphorylates myosin regulatory light chain (MRLC). In turn, phosphorylated myosin light chain (MRLC-P) activates contraction.**B**. Rho-kinase pathway. Rho-kinase is activated by GPCR and inhibits myosin phosphatase and thus phosphorylation and activation of MRLC which results in less relaxation of the cell. Furthermore, Rho-kinase phosphorylates MRLC, resulting in contraction. **C**. Phospholipase C (PLC). Activation of PLC results in the hydrolysis of phosphatidylinositol 4,5-bisphosphate (PIP2) and the production of inositol 1,4,5-trisphosphate (IP3) and diacylglycerol (DAG). IP3 elevates intracellular Ca^{2+} by releasing Ca^{2+} from intracellular stores and DAG activates protein kinase C (PKC). Both mechanisms will result in increased contractility.

Calcium Channels

At least two different types of Ca^{2+} channels have been described in activated HSCs: Voltage operated calcium channels and store operated channels (Figure 4A).

It has been demonstrated that the activation of HSCs is associated with both an up-regulation of L-type voltage-operated Ca^{2+} channels that mediate Ca^{2+} influx and KCl-induced contraction.[57] However, as HSCs have not been shown to be excitable, it will be important to establish the physiological relevance of these channels. Some of the changes in $[Ca^{2+}]_i$ are mediated via store operated calcium channels. [58] Depletion of Ca^{2+} in the $[Ca^{2+}]i$ -stores will lead to activation of these calcium channels, with increased levels of $[Ca^{2+}]_i$. Furthermore, some G-protein coupled receptors, such as endothelin can directly activate receptor gated Ca^{2+}-channels, but this mechanism has not been proven to be present in HSCs. Whatever the mechanism of increased $[Ca^{2+}]_i$, it will result in cell contraction. Indeed, it has been demonstrated that reductions in HSC area, a marker of contractile force generation, correlate with the height of the increased $[Ca^{2+}]_i$ peak.[5, 59]

Rho (Figure 4B)

Rho is a member of the Ras superfamily and recent data demonstrate that activation of Rho-dependent responses is primarily mediated through G-proteins of the Gα12/13 family.[60] A number of Rho effectors has been identified and the two serine/threonine kinases (Rho kinase/ROKα/ROCK-II and p160ROCK/ROCKß), commonly referred to as Rho kinase, are the best characterized.[60] Rho regulates cell morphology through organizing the actin cytoskeleton and control of actomyosin-dependent cellular processes.[61] Rho kinase has been shown to participate in the induction of stress fibers and focal adhesion formation and cell contraction.[49, 62] Furthermore, Rho kinase also phophorylates intermediate filaments, such as glial fibrillary acidic protein and vimentin.[49] In HSCs, Rho and Rho kinase have been shown to enhance myosin activation suggesting a role in the generation of contractile force.[63] This has been supported by the demonstration that Rho signaling pathways regulate agonist (e.g. endothelin-1, lysophosphatidic acid) induced shrinkage of collagen gels.[63, 64] Moreover, HSCs activation was accompanied by Rho-induced formation of actin stress fibers and focal adhesions.[65]

Phospholipase C

Activation of phospholipase C results in the hydrolysis of phosphatidylinositol 4,5-bisphosphate and the production of IP3 and diacylglycerol (Figure 4C). IP3 elevates $[Ca^{2+}]_i$ by releasing Ca^{2+} from intracellular stores and diacylglycerol activates protein kinase C. Thus the hydrolysis of phosphatidylinositol 4,5-bisphosphate generates two important second messengers: Ca^{2+} and protein kinase C.[66] The effects of increased Ca^{2+} have been discussed above. Activation of protein kinase C in smooth muscle by phorbol ester results in a slowly developing and sustained contractile response.[67] The time of initiation is shortened, rate of rise in tension is increased and magnitude of response enhanced by agents (e.g. ionomycin) that increase Ca^{2+} influx. Moreover, in chemically skinned vascular smooth muscle, phorbol ester induces a slowly developing contractile response at constant Ca^{2+} without any change in myosin light chain phosphorylation.[68] The production of a sustained response by protein kinase C appears to involve phosphorylation of intermediate filaments (e.g. desmin, synemin), caldesmon and a small number of unidentified low molecular weight proteins.[69] The role of protein kinase C in HSCs contraction has received very little attention although its involvement is supported by the demonstration that inhibition of protein kinase C prevents the response to endothelin-1.[70]

Phospholipase A2 and D

These phospholipases have not been well studied in HSCs and their mechanisms are less well known. The main effect of PLA_2 is the release of arachidonic acid from the plasma membrane which is an important step in the synthesis of prostaglandins. The latter have important cellular functions including cell contraction and relaxation. Stimulation of protein kinase C results in the activation of phospholipase D and production of the second messenger, phosphatidic acid.[71] Addition of exogenous phospholipase D or phosphatidic acid to quiescent fibroblasts elicits the formation of actin stress fibers and phospholipase D mediates phosphatidic acid-induced stress fiber formation in these cells.[72, 73] Moreover, phospholipase D co-localizes with F-actin and three proteins, vinculin, talin and α-actinin found on the cytoplasmic face of focal adhesions suggesting a role in the assembly/regulation of these structures.[74] Overexpression of phospholipase D results in cytoskeletal reorganisation consistent with a regulatory role in contraction.[75] Interestingly, phosphatidic acid is regulated by both of the major pathways implicated in the control of contraction: a Ca^{2+}-dependent kinase i.e. protein kinase C, and Rho.

Intracellular Signaling of HSC Relaxation (Figure 5)

In comparison to contraction, little is known of the signaling pathways which regulate HSC relaxation. In view of the proposed role of HSC contraction in portal hypertension, a detailed investigation into the mechanisms underlying HSC relaxation may ultimately have major clinical implications.

Cyclic Adenosine Monophosphate (cAMP)

An increase in cAMP appears to reduce HSC contraction. A cAMP-dependent protein kinase has been reported to inactivate myosin light chain kinase by phosphorylating two sites of the protein [76]and, moreover, the cell permeable cAMP analog, dibutyryl cAMP, induces the disappearance of actin stress fibres in contracted HSCs.[70] At high concentration, cAMP can activate a cGMP-dependent kinase (G kinase). Moreover, cAMP reduces Ca^{2+} influx, possibly by a direct effect on L-type Ca^{2+} channels (Figure 5A).[77]

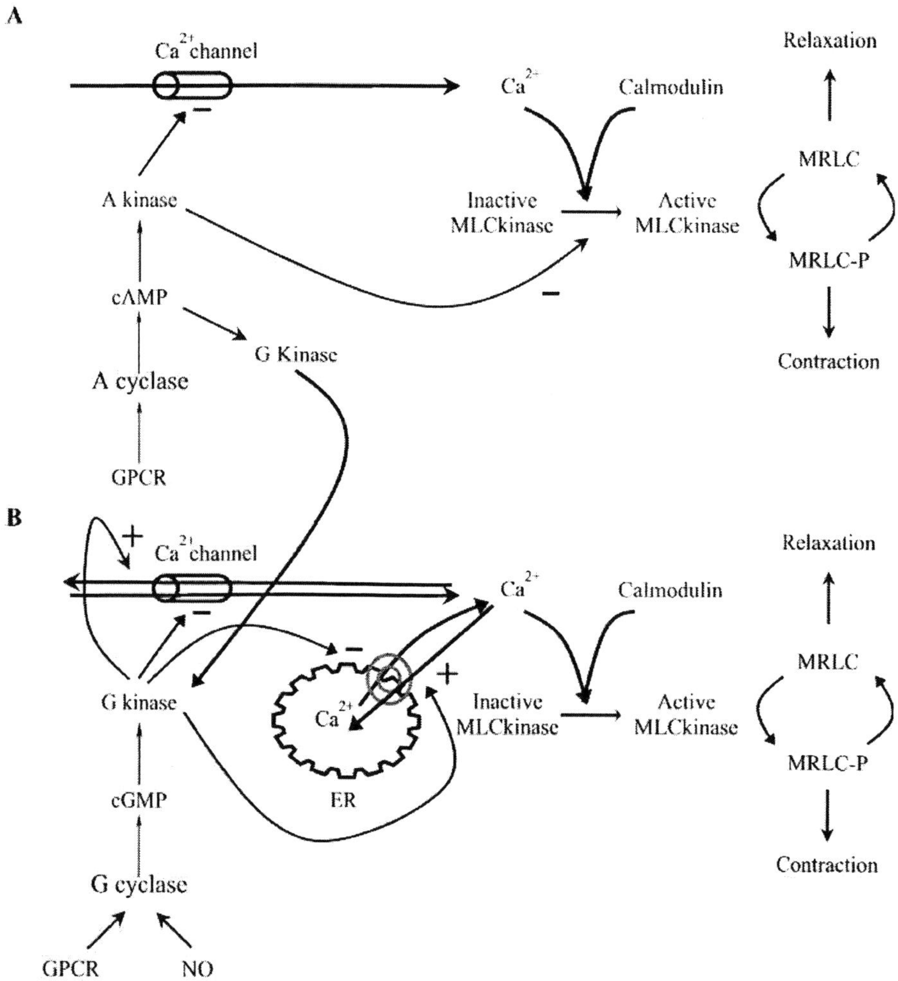

Figure 5: HSCs: mechanisms of relaxation
A. Cyclic adenosine monophosphate (cAMP). Activation of adenyl cyclase results in production of cAMP which activates cAMP dependent A kinase. In turn, A kinase inactivates MLC kinase. At high concentration, cAMP can also activate a cyclic guanosine monophosphate (cGMP)-dependent kinase (G kinase). Cyclic AMP also reduces Ca^{2+} influx, possibly by a direct effect on L-type Ca^{2+} channels.
B. Cyclic guanosine monophosphate. Both GPCR and Nitric oxide (NO) can activate guanylate cyclase (G cyclase), resulting in production of cGMP. An increase in cGMP and activation of G kinase decreases intracellular Ca^2+. Calcium influx is decreased by inhibition of L-type Ca^{2+} channels. Calcium release from intracellular stores is reduced via attenuation of IP3-induced Ca^{2+} release. Calcium efflux is increased by activation of Ca^{2+} ATPase.

Cyclic Guanosine Monophosphate (CGMP)

The elevation of NO, causing activation of guanylate cyclase, an increase in cGMP and activation of G kinase appear to promote HSC relaxation.[28, 70] In smooth muscle cells, G kinase has been shown to decrease $[Ca^{2+}]_i$ by several mechanisms (Figure 5B): (i) decreasing Ca^{2+} influx by inhibiting L-type Ca^{2+} channels, (ii) attenuation of IP3-induced Ca^{2+} release from intracellular stores, and (iii) increasing Ca^{2+} efflux by activation of Ca^{2+} ATPase.[77].Moreover, sodium nitroprusside also induces disappearance of actin stress fibers in contracted HSCs and NO has been reported to disrupt focal adhesion complexes.[78]

It is clear that relaxation of HSCs is also caused by inhibition of contractile mechanisms, for instance inhibition of the activation of Rho. The state of contraction/relaxation will be the result of the sum of contractile and relaxing mechanisms and their inhibition.

Vasoactive Modulators in Portal Hypertension with an Effect on HSCs

The effects of a number of vasoactive substances have been extensively studied in activated HSCs. One of the most potent and certainly most studied vasoactive modulators of HSCs are endothelins. Endothelins comprise a family of 3 homologous oligopeptides of 21 amino acid polypeptides: endothelin-1, endothelin-2 and endothelin-3, which are cleavage products of larger precursor proteins.[79, 80] Preproendothelin is cleaved in big endothelins which have only marginal biologic activity. Endothelin converting enzymes 1 and 2 (ECE-1 and ECE-2) then specifically cleave the big endothelins into the active peptides. Endothelins act through at least 2 G-protein coupled receptors, termed endothelin receptor subtype A (ET_A) and B (ET_B). Moreover, the ET_B receptor has two isoforms: ET_{B1} and ET_{B2}.[81, 82] The affinity of endothelin-1 for the ET_A receptor is higher than that of endothelin-2 and is 100-fold higher than that of endothelin-3, whereas the ET_B receptor has equal affinity for endothelin-1, endothelin-2 and endothelin-3.[82] Endothelin A receptors are mainly localized on smooth muscle cells and predominantly mediate vasoconstriction via activation of phospholipase C, while ET_B receptors are expressed by a variety of cells and have various biological effects. The ET_{B1} receptor induces endothelial cell nitric oxide synthetase (eNOS) resulting in NO release and cell relaxation, whereas ET_{B2} receptors cause vasoconstriction.[21, 81, 83] Both ET_A and ET_B receptors were expressed by HSCs and hepatocytes, while only ET_B receptors were present on sinusoidal endothelial cells and Kupffer cells.[84-87]

There are several arguments that endothelin and endothelin receptors play an important role in portal hypertension. Compared to normal livers, the number of both ET_A and ET_B is increased in cirrhotic livers.[88] In cirrhotic patients, a direct relationship between ET_A and ET_B mRNA abundance and the degree of portal hypertension has been documented.[89] Endothelin-1 levels in human liver correlated with the degree of liver injury[90] and splanchnic endothelin-1 concentration was proportional to the degree of portal hypertension.[91] In addition, several investigators documented increased plasma levels of endothelin-1 in cirrhotic patients, and the levels of endothelin-1 correlated with severity of cirrhosis, the presence of ascites, and the presence of hepatorenal syndrome.[91-102] Very high levels of endothelin-1 have been measured in the splanchnic vessels, but the highest levels of endothelin-1 have been found in hepatic veins.[91, 97, 102] Furthermore, endothelin-1 elicited a sustained vasoconstriction of the hepatic vasculature.[103] On the other hand, short term blockade of endothelin receptors by mixed endothelin$_A$/endothelin$_B$ receptor antagonists decreased portal hypertension in some models of experimental cirrhosis.[32, 104-106] However, these results could not be confirmed following chronic blockade of endothelin receptors.[107] Indeed, in cirrhotic rats treated with a mixed ET_A/ET_B receptor antagonist for 10 weeks, no differences in portal pressure were found.

In patients with portal hypertension, at least part of endothelin-1 is produced in the gut and spleen.[102] In addition, it has been shown that increased endothelin-1 synthesis occurred within the injured liver. Indeed, both sinusoidal endothelial cells and hepatocytes synthesized more endothelin-1, and hepatocytes had a reduced metabolism of endothelin-1.[87, 108] Furthermore, activated HSCs have been shown to be a major site of endothelin-1 synthesis via differential regulation of endothelin converting enzyme-1 mRNA and protein.[109-111] Moreover, during activation of HSCs, sensitivity to endothelin-1 was increased.[30, 31] Enhanced endothelin-1 synthesis and release, and increased sensitivity to endothelin-1 suggests the possibility of a paracrine or autocrine action of endothelin-1.[110] In the early phase of activation of HSCs, ET_A receptors were predominant, but with increasing activation, ET_B receptors became increasingly more abundant.[109] This shift of receptor densities might be important in view of different effects of endothelin-1 during the process of activation of HSCs. Stimulation of ET_A receptors caused contraction and proliferation of HSCs, whereas ET_B receptor stimulation resulted in antiproliferative effects and relaxation.[109, 112, 113] In cultured HSCs, endothelin-1 induced a dose-dependent increase in $[Ca^{2+}]_i$ both by release of Ca^{2+} from intracellular stores and by stimulating Ca^{2+} influx coupled with contraction of the cells.[5]

Table 3: Substances with contractile effect on hepatic stellate cells

Agent	Mechanism
Endothelin-1	$[Ca^{2+}]_i$
Thrombin	$[Ca^{2+}]_i$
Angiotensin II	$[Ca^{2+}]_i$
Vasopresssin	$[Ca^{2+}]_i$
Adenosine	$[Ca^{2+}]_i$?
Substance P	$[Ca^{2+}]_i$
Leukotriene D_4	$[Ca^{2+}]_i$
PGF_2 / thromboxane	$[Ca^{2+}]_i$
Lysophosphtidic acid	Rho-kinase

Nitric oxide is an omnipresent messenger molecule involved in various cellular processes, including neurotransmission, inflammation, and regulation of vascular tone. It is a potent vasodilator, acting in a paracrine fashion by directly stimulating soluble guanylate cyclase, resulting in increased levels of cGMP and consequently decreased $[Ca^{2+}]_i$ and vasorelaxation. Although NO has a short half-life, it has prolonged effects by metabolites such as peroxynitrate. Nitric oxide is produced from L-arginine by three isoforms of nitric oxide synthetase (NOS). A wide variety of cells, including vascular smooth muscle cells, hepatocytes and HSCs, express the inducible form of NOS (iNOS), whereas endothelial cells (eNOS) and neuronal cells (nNOS) express constitutive NOS forms.[114, 115] Several growth factors (e.g. transforming growth factor-β and vascular endothelial growth factor), hypoxia and shear stress increase eNOS mRNA, while tumor necrosis factor-α decreases its expression. The constitutive isoforms respond to changes in $[Ca^{2+}]_i$ and produce small amounts of NO. The iNOS isoform is modulated by a variety of stimuli including cytokines and lipopolysaccharide. Inducible NOS binds calmodulin at almost all $[Ca^{2+}]_i$ concentrations and NO production is high.[114, 116] In cirrhosis, systemic and splanchnic vascular NO production is increased, resulting in the development of a hyperdynamic syndrome. It appears that eNOS is responsible for the enhanced NO synthesis, but the cause is not entirely clear.[115] It has been demonstrated that NO modulates hepatic vascular tone in normal liver, and that sinusoidal endothelial cells express both *in vitro* and *in vivo* eNOS and produce NO.[117, 118] Not only are sinusoidal endothelial cells responsible for basal NO production, but also for an increased release of NO in response to flow and shear stress.[118] Exogenous NO abolished vasoconstricive effects of endothelin-1 in the *in vitro* perfused rat liver.[18, 119] However, in contrast to the high NO production in the systemic and splanchnic vascular system, intrahepatic NO production is deficient in the cirrhotic liver. In cirrhotic rats, the deficit in intrahepatic NO synthesis was located in the sinusoidal and postsinusoidal areas, whereas presinusoidal production was normal.[120] The endothelial dysfunction with decreased NO synthesis by sinusoidal endothelial cells has been attributed to a decreased enzymatic function of eNOS.[121-123]

Nitric oxide was shown to modulate the contractile effect of endothelin-1 on cultured HSCs.[70, 124] Interleukin-1β, tumor necrosis factor-α, or lipopolysaccharides in combination with interferon-γ, led to increased iNOS mRNA levels in HSCs, and increased nitrite levels, possibly by an autocrine mechanism.[124] However, iNOS mRNA and nitrite were not found in HSCs cultured from CCl_4 treated rat livers.[125] Apart from vasoactive effects, deficient NO production in cirrhosis has some other effects: (i) increased thrombogenesis, (ii) enhanced synthesis and deposition of collagen in the space of Disse, (iii) decreased suppression of specific adhesion molecules, and (iv) reduced protection against free oxygen radicals.[115]

Although endothelins and NO are probably the most important and certainly the most studied vasoactive substances, several other substances have been implicated in HSCs contractility and could play a role in the pathogenesis of portal hypertension.

It is known for many years now that the renin angiotensin system is implicated in portal hypertension and its complications. Additionally, the activity of the renin-angiotensin system correlates with the degree of portal hypertension.[126] More recently, the mechanism of action and the involvement of HSCs have been studied in more detail. Angiotensinogen is synthesized by hepatocytes and released in the blood stream where it is transformed by renin to angiotensin I. Angiotensin converting enzyme, an enzyme that is abundant in endothelial cells, then cleaves angiotensin I to angiotensin II. Angiotensin II is an octapeptide primarily acting through 2 angiotensin receptors (AT_1 and AT_2), which are involved in respectively vasoconstriction and vasodilatation. Infusion of angiotensin II resulted in increased intrahepatic vascular resistance and portal hypertension in experimental cirrhosis. In a recent study, it has been shown that the expression of local renin and angiotensinogen mRNA was upregulated in the liver and splenic blood vessels of cirrhotic patients with portal hypertension.[127] Moreover, several studies have shown the presence of AT_1 receptors in activated rat and human HSCs.[128, 129] Via activation of AT_1 receptors, angiotensin II elicited a marked contraction of activated human HSCs by an increase in intracellular $[Ca^{2+}]_i$.[128] The same group of investigators demonstrated that activated, but not quiescent HSCs express renin, angiotensinogen and angiotensin converting enzyme and that activated

HSCs synthesize angiotensin II.[130] These observations suggested that the local renin angiotensin system could be implicated in portal hypertension, not only by effects on splanchnic vessels, but also through contractile effects on HSCs.

Carbon monoxide is a gaseous molecule produced by degradation of heme, mediated by activity of heme oxygenase (HO). Carbon monoxide activates soluble guanylate cyclase to produce cGMP, thereby causing smooth muscle relaxation. Three isoforms of HO have been described: (i) an inducible form, HO-1 (ii) a constitutive form HO-2 and (iii) HO-3, a form with a low catalytic activity.[131] Isoforms HO-1 and HO-2 are expressed in normal liver: HO-1 in Kupffer cells and HO-2 in hepatocytes. Both isoforms were undetectable in normal rat HSCs.[25] Heme oxygenase-1 gene expression was upregulated in hepatocytes and Kupffer cells of rats and patients with cirrhosis and portal hypertension.[132-134] In rats, increased HO-1 expression resulted in increased CO production and a reduction of hepatic vascular resistance.[135] *In vivo* microscopy demonstrated that HO-1 directly acts via HSCs in rat livers.[136] Thus, whereas HO-2 serves as a regulator of sinusoidal tone in normal liver, HO-1 seems to play a role in counteracting the vasoconstrictor effect of endothelin-1 in the stressed liver. Up to now, it remains unknown whether this mediator system is relevant in patients with portal hypertension.

Table 4: Substances with relaxing effect on hepatic stellate cells

Agent	Mechanism
NO	cGMP
CO	cGMP
Atrial Natriuretic Peptide	cGMP/$[Ca^{2+}]_i$
Adrenomedullin	cAMP
Somatostatin	$[Ca^{2+}]_i$/Rho kinase?
Agents increasing cAMP/cGMP	cAMP/cGMP
PGI_2/ PGE_2	cAMP
Y-27632 (Rho kinase inhibitor)	Rho kinase

In denervated, isolated, perfused rat liver, atrial natriuretic peptide antagonised the increased intrahepatic vascular resistance elicited by phenylephrine.[137] Cultured human HSCs have receptors for atrial natriuretic peptide and activation of these receptors reduced the effects of endothelin-1 on $[Ca^{2+}]_i$ and cell contraction.[138, 139] The relaxing effects were shown to be mediated by C-type natriuretic peptide inducing an increase in cGMP and by blockade of store-operated calcium channels.[139] Adrenomedullin is a potent vasodilator of which circulating plasma levels have been shown to be elevated in cirrhosis, as a function of hemodynamic changes.[140, 141] It has been demonstrated that human HSCs have functional receptors for adrenomedullin, the stimulation of which blunted the contractile effect of endothelin-1.[142] Adrenomedullin exerts its relaxing effects in HSCs through cAMP cascades.[143] Interestingly, both cytokines and shear stress augmented expression of C-type natriuretic peptide and adrenomodullin.[144] Somatostatin is used to treat acute variceal bleeding. Somatostatin inhibits the secretion of glucagon, a well known vasodilating agent. Moreover, in the presence of vasoconstrictors involving activation of protein kinase C, octreotide, a somatostatin analogue, had a direct vasoconstrictive effect on vascular smooth muscle of the superior mesenteric artery.[145] We have shown that, on top of the effects on portal blood flow, activation of the somatostatin receptor subtype 1 caused partial inhibition of endothelin-1-induced contraction of stellate cells.[146] Antidiuretic hormone or vasopressin, a potent vasoconstrictor acting through V_1 receptors on vascular smooth muscle cells, was successfully used to treat acute variceal bleeding. Vasopressin also elicited contraction of cultured human HSCs, through V_1 receptors. Stimulation of V_1 receptors is coupled with increased $[Ca^{2+}]_i$ caused by release of Ca^{2+} from intracellular stores.[147]

Several other substances have been investigated *in vitro*, but the *in vivo* significance on portal pressure remains unclear. Vascular endothelial growth factor inhibited contraction of cultured HSCs by attenuating α-smooth muscle actin expression.[148] Agents increasing intracellular cAMP (e.g. adrenomedullin, Iloprost, prostaglandin E2) and cGMP (e.g. lipopolysaccharide, interferon γ, interleukin-β, atrial natriuretic peptide, NO) induce relaxation of stellate cells.[28, 70, 139, 142, 149, 150] Some prostaglandins (e.g. PGI_2, PGE_2) induced relaxation of cultured HSCs, whereas others (e.g. thromboxane, $PGF_{2\alpha}$) induced contraction.[149] Although different effects on portal pressure have been claimed, to date no definite role in portal hypertension has been attributed to most eicosanoids. Administration of leukotriene D_4, a 5-lipoxygenase derived eicosanoid, resulted in marked HSCs contraction coupled with increased $[Ca^{2+}]_i$. Moreover, leukotriene D_4 administration significantly increased portal pressure in rats.[151] Similar to vasopressin, thrombin induced a dose-dependent contraction of activated human HSCs.[5, 139] Thrombin-induced contraction is coupled with a rise in $[Ca^{2+}]_i$ via release of Ca^{2+} from intracellular stores and via store-operated[139] or voltage-operated Ca channels.[5] Substance P caused a dose-dependent contraction of rat HSCs cultured for 24 h.[29] Substance P was increased in decompensated cirrhotic rats and patients, although no direct relation with portal pressure was found.[152, 153] Stellate cells have nucleotide receptors, which are triggered by adenosine, resulting in receptor-mediated contraction of the cells.[154] Lysophosphatidic acid, a product of phospholipid metabolism released by activated platelets, was shown to induce HSCs contraction by a mechanism involving Rho-kinase.[63] Inhibition of Rho signaling by a specific inhibitor of Rho kinase (Y-27632) decreased HSC contraction, proliferation, migration and activation-associated morphologic alterations.[64, 65, 155, 156] It also reduced endothelin-1-induced portal vein constriction in an *ex vivo* liver perfusion model, but no *in vivo* experiments have been published so far.[64]

Although activated HSCs contract in response to vasoactive substances, both *in vivo* and *in vitro*, there has been some debate whether stellate cell contraction is forceful enough to produce sinusoidal constriction. This issue was resolved in a recent study in which stellate cell contraction was directly quantified.[157] It was demonstrated that the average force generated by endothelin-1 induced contraction of a single HSCs was ~ 0.69 dyn, or 14000 dyn/cm^2, which is greater than the sinusoidal pressure in cirrhotic rats, indicating that HSCs can constrict sinusoids and thus contribute to increased sinusoidal resistance.

Pharmacological Treatment Options Directed Towards HSCs

Fibrosis remains the principal cause of increased vascular resistance in liver disease. Because HSCs play a key role in liver fibrogenesis, much effort has been made in the development of drugs acting on HSCs in order to prevent or even revert the process of fibrosis. Potential therapies are currently under investigation.[12, 158] Although clinical experimental studies indicate that hepatic fibrosis is partially reversible, complete resolution of cirrhosis with re-establishment of normal liver histology, will probably not be possible in all situations. Hence, portal hypertension and its complications will continue to be a major challenge for clinicians. Therefore, effective anti-portal hypertensive drugs are needed. Currently, most drugs are directed towards lowering portal blood flow, but new drugs acting on HSCs contractility are being investigated. Ideally, a drug should be antifibrotic, induce stellate cell relaxation and decrease portal blood flow. Some potential candidates will be discussed briefly.

In view of the beneficial effects of endothelin via activation of ET_B receptors (antiproliferative and relaxing effect on HSCs) and the harmful effects of ET_A receptor stimulation (contraction and proliferation of HSCs), selective blockade of ET_A or stimulation of ET_B receptors would be a good approach to treating portal hypertension. Oral administration of a selective ET_A receptor antagonist ameliorated portal hypertension in portal vein ligated rats,[159] and reduced fibrosis in a bile duct ligation model.[160] So far no solid clinical data are available in cirrhotic patients. Although ET_B receptor agonists and endothelin converting enzyme inhibitors are theoretically very interesting molecules, up to now no *in vivo* data are available.

Apart from relaxing effects of NO on HSCs, antiproliferative effects of NO have been demonstrated *in vitro*.[161] Although NO causes relaxation of HSCs, it also increases splanchnic and systemic vasodilatation, thereby increasing splanchnic blood flow which aggravates portal hypertension. Therefore, non-specific NO donors will probably not be clinically useful to treating portal hypertension. Because of the local, intrahepatic NO deficiency, liver-specific NO donors are theoretically interesting drugs. It has been shown recently in cirrhotic rats that a liver-specific NO donor (NCX-1000) decreased enhanced intrahepatic response to vasoconstrictors, and improved adaptability of the portal system to increased portal blood flow.[162] This agonist inhibited HSC contraction *in vitro* and reduced portal pressure in cirrhotic rats.[163] Furthermore, NCX-1000 had no deleterious effect on systemic hemodynamics. No human studies are available as yet. Another approach to increase local intrahepatic NO production is transduction of livers with recombinant adenoviruses carrying NOS gene. Gene transfer of both nNOS and constitutive endothelial NOS was feasible and significantly reduced intrahepatic resistance and portal pressure in different *in vivo* rat models of cirrhosis and portal hypertension.[164, 165] No human data are available.

Losartan, a specific AT_1 receptor antagonist, completely blocked the effects of angiotensin II on HSCs contraction and proliferation.[128] Furthermore, low dose losartan, lowered portal pressure in cirrhotic rats without side effects, whereas higher doses had deleterious effects.[166, 167] Short term administration of losartan and irbesartan, another AT_1 receptor antagonist, induced a significant decrease in portal hypertension in cirrhotic patients, but caused hypotension in some patients, especially those with advanced disease and high plasma renin levels.[168-170] Only recently long term effects have been published. After 6 weeks of treatment with losartan, portal pressure was not significantly reduced in cirrhotic patients. Moreover, it caused hypotension and reduced renal function.[171] Irbesartan, failed to decrease portal pressure in the majority of cirrhotic patients after 2 months of treatment. Like losartan it reduced mean arterial pressure and creatinine clearance.[172] Therefore caution is warranted before treating portal hypertensive patients with AT_1 receptor antagonists. Whether blockade of the renin-angiotensin system has anti-fibrotic properties in the liver as it has been shown for the kidney and heart remains to be proven.

Somatostatin is an efficient drug to treat acute variceal hemorrhage in patients with cirrhosis. The mechanism by which somatostatin lowers portal pressure is incompletely elucidated, but a number of mechanisms which decrease portal venous inflow and intrahepatic vascular resistance have been proposed.[173] Apart from vasoconstrictive effects on mesenteric arteries,[145] and relaxing effect on rat stellate cells,[146] antifibrotic effects have been attributed to somatostatin. The somatostatin analogue octreotide reduced the degree of fibrosis in different animal models.[174-176] Moreover, we have demonstrated decreased production of collagen I and III by cultured HSCs in the presence of somatostatin, suggesting that somatostatin has a direct antifibrotic effect mediated by HSCs.[177]

CONCLUSION

Hepatic stellate cells are key players in the pathogenesis of fibrosis and portal hypertension. Hence, HSCs have become therapeutic targets to treat these dreadful complications of chronic liver disease. HSCs probably also play a role in normal liver microcirculation. The contractile apparatus of HSCs, and the signaling pathways that control contraction or relaxation, require further in depth studies. Antifibrotic and vasomotor effects of multiple agents have been exhaustively investigated, predominantly *in vitro* and in experimental animal models. These studies have led to the identification of drugs causing inhibition of activation and relaxation of HSCs, thereby decreasing fibrosis and portal pressure. Based on this experimental work, clinical studies in patients will have to be undertaken.

REFERENCES

[1] Gupta TK, Chen L, Groszmann RJ. Pathophysiology of portal hypertension. Baillieres *Clin Gastroenterol* 1997;11:203-219.

[2] Bhathal PS, Grossmann HJ. Reduction of the increased portal vascular resistance of the isolated perfused rat liver by vasodilators. *J Hepatol* 1985;1:325-337.

[3] Reichen J, Le M. Verapamil favorably influences hepatic microvascular exchange and function in rats with cirrhosis of the liver. *J Clin Invest* 1986;78:448-455.

[4] Ramadori G. The stellate cell of the liver. *Virchows Arch B Cell Pathol* 1991;61:147-158.

[5] Pinzani M, Failli P, Ruocco C, Casini A, Milani S, Baldi E, Giotti A, Gentilini P. Fat-storing cells as liver-specific pericytes. Spatial dynamics of agonist-stimulated intracellular calcium transients. *J Clin Invest* 1992;90:642-646.

[6] Pinzani M. Hepatic stellate (ITO) cells: expanding roles for a liver-specific pericyte. *J Hepatol* 1995;22:700-706.

[7] Friedman SL. Molecular regulation of hepatic fibrosis, an integrated cellular response to tissue injury. *J Biol Chem* 2000;275:2247-2250.

[8] Burt AD, Le Bail B, Balabaud C, Bioulac-Sage P. Morphologic investigation of sinusoidal cells. *Semin Liver Dis* 1993;13:21-38.

[9] Stoyanova II, Gulubova MV. Immunocytochemical study on the liver innervation in patients with cirrhosis. *Acta Histochem* 2000;102:391-402.

[10] Geerts A. History, heterogeneity, developmental biology, and functions of quiescent hepatic stellate cells. *Semin Liver Dis* 2001;21:311-335.

[11] Pinzani M, Marra F. Cytokine receptors and signaling in hepatic stellate cells. *Semin Liver Dis* 2001;21:397-416.

[12] Bataller R, Brenner DA. Hepatic stellate cells as a target for the treatment of liver fibrosis. *Semin Liver Dis* 2001;21:437-451.

[13] Neaud V, Faouzi S, Guirouilh J, Le Bail B, Balabaud C, Bioulac-Sage P, Rosenbaum J. Human hepatic myofibroblasts increase invasiveness of hepatocellular carcinoma cells: evidence for a role of hepatocyte growth factor. *Hepatology* 1997;26:1458-1466.

[14] Theret K, Musso O, Turlin B, Lotrian D, Bioulac-Sage P, Campion JP, Boudjema K, Clement B. Increased extracellular matrix remodeling is associated with tumor progression in human hepatocellular carcinomas. *Hepatology* 2001;34:82-88.

[15] McCuskey RS. Morphological mechanisms for regulating blood flow through hepatic sinusoids. *Liver* 2000;20:3-7.

[16] Bhunchet E, Wake K. The portal lobule in rat liver fibrosis: a re-evaluation of the liver unit. *Hepatology* 1998;27:481-487.

[17] Nakata K, Leong GF, Brauer RW. Direct measurements of blood pressures in minute vessels of the liver. *Am J Physiol* 1960;199:1181-1188.

[18] Zhang JX, Pegoli WJ, Clemens MG. Endothelin-1 induces direct constriction of hepatic sinusoids. *Am J Physiol* 1994;266:G624-G632.

[19] Zhang JX, Bauer M, Clemens MG. Vessel- and target cell-specific actions of endothelin-1 and endothelin- 3 in rat liver. *Am J Physiol* 1995;269:G269-G277.

[20] Bauer M, Zhang JX, Bauer I, Clemens MG. ET-1 induced alterations of hepatic microcirculation: sinusoidal and extrasinusoidal sites of action. *Am J Physiol* 1994;267:G143-G149.

[21] Bauer M, Bauer I, Zhang JX, Kresge N, Baveja R, Yokoyama Y, Harding D, Clemens MG. Functional significance of endothelin B receptors in mediating sinusoidal and extrasinusoidal effects of endothelins in the intact rat liver. *Hepatology* 2000;31:937-947.

[22] Clemens MG, Zhang JX. Regulation of sinusoidal perfusion: In vivo methodology and control by endothelins. *Semin Liver Dis* 1999;19:383-396.

[23] Suematsu M, Wakabayashi Y, Ishimura Y. Gaseous monoxides: a new class of microvascular regulator in the liver. *Cardiovasc Res* 1996;32:679-686.

[24] Suematsu M, Goda N, Sano T, Kashiwagi S, Egawa T, Shinoda Y, Ishimura Y. Carbon monoxide: an endogenous modulator of sinusoidal tone in the perfused rat liver. *J Clin Invest* 1995;96:2431-2437.

[25] Goda N, Suzuki K, Naito M, Takeoka S, Tsuchida E, Ishimura Y, Tamatani T, Suematsu M. Distribution of heme oxygenase isoforms in rat liver. Topographic basis for carbon monoxide-mediated microvascular relaxation. *J Clin Invest* 1998;101:604-612.

[26] Kaneda K, Ekataksin W, Sogawa M, Matsumura A, Cho A, Kawada N. Endothelin-1-induced vasoconstriction causes a significant increase in portal pressure of rat liver:

localized constrictive effect on distal segment of preterminal portal venules as revealed by light and electron microscopy and serial reconstruction. *Hepatology* 1998;27:735-747.

[27] McCuskey RS, Ito Y, McCuskey M, Ekataksin W, Wake K. Morphological mechanisms for regulating blood flow through hepatic sinusoids: 1998 update and review. In: Wisse E, Knook DL, and Fraser R, eds. Cells of the hepatic sinusoid. 7th ed. Leiden: *Kupffer cell foundation,* 1999:129-134.

[28] Sakamoto M, Ueno T, Sugawara H, Torimura T, Tsuji R, Sujaku K, Sata M, Tanikawa K. Relaxing effect of interleukin-1 on rat cultured Ito cells. *Hepatology* 1997;25:1412-1417.

[29] Sakamoto M, Ueno T, Kin M, Ohira H, Torimura T, Inuzuka S, Sata M, Tanikawa K. Ito cell contraction in response to endothelin-1 and substance P. *Hepatology* 1993;18:978-983.

[30] Reinehr RM, Kubitz R, Peters-Regehr T, Bode JG, Haussinger D. Activation of rat hepatic stellate cells in culture is associated with increased sensitivity to endothelin 1. *Hepatology* 1998;28:1566-1577.

[31] Rockey DC, Housset CN, Friedman SL. Activation-dependent contractility of rat hepatic lipocytes in culture and in vivo. *J Clin Invest* 1993;92:1795-1804.

[32] Rockey DC, Weisiger RA. Endothelin induced contractility of stellate cells from normal and cirrhotic rat liver: implications for regulation of portal pressure and resistance. *Hepatology* 1996;24:233-240.

[33] Ekataksin W, Kaneda K. Liver microvascular architecture: an insight into the pathophysiology of portal hypertension. *Semin Liver Dis* 1999;19:359-382.

[34] Fuchs E, Cleveland DW. A structural scaffolding of intermediate filaments in health and disease. *Science* 1998;279:514-519.

[35] Herrmann H, Aebi U. Intermediate filaments and their associates: multi-talented structural elements specifying cytoarchitecture and cytodynamics. *Curr Opin Cell Biol* 2000;12:79-90.

[36] Lehman W, Graig R, Vibert P, Barany M. Actin and the structure of smooth muscle thin filaments. In: Barany M, ed. Biochemistry of smooth muscle contraction. first ed. *London: Academic press*, 1995:47-60.

[37] Berg JS, Powell BC, Cheney RE. A millennial myosin census. *Mol Biol Cell* 2001;12:780-794.

[38] Dai J, Ting-Beall HP, Hochmuth RM, Sheetz MP, Titus MA. Myosin I contributes to the generation of resting cortical tension. *Biophys J* 1999;77:1168-1176.

[39] Raposo G, Cordonnier MN, Tenza D, Menichi B, Durrbach A, Louvard D, Coudrier E. Association of myosin I alpha with endosomes and lysosomes in mammalian cells. *Mol Biol Cell* 1999;10:1477-1494.

[40] Tang N, Ostap EM. Motor domain-dependent localization of myo1b (myr-1). *Curr Biol* 2001;11:1131-1135.

[41] Novak KD, Titus MA. Myosin I overexpression impairs cell migration. *J Cell Biol* 1997;136:633-647.

[42] Reck-Peterson SL, Provance DW, Jr., Mooseker MS, Mercer JA. Class V myosins. *Biochim Biophys Acta* 2000;1496:36-51.

[43] Vale RD. Myosin V motor proteins: marching stepwise towards a mechanism. *J Cell Biol* 2003;163:445-450.

[44] Ogata I, Saez CG, Greenwel P, Ponce ML, Geerts A, Leinwand LA, Rojkind M. Rat liver fat-storing cell lines express sarcomeric myosin heavy chain mRNA and protein. *Cell Motil Cytoskeleton* 1993;26:125-132.

[45] Mayer DC, Leinwand LA. Sarcomeric gene expression and contractility in myofibroblasts. *J Cell Biol* 1997;139:1477-1484.

[46] Somlyo AP, Somlyo AV. Signal transduction and regulation in smooth muscle. *Nature* 1994;372:231-236.

[47] Somlyo AP, Somlyo AV. Signal transduction by G-proteins, rho-kinase and protein phosphatase to smooth muscle and non-muscle myosin II. *J Physiol* 2000;522 Pt 2:177-185.

[48] Kureishi Y, Kobayashi S, Amano M, Kimura K, Kanaide H, Nakano T, Kaibuchi K, Ito M. Rho-associated kinase directly induces smooth muscle contraction through myosin light chain phosphorylation. *J Biol Chem* 1997;272:12257-12260.

[49] Amano M, Fukata Y, Kaibuchi K. Regulation and functions of Rho-associated kinase. *Exp Cell Res* 2000;261:44-51.

[50] Yee HFJ. Ca2+ and rho signaling pathways: two paths to hepatic stellate cell contraction. *Hepatology* 2001;33:1007-1008.

[51] Yanase M, Ikeda H, Ogata I, Matsui A, Noiri E, Tomiya T, Arai M, Inoue Y, Tejima K, Nagashima K, Nishikawa T, Shibata M, Ikebe M, Rojkind M, Fujiwara K. Functional diversity between Rho-kinase- and MLCK-mediated cytoskeletal actions in a myofibroblast-like hepatic stellate cell line. *Biochem Biophys Res Commun* 2003;305:223-228.

[52] Carloni V, Romanelli RG, Pinzani M, Laffi G, Gentilini P. Expression and function of integrin receptors for collagen and laminin in cultured human hepatic stellate cells. *Gastroenterology* 1996;110:1127-1136.

[53] Cary LA, Guan JL. Focal adhesion kinase in integrin-mediated signaling. *Front Biosci* 1999;4:D102-D113.

[54] Pinzani M, Marra F, Carloni V. Signal transduction in hepatic stellate cells. *Liver* 1998;18:2-13.

[55] Holly SP, Larson MK, Parise LV. Multiple roles of integrins in cell motility. *Exp Cell Res* 2000;261:69-74.

[56] Schmitz AA, Govek EE, Bottner B, Van Aelst L. Rho GTPases: signaling, migration, and invasion. *Exp Cell Res* 2000;261:1-12.

[57] Bataller R, Gasull X, Gines P, Hellemans K, Gorbig MN, Nicolas JM, Sancho-Bru P, De Las H, Gual A, Geerts A, Arroyo V, Rodes J. In vitro and in vivo activation of rat hepatic stellate cells results in de novo expression of L-type voltage-operated calcium channels. *Hepatology* 2001;33:956-962.

[58] Tao J, Mallat A, Gallois C, Belmadani S, Mery PF, Tran-Van Nhieu J, Pavoine C, Lotersztajn S. Biological effects of C-type natriuretic peptide in human myofibroblastic stellate cells. *J Biol Chem* 1999;274:23761-23769.

[59] Bataller R, Nicolas JM, Ginees P, Gorbig MN, Garcia-Ramallo E, Lario S, Tobias E, Pinzani M, Thomas AP, Arroyo V, Rodes J. Contraction of human hepatic stellate cells activated in culture: a role for voltage-operated calcium channels. *J Hepatol* 1998;29:398-408.

[60] Sah VP, Seasholtz TM, Sagi SA, Brown JH. The role of Rho in G protein-coupled receptor signal transduction. *Annu Rev Pharmacol Toxicol* 2000;40:459-489.

[61] Ridley AJ, Hall A. The small GTP-binding protein rho regulates the assembly of focal adhesions and actin stress fibers in response to growth factors. *Cell* 1992;70:389-399.

[62] Uehata M, Ishizaki T, Satoh H, Ono T, Kawahara T, Morishita T, Tamakawa H, Yamagami K, Inui J, Maekawa M, Narumiya S. Calcium sensitization of smooth muscle mediated by a Rho-associated protein kinase in hypertension. *Nature* 1997;389:990-994.

[63] Yanase M, Ikeda H, Matsui A, Maekawa H, Noiri E, Tomiya T, Arai M, Yano T, Shibata M, Ikebe M, Fujiwara K, Rojkind M, Ogata I. Lysophosphatidic acid enhances collagen gel contraction by hepatic stellate cells: association with rho-kinase. *Biochem Biophys Res Commun* 2000;277:72-78.

[64] Kawada N, Seki S, Kuroki T, Kaneda K. ROCK inhibitor Y-27632 attenuates stellate cell contraction and portal pressure increase induced by endothelin-1. *Biochem Biophys Res Commun* 1999;266:296-300.

[65] Yee HFJ. Rho directs activation-associated changes in rat hepatic stellate cell morphology via regulation of the actin cytoskeleton. *Hepatology* 1998;28:843-850.

[66] Berridge MJ. Inositol trisphosphate and diacylglycerol: two interacting second messengers. *Annu Rev Biochem* 1987;56:159-193.

[67] Forder J, Scriabine A, Rasmussen H. Plasma membrane calcium flux, protein kinase C activation and smooth muscle contraction. *J Pharmacol Exp Ther* 1985;235:267-273.

[68] Chatterjee M, Tejada M. Phorbol ester-induced contraction in chemically skinned vascular smooth muscle. *Am J Physiol* 1986;251:C356-C361.

[69] Rasmussen H, Takuwa Y, Park S. Protein kinase C in the regulation of smooth muscle contraction. *FASEB J* 1987;1:177-185.

[70] Kawada N, Tran-Thi TA, Klein H, Decker K. The contraction of hepatic stellate (Ito) cells stimulated with vasoactive substances. Possible involvement of endothelin 1 and nitric oxide in the regulation of the sinusoidal tonus. *Eur J Biochem* 1993;213:815-823.

[71] Liscovitch M, Czarny M, Fiucci G, Tang X. Phospholipase D: molecular and cell biology of a novel gene family. *Biochem J* 2000;345 Pt 3:401-415.

[72] Cross MJ, Roberts S, Ridley AJ, Hodgkin MN, Stewart A, Claesson-Welsh L, Wakelam MJ. Stimulation of actin stress fibre formation mediated by activation of phospholipase D. *Curr Biol* 1996;6:588-597.

[73] Ha KS, Exton JH. Activation of actin polymerization by phosphatidic acid derived from phosphatidylcholine in IIC9 fibroblasts. *J Cell Biol* 1993;123:1789-1796.

[74] Iyer SS, Kusner DJ. Association of phospholipase D activity with the detergent-insoluble cytoskeleton of U937 promonocytic leukocytes. *J Biol Chem* 1999;274:2350-2359.

[75] Colley WC, Sung TC, Roll R, Jenco J, Hammond SM, Altshuller Y, Bar-Sagi D, Morris AJ, Frohman MA. Phospholipase D2, a distinct phospholipase D isoform with novel regulatory properties that provokes cytoskeletal reorganization. *Curr Biol* 1997;7:191-201.

[76] Adelstein RS, Conti MA, Hathaway DR, Klee CB. Phosphorylation of smooth muscle myosin light chain kinase by the catalytic subunit of adenosine 3': 5'-monophosphate-dependent protein kinase. *J Biol Chem* 1978;253:8347-8350.

[77] Rembold CM. Electromechanical and pharmacomechanical coupling. In: Bárány M, ed. Biochemistry of smooth muscle contraction. First ed. San Diego, *CA: Academic Press, Inc.,* 1996:227-239.

[78] Clancy RM, Rediske J, Tang X, Nijher N, Frenkel S, Philips M, Abramson SB. Outside-in signaling in the chondrocyte. Nitric oxide disrupts fibronectin-induced assembly of a subplasmalemmal actin/rho A/focal adhesion kinase signaling complex. *J Clin Invest* 1997;100:1789-1796.

[79] Inoue M, Yanagiasawa M, Kimura S, Kasuya Y, Miyauchi T, Goto K, Masaki T. The human endothelin family: three structurally and pharmacologically distinct isopeptides predicted by three separate genes. *Poc Natl Acad Sci* (USA) 1989;86:2863-2867.

[80] Xu D, Emoto N, Giaid A, Slaughter C, Kaw D, deWit D, Yanagiasawa M. ECE-1: a membrane-bound metalloprotease that catalyzes the proteolytic activation of big endothelin-1. *Cell* 1994;78:473-485.

[81] Clozel M, Gray GA, Breu V, Loffler BM, Osterwalder R. The endothelin ETB receptor mediates both vasodilation and vasoconstriction in vivo. *Biochem Biophys Res Commun* 1992;186:867-873.

[82] Sakurai T, Yanagiasawa M, Masaki T. Molecular characterization of endothelin receptors. *Trends Pharmacol Sci* 1992;13:103-108.

[83] Higuchi H, Satoh T. Endothelin-1 induces vasoconstriction and nitric oxide release via endothelin ET(B) receptors in isolated perfused rat liver. *Eur J Pharmacol* 1997;328:175-182.

[84] Housset C, Rockey DC, Bissell DM. Endothelin receptors in rat liver: lipocytes as a contractile target for endothelin 1. *Proc Natl Acad Sci* U S A 1993;90:9266-9270.

[85] Jouneaux C, Mallat A, Serradeil-Le GC, Goldsmith P, Hanoune J, Lotersztajn S. Coupling of endothelin B receptors to the calcium pump and phospholipase C via Gs and Gq in rat liver. *J Biol Chem* 1994;269:1845-1851.

[86] Serradeil-Le GC, Jouneaux C, Sanchez-Bueno A, Raufaste D, Roche B, Preaux AM, Maffrand JP, Cobbold PH, Hanoune J, Lotersztajn S. Endothelin action in rat liver. Receptors, free Ca2+ oscillations, and activation of glycogenolysis. *J Clin Invest* 1991;87:133-138.

[87] Kuddus RH, Nalesnik MA, Subbotin VM, Rao AS, Gandhi CR. Enhanced synthesis and reduced metabolism of endothelin-1 (ET-1) by hepatocytes--an important mechanism of increased endogenous levels of ET-1 in liver cirrhosis. *J Hepatol* 2000;33:725-732.

[88] Yokomori H, Oda M, Ogi M, Kamegaya Y, Tsukada N, Nakamura M, Ishii H. Enhanced expression of endothelin receptor subtypes in cirrhotic rat liver. *Liver* 2001;21:114-122.

[89] Leivas A, Jimenez W, Bruix J, Boix L, Bosch J, Arroyo V, Rivera F, Rodes J. Gene expression of endothelin-1 and ET(A) and ET(B) receptors in human cirrhosis: relationship with hepatic hemodynamics. *J Vasc Res* 1998;35:186-193.

[90] Alam I, Bass NM, Bacchetti P, Gee L, Rockey DC. Hepatic tissue endothelin-1 levels in chronic liver disease correlate with disease severity and ascites. *Am J Gastroenterol* 2000;95:199-203.

[91] Gerbes AL, Moller S, Gulberg V, Henriksen JH. Endothelin-1 and -3 plasma concentrations in patients with cirrhosis: role of splanchnic and renal passage and liver function. *Hepatology* 1995;21:735-739.

[92] Moore K, Wendon J, Frazer M, Karani J, Williams R, Badr K. Plasma endothelin immunoreactivity in liver disease and the hepatorenal syndrome. *N Engl J Med* 1992;327:1774-1778.

[93] Uchihara M, Izumi N, Sato C, Marumo F. Clinical significance of elevated plasma endothelin concentration in patients with cirrhosis. *Hepatology* 1992;16:95-99.

[94] Asbert M, Gines A, Gines P, Jimenez W, Claria J, Salo J, Arroyo V, Rivera F, Rodes J. Circulating levels of endothelin in cirrhosis. *Gastroenterology* 1993;104:1485-1491.

[95] Moller S, Emmeluth C, Henriksen JH. Elevated circulating plasma endothelin-1 concentrations in cirrhosis. *J Hepatol* 1993;19:285-290.

[96] Matsumoto H, Uemasu J, Kitano M, Kawasaki H. Clinical significance of plasma endothelin-1 in patients with chronic liver disease. *Dig Dis Sci* 1994;39:2665-2670.

[97] Moller S, Gulberg V, Henriksen JH, Gerbes AL. Endothelin-1 and endothelin-3 in cirrhosis: relations to systemic and splanchnic haemodynamics. *J Hepatol* 1995;23:135-144.

[98] Salo J, Francitorra A, Follo A, Navasa M, Gines A, Jimenez W, Gines P, Arroyo V, Rivera F, Rodes J. Increased plasma endothelin in cirrhosis. Relationship with systemic endotoxemia and response to changes in effective blood volume. *J Hepatol* 1995;22:389-398.

[99] Tsai YT, Lin HC, Yang MC, Lee FY, Hou MC, Chen LS, Lee SD. Plasma endothelin levels in patients with cirrhosis and their relationships to the severity of cirrhosis and renal function. *J Hepatol* 1995;23:681-688.

[100] Martinet JP, Legault L, Cernacek P, Roy L, Dufresne MP, Spahr L, Fenyves D, Pomier-Layrargues G. Changes in plasma endothelin-1 and Big endothelin-1 induced by transjugular intrahepatic portosystemic shunts in patients with cirrhosis and refractory ascites. *J Hepatol* 1996;25:700-706.

[101] Bernardi M, Gulberg V, Colantoni A, Trevisani F, Gasbarrini A, Gerbes AL. Plasma endothelin-1 and -3 in cirrhosis: relationship with systemic hemodynamics, renal function and neurohumoral systems. *J Hepatol* 1996;24:161-168.

[102] Nagasue N, Dhar DK, Yamanoi YE, Udagawa J, Yamamoto A, Tachibana M, Kubota H, Kohno H, Harada T. Production and release of endothelin-1 from the gut and spleen in portal hypertension due to cirrhosis. *Hepatology* 2000;31:1107-1114.

[103] Gandhi CR, Stephenson K, Olson MS. Endothelin, a potent peptide agonist in the liver. *J Biol Chem* 1990;265:17432-17435.

[104] Sogni P, Moreau R, Gomola A, Gadano A, Cailmail S, Calmus Y, Clozel M, Lebrec D. Beneficial hemodynamic effects of bosentan, a mixed ET(A) and ET(B) receptor antagonist, in portal hypertensive rats. *Hepatology* 1998;28:655-659.

[105] Reichen J, Gerbes AL, Steiner MJ, Sagesser H, Clozel M. The effect of endothelin and its antagonist Bosentan on hemodynamics and microvascular exchange in cirrhotic rat liver. *J Hepatol* 1998;28:1020-1030.

[106] Kojima H, Yamao J, Tsujimoto T, Uemura M, Takaya A, Fukui H. Mixed endothelin receptor antagonist, SB209670, decreases portal pressure in biliary cirrhotic rats in vivo by reducing portal venous system resistance. *J Hepatol* 2000;32:43-50.

[107] Poo JL, Jimenez W, Maria MR, Bosch-Marce M, Bordas N, Morales-Ruiz M, Perez M, Deulofeu R, Sole M, Arroyo V, Rodes J. Chronic blockade of endothelin receptors in cirrhotic rats: hepatic and hemodynamic effects. *Gastroenterology* 1999;116:161-167.

[108] Rieder H, Ramadori G, Meyer zum Buschenfelde KH. Sinusoidal endothelial liver cells in vitro release endothelin: augmentation by transforming growth factor ß and Kupffer cell-conditioned media. *Klin Wochenschr* 1991;69:387-391.

[109] Pinzani M, Milani S, De Franco R, Grappone C, Caligiuri A, Gentilini A, Tosti-Guerra C, Maggi M, Failli P, Ruocco C, Gentilini P. Endothelin 1 is overexpressed in human cirrhotic liver and exerts multiple effects on activated hepatic stellate cells. *Gastroenterology* 1996;110:534-548.

[110] Rockey D, Fouassier L, Chung JJ, Carayon A, Vallee P, Rey C, Housset C. Cellular localization of endothelin-1 and increased production in liver injury in the rat: Potential for autocrine and paracrine effects on stellate cells. *Hepatology* 1998;27:472-480.

[111] Shao R, Rockey DC. Regulation of endothelin-1 synthesis by endothelin-converting enzyme-1 during wound healing. *J Biol Chem* 1999;274:3228-3234.

[112] Mallat A, Fouassier L, Preaux AM, Gal CS, Raufaste D, Rosenbaum J, Dhumeaux D, Jouneaux C, Mavier P, Lotersztajn S. Growth inhibitory properties of endothelin-1 in human hepatic myofibroblastic Ito cells. An endothelin B receptor-mediated pathway. *J Clin Invest* 1995;96:42-49.

[113] Mallat A, Preaux AM, Serradeil-Le GC, Raufaste D, Gallois C, Brenner DA, Bradham C, Maclouf J, Iourgenko V, Fouassier L, Dhumeaux D, Mavier P, Lotersztajn S. Growth inhibitory properties of endothelin-1 in activated human hepatic stellate cells: a cyclic adenosine monophosphate-mediated pathway. Inhibition of both extracellular signal-regulated kinase and c-Jun kinase and upregulation of endothelin B receptors. *J Clin Invest* 1996;98:2771-2778.

[114] Moncada S, Higgs A. The L-arginine-nitric oxide pathway. *N Engl J Med* 1993;329:2002-2012.

[115] Wiest R, Groszmann RJ. Nitric oxide and portal hypertension: its role in the regulation of intrahepatic and splanchnic vascular resistance. *Semin Liver Dis* 1999;19:411-426.

[116] Sessa WC. The nitric oxide synthetase family of proteins. *J Vasc Res* 1994;31:131-143.

[117] Mittal MK, Gupta TK, Lee FY, Sieber CC, Groszmann RJ. Nitric oxide modulates hepatic vascular tone in normal rat liver. *Am J Physiol* 1994;267:G416-G422.

[118] Shah V, Haddad FG, Garcia-Cardena G, Frangos JA, Mennone A, Groszmann RJ, Sessa WC. Liver sinusoidal endothelial cells are responsible for nitric oxide modulation of resistance in the hepatic sinusoids. *J Clin Invest* 1997;100:2923-2930.

[119] Tran-Thi TA, Kawada N, Decker K. Regulation of endothelin-1 action on the perfused rat liver. *FEBS Lett* 1993;318:353-357.

[120] Loureiro-Silva MR, Cadelina GW, Groszmann RJ. Deficit in nitric oxide production in cirrhotic rat livers is located in the sinusoidal and postsinusoidal areas. *Am J Physiol Gastrointest Liver Physiol* 2003;284:G567-G574.

[121] Gupta TK, Toruner M, Chung MK, Groszmann RJ. Endothelial dysfunction and decreased production of nitric oxide in the intrahepatic microcirculation of cirrhotic rats. *Hepatology* 1998;28:926-931.

[122] Rockey DC, Chung JJ. Reduced nitric oxide production by endothelial cells in cirrhotic rat liver: endothelial dysfunction in portal hypertension. *Gastroenterology* 1998;114:344-351.

[123] Shah V, Toruner M, Haddad FG, Cadelina G, Papapetropoulos A, Choo K, Sessa WC, Groszmann RJ. Impaired endothelial nitric oxide synthase activity associated with enhanced caveolin binding in experimental cirrhosis in the rat. *Gastroenterology* 1999;117:1222-1228.

[124] Rockey DC, Chung JJ. Inducible nitric oxide synthase in rat hepatic lipocytes and the effect of nitric oxide on lipocyte contractility. *J Clin Invest* 1995;95:1199-1206.

[125] Rockey DC, Chung JJ. Regulation of inducible nitric oxide synthase and nitric oxide during hepatic injury and fibrogenesis. *Am J Physiol* 1997;273:G124-G130.

[126] Bosch J, Arroyo V, Betrui A, Mas A, Carrilho F, Navarro-Lopez F, Rodes J. Hepatic hemodynamics and the renin-angiotensin system in cirrhosis. *Gastroenterology* 1980;78:92-99.

[127] Zhang L, Yang Z, Shi BM, Li DP, Fang CY, Qiu FZ. Expression of local renin and angiotensinogen mRNA in cirrhotic portal hypertensive patient. *World J Gastroenterol* 2003;9:1584-1588.

[128] Bataller R, Gines P, Nicolas JM, Gorbig MN, Garcia-Ramallo E, Gasull X, Bosch J, Arroyo V, Rodes J. Angiotensin II induces contraction and proliferation of human hepatic stellate cells. *Gastroenterology* 2000;118:1149-1156.

[129] Zhang Y, Yang X, Wu P, Xu L, Liao G, Yang G. Expression of angiotensin II type 1 receptor in rat hepatic stellate cells and its effects on cell growth and collagen production. *Horm Res* 2003;60:105-110.

[130] Bataller R, Sancho-Bru P, Gines P, Lora JM, Al Garawi A, Sole M, Colmenero J, Nicolas JM, Jimenez W, Weich N, Gutierrez-Ramos JC, Arroyo V, Rodes J. Activated human hepatic stellate cells express the renin-angiotensin system and synthesize angiotensin II. *Gastroenterology* 2003;125:117-125.

[131] Suematsu M, Ishimura Y. The heme oxygenase-carbon monoxide system: A regulator of hepatobiliary function. *Hepatology* 2000;31:3-6.

[132] Fernandez M, Bonkovsky HL. Increased heme oxygenase-1 gene expression in liver cells and splanchnic organs from portal hypertensive rats. *Hepatology* 1999;29:1672-1679.

[133] Matsumi M, Takahashi T, Fujii H, Ohashi I, Kaku R, Nakatsuka H, Shimizu H, Morita K, Hirakawa M, Inagaki M, Sadamori H, Yagi T, Tanaka N, Akagi R. Increased heme oxygenase-1 gene expression in the livers of patients with portal hypertension due to severe hepatic cirrhosis. *J Int Med Res* 2002;30:282-288.

[134] Makino N, Suematsu M, Sugiura Y, Morikawa H, Shiomi S, Goda N, Sano T, Nimura Y, Sugimachi K, Ishimura Y. Altered expression of heme oxygenase-1 in the livers of patients with portal hypertensive diseases. *Hepatology* 2001;33:32-42.

[135] Wakabayashi Y, Takamiya R, Mizuki A, Kyokane T, Goda N, Yamaguchi T, Takeoka S, Tsuchida E, Suematsu M, Ishimura Y. Carbon monoxide overproduced by heme oxygenase-1 causes a reduction of vascular resistance in perfused rat liver. *Am J Physiol* 1999;277:G1088-G1096.

[136] Rensing H, Bauer I, Zhang JX, Paxian M, Pannen BH, Yokoyama Y, Clemens MG, Bauer M. Endothelin-1 and heme oxygenase-1 as modulators of sinusoidal tone in the stress-exposed rat liver. *Hepatology* 2002;36:1453-1465.

[137] Bilzer M, Paumgartner G, Gerbes AL. Prolonged antagonism of adrenergic vasoconstriction in the rat liver by atrial natriuretic peptide. *Gastroenterology* 1995;108:803-811.

[138] Gorbig MN, Gines P, Bataller R, Nicolas JM, Garcia-Ramallo E, Tobias E, Titos E, Rey MJ, Claria J, Arroyo V, Rodes J. Atrial natriuretic peptide antaginizes endothelin-induced calcium increase and cell contraction in cultured human hepatic stellate cells. *Hepatology* 1999;30:501-509.

[139] Tao J, Mallat A, Gallois C, Belmadani S, Mery PF, Tran-Van Nhieu J, Pavoine C, Lotersztajn S. Biological effects of C-type natriuretic peptide in human myofibroblastic stellate cells. *J Biol Chem* 1999;274:23761-23769.

[140] Guevara M, Gines P, Jimenez W, Sort P, Fernandez-Esparrach G, Escorsell A, Bataller R, Bosch J, Arroyo V, Rivera F, Rodes J. Increased adrenomedullin levels in cirrhosis: Relationship with hemodynamic abnormalities and vasoconstrictor systems. *Gastroenterology* 1998;114:336-343.

[141] Fernandez-Rodriguez CM, Prada IR, Prieto J, Montuenga LM, Elssasser T, Quiroga J, Moreiras M, Andrade A, Cuttitta F. Circulating adrenomedullin in cirrhosis: relationship to hyperdynamic circulation. *J Hepatol* 1998;29:250-256.

[142] Gorbig MN, Gines P, Bataller R, Nicolas JM, Garcia-Ramallo E, Cejudo P, Sancho-Bru P, Jimenez W, Arroyo V, Rodes J. Human hepatic stellate cells secrete adrenomedullin: potential autocrine factor in the regulation of cell contractility. *J Hepatol* 2001;34:222-229.

[143] Kawada N, Inoue M. Effect of adrenomedullin on hepatic pericytes (stellate cells) of the rat. *FEBS Lett* 1994;356:109-113.

[144] Chun TH, Itoh H, Ogawa Y, Tamura N, Takaya K, Igaki T, Yamashita J, Doi K, Inoue M, Masatsugu K, Korenaga R, Ando J, Nakao K. Shear stress augments expression of C-type natriuretic peptide and adrenomedullin. *Hypertension* 1997;29:1296-1302.

[145] Wiest R, Tsai MH, Groszmann RJ. Octreotidepotentiates PKC-dependent vasoconstrictors in portal-hypertensive and control rats. *Gastroenterology* 2001;120:975-983.

[146] Reynaert H, Vaeyens F, Qin H, Hellemans K, Chatterjee N, Winand D, Quartier E, Schuit F, Urbain D, Kumar U, Patel YC, Geerts A. Somatostatin suppresses endothelin-1-induced rat hepatic stellate cell contraction via somatostatin receptor subtype 1. *Gastroenterology* 2001;121:915-930.

[147] Bataller R, Nicolas JM, Gines P, Esteve A, Gorbig MN, Garcia-Ramallo E, Pinzani M, Ros J, Jimenez W, Thomas AP, Arroyo V, Rodes J. Arginine vasopressin induces contraction and stimulates growth of cultured human hepatic stellate cells. *Gastroenterology* 1997;113:615-624.

[148] Mashiba S, Mochida S, Ishikawa K, Inao M, Matsui A, Ohno A, Ikeda H, Nagoshi S, Shibuya M, Fujiwara K. Inhibition of hepatic stellate cell contraction during activation in vitro by vascular endothelial growth factor in association with upregulation of FLT tyrosine kinase receptor family, FLT-1. *Biochem Biophys Res Commun* 1999;258:674-678.

[149] Kawada N, Klein H, Decker K. Eicosanoid-mediated contractility of hepatic stellate cells. *Biochem J* 1992;285 (Pt 2):367-371.

[150] Kawada N, Kuroki T, Uoya M, Inoue M, Kobayashi K. Smooth muscle alpha-actin expression in rat hepatic stellate cell is regulated by nitric oxide and cGMP production. *Biochem Biophys Res Commun* 1996;229:238-242.

[151] Titos E, Claria J, Bataller R, Bosch-Marce M, Gines P, Jimenez W, Arroyo V, Rivera F, Rodes J. Hepatocyte-derived cysteinyl leukotrienes modulate vascular tone in experimental cirrhosis. *Gastroenterology* 2000;119:794-805.

[152] Fernandez-Rodriguez CM, Prieto J, Quiroga J, Zozoya JM, Andrade A, Nunez M, Sangro B, Penas J. Plasma levels of substance P in liver cirrhosis: relationship to the

activation of vasopressor systems and urinary sodium excretion. *Hepatology* 1995;21:35-40.

[153] Chu CJ, Lee FY, Wang SS, Chang FY, Tsai YT, Lin HC, Hou MC, Wu SL, Tai CC, Lee SD. Hyperdynamic circulation of cirrhotic rats: role of substance P and its relationship to nitric oxide. *Scand J Gastroenterol* 1997;32:841-846.

[154] Takemura S, Kawada N, Hirohashi K, Kinoshita H, Inoue M. Nucleotide receptors in hepatic stellate cells of the rat. *FEBS Lett* 1994;354:53-56.

[155] Iwamoto H, Nakamuta M, Tada S, Sugimoto R, Enjoji M, Nawata H. A p160ROCK-specific inhibitor, Y-27632, attenuates rat hepatic stellate cell growth. *J Hepatol* 2000;32:762-770.

[156] Tangkijvanich P, Tam SP, Yee HFJ. Wound-induced migration of rat hepatic stellate cells is modulated by endothelin-1 through rho-kinase-mediated alterations in the acto-myosin cytoskeleton. *Hepatology* 2001;33:74-80.

[157] Thimgan MS, Yee HF. Quantitation of rat hepatic stellate cell contraction: stellate cells' contribution to sinusoidal resistance. *Am J Physiol* 1999;277:G137-G143.

[158] Friedman SL, Maher JJ, Bissell DM. Mechanisms and therapy of hepatic fibrosis: report of the AASLD Single Topic Basic Research Conference. *Hepatology* 2000;32:1403-1408.

[159] De Gottardi A, Shaw S, Sagesser H, Reichen J. Type A, but not type B, endothelin receptor antagonists significantly decrease portal pressure in portal hypertensive rats. *J Hepatol* 2000;33:733-737.

[160] Cho JJ, Hocher B, Herbst H, Jia JD, Ruehl M, Hahn EG, Riecken EO, Schuppan D. An oral endothelin-A receptor antagonist blocks collagen synthesis and deposition in advanced rat liver fibrosis. *Gastroenterology* 2000;118:1169-1178.

[161] Failli P, De Franco R, Caligiuri A, Gentilini A, Romanelli RG, Marra F, Batignani G, Guerra CT, Laffi G, Gentilini P, Pinzani M. Nitrovasodilators inhibit platelet-derived growth factor-induced proliferation and migration of activated human hepatic stellate cells. *Gastroenterology* 2000;119:479-492.

[162] Loureiro-Silva MR, Cadelina GW, Iwakiri Y, Groszmann RJ. A liver-specific nitric oxide donor improves the intra-hepatic vascular response to both portal blood flow increase and methoxamine in cirrhotic rats. *J Hepatol* 2003;39:940-946.

[163] Fiorucci S, Antonelli E, Morelli O, Mencarelli A, Casini A, Mello T, Palazzetti B, Tallet D, del Soldato P, Morelli A. NCX-1000, a NO-releasing derivative of ursodeoxycholic acid, selectively delivers NO to the liver and protects against development of portal hypertension. *Proc Natl Acad Sci* U S A 2001;98:8897-8902.

[164] Yu Q, Shao R, Qian HS, George SE, Rockey DC. Gene transfer of the neuronal NO synthase isoform to cirrhotic rat liver ameliorates portal hypertension. *J Clin Invest* 2000;105:741-748.

[165] Van de Casteele M, Omasta A, Janssens S, Roskams T, Desmet V, Nevens F, Fevery J. In vivo gene transfer of endothelial nitric oxide synthase decreases portal pressure in anaesthetised carbon tetrachloride cirrhotic rats. *Gut* 2002;51:440-445.

[166] Croquet V, Moal F, Veal N, Wang J, Oberti F, Roux J, Vuillemin E, Gallois Y, Douay O, Chappard D, Cales P. Hemodynamic and antifibrotic effects of losartan in rats with liver fibrosis and/or portal hypertension. *J Hepatol* 2002;37:773-780.

[167] Heller J, Shiozawa T, Trebicka J, Hennenberg M, Schepke M, Neef M, Sauerbruch T. Acute haemodynamic effects of losartan in anaesthetized cirrhotic rats. *Eur J Clin Invest* 2003;33:1006-1012.

[168] Schneider AW, Kalk JF, Klein CP. Effect of losartan, an angiotensin II receptor antagonist, on portal pressure in cirrhosis. *Hepatology* 1999;29:334-339.

[169] De BK, Bandyopadhyay K, Das TK, Das D, Biswas PK, Majumdar D, Mandal SK, Ray S, Dasgupta S. Portal pressure response to losartan compared with propranolol in patients with cirrhosis. *Am J Gastroenterol* 2003;98:1371-1376.

[170] Schepke M, Werner E, Biecker E, Schiedermaier P, Heller J, Neef M, Stoffel-Wagner B, Hofer U, Casselmann WH, Sauerbruch T. Hemodynamic effects of the angiotensin II receptor antagonist irbesartan in patients with cirrhosis and portal hypertension. *Gastroenterology* 2001;121:389-395.

[171] Gonzalez-Abraldes J, Albillos A, Banares R, Del Arbol LR, Moitinho E, Rodriguez C, Gonzalez M, Escorsell A, Garcia-Pagan JC, Bosch J. Randomized comparison of long-term losartan versus propranolol in lowering portal pressure in cirrhosis. *Gastroenterology* 2001;121:382-388.

[172] Venon WD, Baronio M, Leone N, Rolfo E, Fadda M, Barletti C, Todros L, Saracco G, Rizzetto M. Effects of long-term Irbesartan in reducing portal pressure in cirrhotic patients: comparison with propranolol in a randomised controlled study. *J Hepatol* 2003;38:455-460.

[173] Reynaert H, Geerts A. Pharmacological rationale for the use of somatostatin and analogues in portal hypertension. *Aliment Pharmacol Ther* 2003;18:375-386.

[174] Fort J, Oberti F, Pilette C, Veal N, Gallois Y, Douay O, Rousselet MC, Rosenbaum J, Cales P. Antifibrotic and hemodynamic effects of the early and chronic administration of octreotide in two models of liver fibrosis in rats. *Hepatology* 1998;28:1525-1531.

[175] Mansy SS, Yehia HA, Hassan MM, Hassan EA, Youssef MM, Hadi AA, Mackenzie CD. Effect of octreotide on the pathology of hepatic schistosomiasis. *Arzneimittelforschung* 1998;48:855-861.

[176] Tracy TFJ, Tector AJ, Goerke ME, Kitchen S, Lagunoff D. Somatostatin analogue (octreotide) inhibits bile duct epithelial cell proliferation and fibrosis after extrahepatic biliary obstruction. *Am J Pathol* 1993;143:1574-1578.

[177] Reynaert H, Vaeyens F, Rombouts K, Hellemans K, Chatterjee N, Urbain D, Geerts A. Effect of Somatostatin-14 on Extracellular Matrix Expression by Activated Rat hepatic stellate cells. *J Hepatol* 2001;34 Suppl 1:6.

In: Hypertension: New Research
Editor: Elwood F. Benhagen, pp. 141-163
ISBN: 1-59454-204-X

Chapter V

REMODELING OF RESISTANCE ARTERIES IN HYPERTENSION

Hope D. I. Anderson
National Centre for Agri-Food Research in Medicine,
St. Boniface Hospital Research Centre
And Faculty of Pharmacy, University of Manitoba

ABSTRACT

During the pathogenesis of hypertension, blood pressure may rise as a result of genetic or environmental determinants of increased neurohumoral and hormonal drive. The incidental induction of growth and other processes such as oxidative stress, inflammation, mechanosensing, extracellular matrix components deposition and turnover, as well as apoptosis may contribute to vascular fibrosis and remodeling. Importantly, vascular remodeling may perpetuate a cycle in which blood pressure elevation is amplified to further drive these modulators of remodeling (for example, hypertension-induced inflammation). Oxidative stress or excess generation of reactive oxygen species has been described both in animal models of hypertension and in human essential hypertensive patients. Inflammation in the vascular wall likewise plays a major role in the pathogenesis of vascular disease. Vascular cells and inflammatory cells interact leading to increased expression of adhesion molecule, cytokines, chemokines, matrix metalloproteinases, and growth factors. Fibrosis also occurs, where extracellular matrix components such as collagen, elastin, and/or fibronectin accumulate in the vessel wall, whether by increased deposition or by reduced degradation via diminished matrix metalloproteinase/protease activity. Apoptosis or gene-regulated cell death also appears to be a modulator of hypertension-related resistance artery remodeling, whether increased or decreased in various tissues. The combined effect of all of these processes is remodeling of resistance arteries. Initially adaptive, resistance artery remodeling must be addressed therapeutically before it becomes maladaptive, compromises organ function, and contributes to the complications of hypertension. Understanding the mechanisms underlying vascular remodeling provides attractive therapeutic targets to this end.

INTRODUCTION

Hypertension is associated with increased risk of cardiovascular complications, including stroke, coronary artery disease, and congestive heart failure [1]. In developed countries such as the United States, more than 20 per cent of individuals have elevated blood pressure [2]. In general, the etiology of elevated blood pressure is not understood; only 5 per cent of cases have an identifiable cause [3], and the remaining cases are termed *essential hypertension.*

There is one parameter that is consistently abnormal in all forms of hypertension, and that is an augmentation of peripheral resistance [4]. Mean arterial pressure = cardiac output x total peripheral vascular resistance. By measuring intraluminal pressures, it is known that larger vessels contribute negligibly to peripheral resistance, whereas pressure drops significantly in the small "resistance" artery and arteriolar level of the vascular tree [5-7].

Currently, the evidence suggests that this increased peripheral resistance is due to narrowing of resistance arteries as well as rarefaction of arterioles (that is, a diminution in the number of arterioles) [8].

RESISTANCE ARTERIES

Resistance arteries consist of three layers: intima (innermost), media (middle), and adventitia (outermost). Endothelial cells of the intima line the arterial lumen as a monolayer of cells, and are adjacent to an internal elastic lamina that borders between the intima the media. The media consists of smooth muscle cells and connective tissue, whereas the adventitia contains extracellular matrix proteins, fibroblasts, and sympathetic nerves. In terms of resistance, diameter of the lumen is most relevant, contributing exponentially to the fourth power, according to Poiseuille's equation [8]. Lumen diameter is determined by the function (contractile state), mechanical properties (stiffness), and structure (lumen diameter and media thickness) of the artery. This chapter will focus on events taking place in the media of the vessel wall during the pathogenesis of hypertension, in particular remodeling of vascular structure. Though the endothelium may participate in some of these effects to an important degree, its contribution will only be addressed peripherally, and the reader is directed to the many reviews on the subject.

RESISTANCE ARTERY REMODELING IN HYPERTENSION

There are two types of remodeling which, to varying degrees and not exclusively from each other, resistance arteries undergo in the development of hypertension: eutrophic and hypertrophic [9]. In inward eutrophic remodeling, outer and lumen diameters are reduced, media cross-sectional area is unaltered, and media/lumen ratio is increased, in the absence of vascular stiffening. Eutrophic remodeling of resistance arteries is the predominant form in patients with mild essential hypertension [10, 11], as well as animal models of hypertension such as the spontaneously hypertensive rat (SHR) [12] and the 2-kidney, 1 clip Goldblatt rat [13]. In contrast, hypertrophic remodeling involves an increase in cross-sectional area of the media so that the growing media encroaches on the lumen to increase media/lumen ratio. Hypertrophic remodeling prevails in more severe forms of hypertension, including patients with secondary hypertension [14], deoxycorticosterone acetate (DOCA)-salt rats [15], 1-kidney, 1clip (1K1C) Goldblatt rats [16, 17], and Dahl salt-sensitive hypertensive rats [18].

OXIDATIVE STRESS

Enhanced Oxidative Stress in Hypertension

Overproduction of reactive oxygen species in the endothelium may contribute to vascular remodeling [19]. Indeed, overproduction of free radicals has been described both in animal models of hypertension and in human essential hypertensive patients (for review, see [20]). Augmented superoxide generation [21], particularly in the microvasculature [22, 23] was first reported in SHR, where introducing superoxide dismutase reduced blood pressure in SHR but not Wistar-Kyoto normotensive control rats [21]. Oxidative stress is also marked in the mesenteric microvasculature of the Dahl salt-sensitive hypertensive rat [24]. In humans, not only is oxidative stress enhanced in patients with essential hypertension [25], but it is also significantly increased in normotensive individuals with only a genetic predisposition or risk for development of hypertension [26].

Generation of Reactive Oxygen Species

Under normal conditions, approximately 5 per cent of the total amount of molecular oxygen consumed is used to generate superoxide anion, hydrogen peroxide, nitric oxide, and carbon monoxide [20]. Superoxide anion is generated through several enzyme systems including but not limited to reduced nicotinamide adenine dinucleotide (phosphate) (NAD(P)H) oxidase and xanthine oxidase [27, 28]. Since superoxide anion is purported to contribute to the development of vascular abnormalities in hypertension [29], it follows that treating hypertensive rats with a superoxide dismutase mimetic prevents vascular remodeling in stroke-prone SHR [30]. Furthermore, therapies that regress vascular hypertrophy also reduce oxidative stress in the vasculature, as shown with endothelin receptor blockade [31] or peroxisome proliferator-activated receptor-alpha and –gamma agonists [32] in DOCA-salt rats.

Superoxide anion might be exerting vascular effects through a variety of mechanisms. First, superoxide anion is critically involved in the breakdown of nitric oxide [33]. In addition to being a potent vasodilator [34-36], endogenous nitric oxide mediates anti-proliferative effects on vascular smooth muscle cells [37], inhibits platelet aggregation, and modulates leukocyte adhesion to the endothelium [38]. Thus, interference with nitric oxide bioavailability is thought to contribute to the vasomotor dysregulation, prothrombotic and hyperproliferative states that exist in the vasculature of patients with hypertension. In addition, the presence of unpaired electrons causes superoxide anion to be highly reactive, and when it reacts with nitric oxide, it generates peroxynitrite [39]. Peroxynitrite is a potent oxidant believed to be responsible for vascular injury via oxidation of proteins, DNA, and lipids in vascular cells [40].

In addition to quenching nitric oxide, superoxide anion may also serve as a substrate of other biologically active reactive oxygen species, and most notably, of hydrogen peroxide.

Hydrogen peroxide plays an important role in stimulating vascular smooth muscle proliferation [41] and hypertrophy [42].

i. Vascular NAD(P)H Oxidase

Vascular NAD(P)H oxidase is the most important source of superoxide anion in vascular cells [43-47], and it is known to contribute to the regulation of proliferation of vascular smooth muscle cells and to the onset of hypertension [46, 48].

NAD(P)H oxidase has been implicated in various rat models of hypertension, including angiotensin II-induced hypertension, DOCA-salt and renovascular hypertension, genetic models such as SHR or stroke-prone SHR, as well as in humans with essential hypertension [29]. With respect to angiotensin II-induced hypertension, angiotensin II has been shown specifically to elicit generation of superoxide anion in smooth muscle cells from resistance arteries of hypertensive patients via phospholipase D-dependent, NAD(P)H oxidase-sensitive pathways [49]. Furthermore, human vascular smooth muscle cells express a neutrophil-like NAD(P)H oxidase, wherein angiotensin II regulates the enzyme by inducing phosphorylation of p47phox, translocation of cytosolic subunits, and de novo protein synthesis [50]. These actions of angiotensin II appear to be dependent on activation of the p42/44 ERK-MAPK pathway activation [51], c-Src [52, 53], as well as epidermal growth factor receptor transactivation, phosphatidylinositol-3-kinase, and Rac [52], as delineated in vascular smooth muscle cells. Downstream from NAD(P)H oxidase activation, evidence exists to suggest that angiotensin II activates a number of signal transduction pathways, including for example, JNK and p38 MAPK activation [54], which may in turn contribute to the vascular remodeling process [55].

Increased superoxide anion production also occurs in DOCA-salt rats [56] and renovascular hypertension models such as the 2-kidney, 1-clip rat [57], and in both animal models, NAD(P)H oxidase activity has been implicated [58, 59]. Likewise, in SHR, superoxide anion generation is increased in arterioles [22], and introducing superoxide dismutase into the vessel wall normalizes blood pressure in these animals [21]. Upregulation of NAD(P)H oxidase and subsequent superoxide anion generation in SHR appears to be independent of high blood pressure per se but rather, overactivity of the renin-angiotensin system seems to play a critical role [48].

In humans with essential hypertension, NAD(P)H oxidase is a source of basal superoxide anion production in internal mammary arteries and saphenous veins, ostensibly from vascular smooth muscle cells [60]. The expression of NAD(P)H oxidase in these arteries in angiotensin II-dependent [60]; likewise, angiotensin II has been shown specifically in resistance arteries to elicit generation of superoxide in smooth muscle cells from subcutaneous resistance arteries of patients with hypertension [49]. It is not yet clear whether vascular NAD(P)H oxidase activity plays a role in human hypertension.

ii. Vascular Xanthine Oxidase

Xanthine oxidase (XO) represents an important candidate as a superoxide anion-producing system and has long been considered a critical player in the pathogenesis of reoxygenation-induced microvascular changes and tissue injury [61-64]. In the microvasculature, endothelial cells are the major source of the XO system [65], and in SHR, XO activity is significantly elevated vs. WKY rats, thereby contributing to reduced nitric oxide-dependent vasorelaxation of microvessels [66]. Superoxide anion formation in the microvasculature of Dahl hypertensive rats also involves XO activity [67], and thus it seems that XO-mediated superoxide generation may elevate vascular tone in these hypertensive models.

iii. Cytochrome P450s and the Heme Oxygenase-CO System

Cytochrome P450 monooxygenases also contribute significantly to elevation of vascular tone in hypertensive patients [68] through various mechanisms including generation of adrenocortical hormones (for example, aldosterone) [69], and vasoactive arachidonic acid metabolites (for example, hydroxyeicosatetraenoic acid (HETE)) [70-72].

Carbon monoxide, generated by heme oxygenase (HO), is likewise purported to be a modulator of vascular tone [73] and smooth muscle cell growth [74, 75]. There is contradictory evidence as to whether carbon monoxide overproduction diminishes or augments vascular resistance in hypertensives [20]. Upregulation of HO-1 suppresses hypertensive responses through the action of carbon monoxide [76, 77]. In contrast, carbon monoxide could serve as a partial antagonist for soluble guanylate cyclase, the enzyme targeted by nitric oxide. Indeed, induction of CO could interfere via competition with nitric oxide-mediated guanylate cyclase activation. Overexpression of HO-1 in vascular smooth muscle cells increases blood pressure and reduces sensitivity to exogenous nitro-based vasodilators [78].

INFLAMMATION

Inflammation in the vascular wall plays a major role in the pathogenesis of vascular disease [79]. Interactions between vascular cells and inflammatory cells (for example, neutrophils, lymphocytes, and monocytes) trigger inflammatory responses including increased expression of adhesion molecule, cytokines, chemokines, matrix metalloproteinases, and growth factors [80]. In the vasculature, NF-κB is a major signaling pathway involved in the inflammatory response [81]. Upon activation by various stimuli including cytokines and reactive oxygen species [81], NF-κB in turn upregulates adhesion molecules (for example, intercellular adhesion molecule 1 [ICAM-1] and vascular cell adhesion molecule 1 [VCAM-1]), cytokines (for example, tumor necrosis factor-alpha and interleukin 6), as well as the production of chemokines (for example, monocyte chemotactic protein 1 [MCP-1]) [81]. Vasoactive proteins such as angiotensin II [82] and endothelin-1 [83] invoke these inflammatory mechanisms and as such, can predispose to atherosclerosis [79]. In apparently healthy men, blood pressure level is associated with augmented circulating levels of ICAM-1 and interleukin 6 [84]. Furthermore, angiotensin II, the AT_1-angiotensin receptor subtype, and angiotensin converting enzyme colocalized with interleukin-6 in human coronary atherosclerotic plaques [85]. The involvement of angiotensin II (and endothelin-1) provides a link between hypertension and atherosclerosis.

It is also likely that inflammation plays a role in the process leading to hypertrophy and/or remodeling of small and large vessels in hypertension [86]. This is not unexpected since vascular inflammatory responses are in large part invoked by angiotensin II and endothelin-1, and both of these are well-known to mediate small artery hypertrophy and remodeling [18, 87-91].

i. Angiotensin II and Inflammation

Rats doubly transgenic for human renin and human angiotensinogen develop a malignant form of hypertension in which inflammatory mediators are activated, adhesion molecules are upregulated, and monocyte-macrophage infiltration is evident in the kidney and heart [92]. The actions of angiotensin II are mediated largely via stimulation of production of superoxide anion and, further downstream, activation of redox-sensitive genes [93]. Of the transcription factors activated by these reactive oxygen species, NF-κB clearly plays an important role [94-96]. Expression of adhesion molecules such as VCAM-1 is increased in aortae of angiotensin II-infused rats [97], and angiotensin II-induced VCAM-1 gene expression in vascular smooth muscle cells [97] and endothelial cells [98] is mediated by NF-κB. Likewise, angiotensin II-dependent augmentation of MCP-1 in vascular smooth muscle cells is attenuated by inhibition of NF-κB [99]. Such a role of NF-κB extends to human vascular smooth muscle cells as well, where angiotensin II stimulates interleukin-6 production, again in an NF-κB-dependent manner [94].

Investigating inflammatory responses has only recently extended to the microvasculature. However, Mervalla *et al.* [100] have reported increased expression of ICAM-1 and VCAM-1 in the interstitium, intima, and adventitia of renal small arteries in the double-transgenic rat carrying human renin and angiotensin genes. Angiotensin II-dependent inflammation in renal small arteries was also dependent on NF-κB [96] and can be observed in mesenteric resistance arteries, where angiotensin II infusion increases VCAM-1 and platelet endothelial cell adhesion molecule [101]. Further study is required to determine how large a contribution inflammatory pathways elicited by angiotensin II make in determining remodeling and hypertrophy of resistance arteries.

ii. Endothelin-1 and Inflammation

There exists overlap between angiotensin II and endothelin-1 with respect to generating vascular inflammation, which is not surprising since angiotensin II potently stimulates endothelin-1 synthesis [83]. As mentioned above, rats doubly transgenic for human renin and human angiotensinogen develop a malignant form of hypertension in which inflammatory mediators are activated, adhesion molecules are upregulated, and monocyte-macrophage infiltration is evident in the kidney and heart [92]. NF-κB and AP-1 activation, perivascular monocyte/macrophage infiltration, as well as upregulation of ICAM-1 and VCAM-1 in these rats were abrogated by blocking endothelin receptors [102]. These data implicate endothelin-1 as a downstream mediator of the inflammatory response invoked by angiotensin II.

In hypertensive patients, elevated levels of inflammatory markers such as MCP-1, soluble ICAM-1, and soluble VCAM-1 correlated with plasma endothelin-1 [103]. In the DOCA-salt hypertensive rat, increases in NF-κB and VCAM-1 are prevented by antagonizing endothelin receptors, albeit in the heart rather than vasculature [104]. These data suggest that endothelin-1 can activate NF-κB and thereby perhaps, increase expression of cytokine and adhesion molecules. Indeed, in human vascular smooth muscle cells, endothelin-1 activation of ET_A-endothelin receptors does trigger release of interleukin-6 via NF-κB [105]. Again, further study is required to determine the combined role of endothelin-1 and inflammation in determining remodeling and hypertrophy of resistance arteries.

MECHANOSENSING

Intraluminal pressure is linked to both hypertrophic and eutrophic remodeling. Protecting a vascular bed from a rise in pressure will prevent changes in vessel structure as observed in resistance arteries from SHR [106]. Reversing blood pressure elevation in 1K1C rats reverses small artery hypertrophy [107]. Current data thus support the hypothesis that increased pressure, through an increase in circumferential wall stress, can account for both hypertrophy and inward, eutrophic remodeling [108].

i. Focal Adhesion Sites

Vascular smooth muscles are attached to the surrounding extracellular matrix via integrins (for review on integrins, see [109]). Whereas mechanical strain of rat vascular smooth muscle cells induced mitogenesis, inhibiting integrins with arginine-glycine-aspartic acid (RGD) peptides abrogated this strain response [110]. The extracellular domain of integrins determines binding specificity to matrix proteins such as collagen, laminin, or fibronectin, which in turn, influence integrin signaling. For example, fibronectin promoted a mitogenic response whereas laminin increased expression of smooth muscle-specific myosin [111]. In some systems, mechanical strain can lead to activation of mitogen-activated protein kinases (MAPKs), extracellular signaling-regulated kinase (Erk1/2), and c-Jun N-terminal kinase (JNK) in an RGD-sensitive manner [112]. Growth responses in response to mechanical stimuli often result from recruitment and activation of focal adhesion kinase (FAK), Src, and downstream cascades (i.e. MAPKs) [113, 114]. Interestingly, in SHR, expression of $\alpha_v\beta_3$ and $\alpha_5\beta_1$ integrins was increased in SHR aged 20 versus 6 weeks. Expression of $\alpha_5\beta_1$ integrins was lower in young SHR, and $\alpha_v\beta_3$ integrins were overexpressed in adult SHR versus WKY rats [115].

ii. Wall Stress

As pressure rises in resistance arteries, myogenic tone opposes the stretch of the vascular wall [116], so that an increase in myogenic tone results in lesser wall stress (defined as rP/WT, where r is the blood vessel radius, P is the transmural pressure, and WT is the wall thickness). Thus, remodeling serves the purpose, where hypertrophy thickens the vessel wall or the media/lumen ratio is increased, to normalize wall stress in the presence of augmented intraluminal pressure. In the absence of a hypertrophic stimulus, resistance arteries may turn over matrix and reform focal adhesion sites to achieve inward eutrophic remodeling [108]. Genes relative to remodeling are certainly invoked by mechanical stimuli. In mesenteric resistance arteries, proto-oncogene expression correlated with wall stress, and in the presence of stress-reducing myogenic responses, pressure-induced expression of c-myc was invoked to a lesser degree [117].

Extracellular Matrix Proteins

Fibrillar extracellular matrix in the vascular wall is comprised of structural proteins (collagen and elastin) and adhesive proteins (for example, laminin and fibronectin). Collagens and elastin are the major protein constituents of blood vessels.

i. Collagen

The basic unit of fibrillar collagens is the 300 nm triple helix, with each chain comprised of about 330 repeats of the amino acid sequence –Gly-X-Y-, where X is often proline and Y is often hydroxyproline. After secretion in the extracellular compartment and removal of N- and C-propeptides, collagen triple helices aggregate in fibrils [118].

There are 19 collagen types known to date. Collagens I and III respectively represent 60 per cent and 30 per cent of vascular collagen [119-121]. The remaining 10 per cent include fibrillar collagen V, fibril-associated collagens with interrupted triple helix types XII and XIV, microfibrillar collagen VI, basement membrane collagen IV, and collagen VIII [118]. In normal arteries, fibrillar collagens I and III are major constituents of the intima, media, and adventitia, whereas types I, III, IV, and V are in endothelial and smooth muscle cell basement membranes [122].

Hypertension-related vascular fibrosis involves deposition and/or accumulation of extracellular matrix proteins in the arterial wall. Collagen is the extracellular fibrillar component that may alter passive pressure/diameter relationships of arteries and induce progressive vascular stiffening [123]. Collagen synthesis is increased in SHR and DOCA-salt rats throughout the vascular bed including their aortae, mesenteric arteries, cerebral microvessels, pial arteries, and basilar arteries [124, 125]. The degree of total collagen accumulation that results following synthesis may be bed-specific, however; it occurs in coronary arteries [126] but less consistently in aortae from SHR [127], stroke-prone SHR [128], and DOCA-salt rats [129]. Despite a lack of obvious change in total collagen, modulation of collagen types is observable. In Japanese and Lyon SHR strains, collagen III but not collagen I is increased in aortae [130], and in stroke-prone SHR, collagens I, III, and IV were upregulated in aortae and mesenteric arteries [131].

With respect to resistance arteries, collagen is increased in SHR mesenteric resistance arteries [115, 132] and notably, in subcutaneous resistance arteries from essential hypertensive humans [133]. In these patients, we surprisingly found that increased collagen deposition was associated with reduced, rather than increased stiffness [133]. These findings suggested that it is not the amount of collagen in the vessel wall but rather the recruitment of collagen fibers and possibly changes in extracellular matrix-smooth muscle anchoring [122] that result in increased stiffness of the vessel wall at higher pressures.

A major modulator of collagen synthesis is angiotensin II. By acting at both AT_1-[134-136] and AT_2-angiotensin receptors [137, 138], it stimulates production of collagen I in human vascular smooth muscle cells [136] at least in part via activation of the MAPK/ERK pathway [139]. Angiotensin II also invokes the involvement of other growth factors such as platelet-derived growth factor, transforming growth factor-β (TGF-β), insulin-like growth factor, and basic fibroblast growth factor [140]. Mechanical strain of vascular smooth muscle cells increased angiotensin II which resulted in TGF-β generation. In turn, TGF-β clearly stimulates collagen synthesis, which is inhibited by TGF-β neutralizing antibody or truncated TGF-β type II receptor [141]. This suggests a linear pathway in which angiotensin II stimulates TGF-β, which then triggers collagen synthesis. Indeed, exogenous TGF-β results in augmented collagen synthesis [141].

Endothelin is also linked to angiotensin II-dependent collagen synthesis. Activation of the collagen I-α^2 chain promoter by angiotensin was attenuated by antagonizing endothelin receptors [142], and collagen I synthesis can be directly stimulated by exogenous endothelin-1 in coronary artery smooth muscle cells [143]. Interplay between endothelin and aldosterone may be involved, too. Aortic collagen accumulation is inhibited by antagonizing aldosterone [144] and in aldosterone-infused rats, arterial collagen deposition is prevented by antagonism of endothelin receptors [145].

ii. Elastin

As mentioned above, in resistance arteries, elastin is found in the internal and external elastic lamina and represents 90 per cent of elastic fibers. Cross-linking of the elastin precursor, tropoelastin, results from the condensation of two or three lysine/allysine residues [146], and it is this process that gives renders elastin "elastic." The total amount of elastin is reportedly unchanged in resistance arteries from hypertensive rats [115, 147] and essential hypertensive patients [133]. Indeed, in mesenteric resistance arteries from SHR, redistribution of elastin within the internal elastic lamina led to smaller fenestrae but no change in fenestrae number or elastin amount. However, incubation with elastase abolished all the structural and mechanical differences between strains, demonstrating that elastin plays a critical role in determining vascular dimensions and mechanical properties in a resistance artery, but this role is not dependent on absolute elastin quantity [148].

iii. Other Proteins

Other structural glycoproteins are integral to the extracellular matrix structure and function in the arterial wall. These include, though not exclusively, fibronectin, laminin, vitronectin, thrombospondin, and tenascin [118].

Fibronectin deposition or expression is certainly increased in large arteries of hypertensive rats, including aortae from SHR [127] and Dahl salt-sensitive rats [134, 149] as well as carotid arteries from SHR [150] and stroke-prone SHR [151]. It is also augmented in resistance arteries of the aldosterone-infused rat model of hypertension [152]. This increase in fibronectin deposition has been linked to upregulation of α_5-integrins [115, 127], at least in SHR. This suggests that fibronectin matrix assembly, which requires the interaction between the RGD site of fibronectin and α_5-integrins [153], is also elevated in SHR vessels.

Smooth muscle cell growth in the arterial wall media may be facilitated by various extracellular proteins. For example, tenascin-C is an extracellular matrix glycoprotein that acts as a ligand for $\alpha_5\beta_3$ integrins. Co localizing with proliferating smooth muscle cells in SHR [154], tenascin-C may serve as a survival factor that protects from apoptosis but promotes proliferation. Another RGD-containing protein associated with smooth muscle cell proliferation is osteopontin [155], which is a ligand for $\alpha_v\beta_3$ integrins [156]. In the angiotensin-infused rat model of hypertension, marked smooth muscle cell expression of osteopontin, along with that of elastin, was observed [157], where it may mediate proliferation.

Extracellular Matrix Proteinases and Inhibitors

In the adult, under normal conditions, turnover of collagen and elastic fibers is slow [158]. Turnover (that is, degradation and/or fragmentation of fibers) may increase in cases where vascular disease presents. Enzymes that degrade collagen are mainly matrix metalloproteinases (MMPs). There are also elastinolytic enzymes, which are comprised of all four classes of proteinases (serine, metallo-, aspartic, and cysteine proteases) [159, 160]. At present, only matrix metalloproteinases and serine proteinases are known to participate in vascular extracellular matrix remodeling [118].

i. Matrix Metalloproteinases

Matrix metalloproteinases are Zn^{2+} and Ca^{2+}-dependent proteolytic enzymes that degrade extracellular matrix proteins and in particular, collagens [161, 162]. Several MMPs are present in the vasculature, either under basal or induced conditions. These include collagenases (interstitial collagenase MMP-1 and MMP-3) that digest structural or fibrillar collagens (types I to III), subendothelial basement membrane gelatinases (MMP-2 and MMP-9) that digest denatured collagen (gelatin) and collagen types IV and V, elastases (MMP-7 and MMP-12), stromelysins (MMP-3) that digest adhesive molecules such as laminin, fibronectin, nonfibrillar collagens and proteoglycans, and finally, membrane type MMPs (MT-MMPs) [118, 123].

MMP activity is tightly regulated by (a) MMP gene expression and protein secretion levels, (b) activation of the inactive pro-enzyme, and (c) inhibition by tissue inhibitors of matrix metalloproteinases (TIMPs). Actually, the two latter mechanisms, activation of MMPs and inhibition by TIMPs appear to play a more crucial role than MMP gene expression [118, 163, 164]. Indeed, even though proMMP-2 is constitutively expressed in the normal arterial wall, no smooth muscle migration or elastin degradation is detectable [118].

MMP-mediated modulation of extracellular matrix could result in cytoskeletal reorganization and vascular remodeling in hypertension. In serum from SHR [165,166] and essential hypertensive patients [167], enhanced synthesis of collagen I was not balanced by its degradation; in fact, serum concentrations of MMP-1 were reduced in hypertensive patients [168], as was MMP-1 activity in young SHR prior to elevation of blood pressure [169]. Interestingly, in patients with essential hypertension, not only is serum MMP-1 reduced, but TIMP-1 is also increased [168], suggesting a shift toward inhibiting degradative capacity. MMP-3 activity was also diminished [169], which may promote accumulation of fibronectin and proteoglycans in SHR [170, 171]. Pro-MMP-2 and activated MMP-2 activities were reduced in mesenteric arteries from adult SHR [169], which could facilitate accumulation of types IV and V collagen and fibronectin [131]. In untreated essential hypertensive patients, plasma concentrations of active MMP-2 and MMP-9, mainly related to vascular extracellular matrix metabolism, are depressed. Furthermore, six-month treatment with amlodipine normalized MMP-9 but not MMP-2 plasma concentrations [172]. These data suggest that changes in MMP activity may contribute to resistance artery remodeling in hypertension by modulating vascular extracellular matrix. This requires further study, however.

Apoptosis

Inward eutrophic remodeling, in which outer and lumen diameters are reduced, media cross-sectional is unaltered, and media/lumen ratio is increased in the absence of vascular stiffening predominates in some forms of hypertension including mild essential hypertensive patients [10]. Since media cross-sectional area is unchanged, this raises the possibility that media growth may be compensated for by apoptosis. Apoptosis, defined as gene-regulated cell death, was first recognized as a developmental mechanism to refine growth processes [173].

Apoptosis is invoked during the pathogenesis of cardiovascular disease. In hypertensive rats, its occurrence has been reported to varying degrees in the heart [174-176], brain [174], kidney [174, 177], and arteries [178, 179]. In large arteries, particularly aortae, apoptosis has been detected in DOCA-salt rats [180], SHR [181], and angiotensin-infused rats [182]. Aortic vascular smooth muscle cells appear to be more vulnerable to apoptotic processes in hypertensive rats versus cells from their normotensive counterparts [183].

In resistance arteries, apoptosis (whether enhanced or diminished) may also be a modulator of vascular structure, but in an age- and bed-specific manner. Apoptosis is actually reduced in young SHR suggesting that reduced cell death may contribute to the apparent growth of the vascular wall [184]. By the age of 8 and 12 weeks, however, SHR not only exhibit increases in blood pressure and small artery media/lumen ratios, but also an increase in apoptosis [185]. Apoptosis is not globally increased and is in fact reduced in small myocardial arteries [186], whereas it is enhanced in arterioles and capillaries, suggesting that apoptosis may also influence vascular resistance via rarefaction.

Though the role of apoptosis in resistance artery remodeling remains to be clarified, its modulators are common to that of remodeling. Candidates include, though not exclusively, reactive oxygen species [187], angiotensin [188], and endothelin [189]. Angiotensin II infusion increases apoptotic rate in aortae [182], and in SHR, blockade of AT_1-angiotensin receptors augments vascular smooth muscle apoptosis via activation of AT_2-angiotensin receptors [190]. Likewise, exogenous endothelin-1 induces apoptosis via ET_B receptors [189], whereas there is some evidence that ET_A receptors may mediate anti-apoptotic effects [179].

Regression of vascular remodeling by anti-hypertensive therapy may involve induction of apoptosis. The mechanisms involved appear to be more complex than mere blood pressure-lowering, since hydralazine has no effect on apoptotic rate of vascular smooth muscle cells in SHR thoracic aortae, as opposed to the stimulatory actions of ACE inhibition, AT_1-angiotensin receptor antagonism and Ca^{2+} channel blockers [191]. Ca^{2+} channel blockers such as nifedipine, amlodipine, or verapamil stimulate apoptosis of smooth muscle cells [181, 192, 193], either in thoracic aortae or coronary arteries. There are data suggesting that therapeutically-induced apoptosis occurs in waves [179, 190, 191]. Other studies, however, have shown continuous elevations in apoptotic rates, persisting through 12 weeks of treatment with enalapril and amlodipine [181, 191] and 16 weeks with quinapril [194]. ET_A-selective endothelin receptor antagonism also enhances apoptosis in aortae of an endothelin-dependent rat model of hypertension (DOCA-salt rat) where hypertrophic remodeling predominates [180]. The effects of anti-hypertensive therapy on apoptotic rates in resistance arteries, rather than large arteries, remains to be clarified.

Concluding Remarks

Vascular remodeling impacts peripheral resistance to blood flow. Thus, it plays an important role in contributing to the pathogenesis, maintenance, and complications of hypertension. Evidence suggests that in addition to growth per se, other processes influence the degree of remodeling that occurs, including oxidative stress, inflammation, mechanosensing, extracellular matrix components and turnover, as well as apoptosis. Remodeling resulting from these processes may initially be compensatory (for example, to chronic vasoconstriction) but with time, becomes maladaptive. The end result is compromised organ function and the complications normally associated with hypertension. Research is ongoing to target each of these processes therapeutically.

Acknowledgements

Dr. Anderson is a recipient of a Senior Fellowship (Phase 2) from the Canadian Institutes of Health Research.

References

[1] 1997 The sixth report of the Joint National Committee on prevention, detection, evaluation, and treatment of high blood pressure. *Arch Intern Med* 157:2413-46

[2] Burt VL, Whelton P, Roccella EJ, et al. 1995 Prevalence of hypertension in the US adult population. Results from the Third National Health and Nutrition Examination Survey, 1988-1991. *Hypertension* 25:305-13

[3] Lever AF SJ 1994 Investigating the hypetensive patient: an overview. In: JD S (ed) *Textbook of hypertension.* Blackwell Scientific Publications, Oxford, pp 1026-1030

[4] Mulvany MJ 2002 Small artery remodeling and significance in the development of hypertension. *News Physiol Sci* 17:105-9

[5] DeLano FA, Schmid-Schonbein GW, Skalak TC, Zweifach BW 1991 Penetration of the systemic blood pressure into the microvasculature of rat skeletal muscle. *Microvasc Res* 41:92-110

[6] Folkow B 1989 The Benjamin W. Zweifach Award lecture. Functional and structural "autoregulation"--some personal considerations concerning the century-old development of these microvascular concepts. *Microvasc Res* 37:242-55

[7] Schiffrin EL, Thibault G 1991 Plasma endothelin in human essential hypertension. Am *J Hypertens* 4:303-8

[8] Mulvany MJ 2002 Small artery remodeling in hypertension. *Curr Hypertens Rep* 4:49-55

[9] Mulvany MJ, Baumbach GL, Aalkjaer C, et al. 1996 Vascular remodeling. *Hypertension* 28:505-6

[10] Korsgaard N, Aalkjaer C, Heagerty AM, Izzard AS, Mulvany MJ 1993 Histology of subcutaneous small arteries from patients with essential hypertension. *Hypertension* 22:523-6

[11] Schiffrin EL, Deng LY, Larochelle P 1993 Morphology of resistance arteries and comparison of effects of vasoconstrictors in mild essential hypertensive patients. *Clin Invest Med* 16:177-86

[12] Deng LY, Schiffrin EL 1992 Effects of endothelin-1 and vasopressin on resistance arteries of spontaneously hypertensive rats. *Am J Hypertens* 5:817-22

[13] Li JS, Knafo L, Turgeon A, Garcia R, Schiffrin EL 1996 Effect of endothelin antagonism on blood pressure and vascular structure in renovascular hypertensive rats. *Am J Physiol* 271:H88-93

[14] Rizzoni D, Porteri E, Castellano M, et al. 1996 Vascular hypertrophy and remodeling in secondary hypertension. *Hypertension* 28:785-90

[15] Deng LY, Schiffrin EL 1992 Effects of endothelin on resistance arteries of DOCA-salt hypertensive rats. *Am J Physiol* 262:H1782-7

[16] Korsgaard N, Mulvany MJ 1988 Cellular hypertrophy in mesenteric resistance vessels from renal hypertensive rats. *Hypertension* 12:162-7

[17] Deng LY, Schiffrin EL 1991 Morphological and functional alterations of mesenteric small resistance arteries in early renal hypertension in rats. *Am J Physiol* 261:H1171-7

[18] d'Uscio LV, Barton M, Shaw S, Moreau P, Luscher TF 1997 Structure and function of small arteries in salt-induced hypertension: effects of chronic endothelin-subtype-A-receptor blockade. *Hypertension* 30:905-11

[19] Griendling KK, Sorescu D, Lassegue B, Ushio-Fukai M 2000 Modulation of protein kinase activity and gene expression by reactive oxygen species and their role in vascular physiology and pathophysiology. *Arterioscler Thromb Vasc Biol* 20:2175-83

[20] Suematsu M, Suzuki H, Delano FA, Schmid-Schonbein GW 2002 The inflammatory aspect of the microcirculation in hypertension: oxidative stress, leukocytes/endothelial interaction, apoptosis. *Microcirculation* 9:259-76

[21] Nakazono K, Watanabe N, Matsuno K, Sasaki J, Sato T, Inoue M 1991 Does superoxide underlie the pathogenesis of hypertension? Proc Natl Acad Sci U S A 88:10045-8

[22] Suzuki H, Swei A, Zweifach BW, Schmid-Schonbein GW 1995 In vivo evidence for microvascular oxidative stress in spontaneously hypertensive rats. Hydroethidine microfluorography. *Hypertension* 25:1083-9

[23] Suzuki H, Zweifach BW, Forrest MJ, Schmid-Schonbein GW 1995 Modification of leukocyte adhesion in spontaneously hypertensive rats by adrenal corticosteroids. *J Leukoc Biol* 57:20-6

[24] Swei A, Lacy F, DeLano FA, Schmid-Schonbein GW 1997 Oxidative stress in the Dahl hypertensive rat. *Hypertension* 30:1628-33

[25] Lacy F, Kailasam MT, O'Connor DT, Schmid-Schonbein GW, Parmer RJ 2000 Plasma hydrogen peroxide production in human essential hypertension: role of heredity, gender, and ethnicity. *Hypertension* 36:878-84

[26] Lacy F, O'Connor DT, Schmid-Schonbein GW 1998 Plasma hydrogen peroxide production in hypertensives and normotensive subjects at genetic risk of hypertension. *J Hypertens* 16:291-303

[27] Babior BM 1999 NADPH oxidase: an update. *Blood* 93:1464-76

[28] Parks DA, Granger DN 1986 Xanthine oxidase: biochemistry, distribution and physiology. *Acta Physiol Scand Suppl* 548:87-99

[29] Zalba G, San Jose G, Moreno MU, et al. 2001 Oxidative stress in arterial hypertension: role of NAD(P)H oxidase. *Hypertension* 38:1395-9

[30] Park JB, Touyz RM, Chen X, Schiffrin EL 2002 Chronic treatment with a superoxide dismutase mimetic prevents vascular remodeling and progression of hypertension in salt-loaded stroke-prone spontaneously hypertensive rats. *Am J Hypertens* 15:78-84

[31] Callera GE, Touyz RM, Teixeira SA, et al. 2003 ETA receptor blockade decreases vascular superoxide generation in DOCA-salt hypertension. *Hypertension* 42:811-7

[32] Iglarz M, Touyz RM, Amiri F, Lavoie MF, Diep QN, Schiffrin EL 2003 Effect of peroxisome proliferator-activated receptor-alpha and -gamma activators on vascular remodeling in endothelin-dependent hypertension. *Arterioscler Thromb Vasc Biol* 23:45-51

[33] Gryglewski RJ, Palmer RM, Moncada S 1986 Superoxide anion is involved in the breakdown of endothelium-derived vascular relaxing factor. *Nature* 320:454-6

[34] Griffith TM, Edwards DH, Davies RL, Harrison TJ, Evans KT 1987 EDRF coordinates the behaviour of vascular resistance vessels. *Nature* 329:442-5

[35] Furchgott RF, Carvalho MH, Khan MT, Matsunaga K 1987 Evidence for endothelium-dependent vasodilation of resistance vessels by acetylcholine. *Blood Vessels* 24:145-9

[36] Palmer RM, Ferrige AG, Moncada S 1987 Nitric oxide release accounts for the biological activity of endothelium-derived relaxing factor. *Nature* 327:524-6

[37] Garg UC, Hassid A 1989 Nitric oxide-generating vasodilators and 8-bromo-cyclic guanosine monophosphate inhibit mitogenesis and proliferation of cultured rat vascular smooth muscle cells. *J Clin Invest* 83:1774-7

[38] Kubes P, Suzuki M, Granger DN 1991 Nitric oxide: an endogenous modulator of leukocyte adhesion. *Proc Natl Acad Sci U S A* 88:4651-5

[39] Beckman JS, Beckman TW, Chen J, Marshall PA, Freeman BA 1990 Apparent hydroxyl radical production by peroxynitrite: implications for endothelial injury from nitric oxide and superoxide. *Proc Natl Acad Sci U S A* 87:1620-4

[40] Ballinger SW, Patterson C, Yan CN, et al. 2000 Hydrogen peroxide- and peroxynitrite-induced mitochondrial DNA damage and dysfunction in vascular endothelial and smooth muscle cells. *Circ Res* 86:960-6

[41] Ushio-Fukai M, Alexander RW, Akers M, Griendling KK 1998 p38 Mitogen-activated protein kinase is a critical component of the redox-sensitive signaling pathways activated by angiotensin II. Role in vascular smooth muscle cell hypertrophy. *J Biol Chem* 273:15022-9

[42] Zafari AM, Ushio-Fukai M, Akers M, et al. 1998 Role of NADH/NADPH oxidase-derived H2O2 in angiotensin II-induced vascular hypertrophy. *Hypertension* 32:488-95

[43] Mohazzab KM, Kaminski PM, Wolin MS 1994 NADH oxidoreductase is a major source of superoxide anion in bovine coronary artery endothelium. *Am J Physiol* 266:H2568-72

[44] Pagano PJ, Ito Y, Tornheim K, Gallop PM, Tauber AI, Cohen RA 1995 An NADPH oxidase superoxide-generating system in the rabbit aorta. *Am J Physiol* 268:H2274-80

[45] Jones SA, O'Donnell VB, Wood JD, Broughton JP, Hughes EJ, Jones OT 1996 Expression of phagocyte NADPH oxidase components in human endothelial cells. *Am J Physiol* 271:H1626-34

[46] Griendling KK, Minieri CA, Ollerenshaw JD, Alexander RW 1994 Angiotensin II stimulates NADH and NADPH oxidase activity in cultured vascular smooth muscle cells. *Circ Res* 74:1141-8

[47] Sorescu D, Somers MJ, Lassegue B, Grant S, Harrison DG, Griendling KK 2001 Electron spin resonance characterization of the NAD(P)H oxidase in vascular smooth muscle cells. *Free Radic Biol Med* 30:603-12

[48] Zalba G, Beaumont FJ, San Jose G, et al. 2000 Vascular NADH/NADPH oxidase is involved in enhanced superoxide production in spontaneously hypertensive rats. *Hypertension* 35:1055-61

[49] Touyz RM, Schiffrin EL 2001 Increased generation of superoxide by angiotensin II in smooth muscle cells from resistance arteries of hypertensive patients: role of phospholipase D-dependent NAD(P)H oxidase-sensitive pathways. *J Hypertens* 19:1245-54

[50] Touyz RM, Chen X, Tabet F, et al. 2002 Expression of a functionally active gp91phox-containing neutrophil-type NAD(P)H oxidase in smooth muscle cells from human resistance arteries: regulation by angiotensin II. *Circ Res* 90:1205-13

[51] Laplante MA, Wu R, El Midaoui A, de Champlain J 2003 NAD(P)H oxidase activation by angiotensin II is dependent on p42/44 ERK-MAPK pathway activation in rat's vascular smooth muscle cells. *J Hypertens* 21:927-36

[52] Seshiah PN, Weber DS, Rocic P, Valppu L, Taniyama Y, Griendling KK 2002 Angiotensin II stimulation of NAD(P)H oxidase activity: upstream mediators. *Circ Res* 91:406-13

[53] Touyz RM, Yao G, Schiffrin EL 2003 c-Src Induces Phosphorylation and Translocation of p47phox: Role in Superoxide Generation by Angiotensin II in Human Vascular Smooth Muscle Cells. *Arterioscler Thromb Vasc Biol* 23:981-7

[54] Viedt C, Soto U, Krieger-Brauer HI, et al. 2000 Differential activation of mitogen-activated protein kinases in smooth muscle cells by angiotensin II: involvement of p22phox and reactive oxygen species. *Arterioscler Thromb Vasc Biol* 20:940-8

[55] Kim S, Iwao H 2003 Stress and vascular responses: mitogen-activated protein kinases and activator protein-1 as promising therapeutic targets of vascular remodeling. *J Pharmacol Sci* 91:177-81

[56] Somers MJ, Mavromatis K, Galis ZS, Harrison DG 2000 Vascular superoxide production and vasomotor function in hypertension induced by deoxycorticosterone acetate-salt. *Circulation* 101:1722-8

[57] Ploth DW 1983 Angiotensin-dependent renal mechanisms in two-kidney, one-clip renal vascular hypertension. *Am J Physiol* 245:F131-41

[58] Wu R, Millette E, Wu L, de Champlain J 2001 Enhanced superoxide anion formation in vascular tissues from spontaneously hypertensive and desoxycorticosterone acetate-salt hypertensive rats. *J Hypertens* 19:741-8

[59] Heitzer T, Wenzel U, Hink U, et al. 1999 Increased NAD(P)H oxidase-mediated superoxide production in renovascular hypertension: evidence for an involvement of protein kinase C. *Kidney Int* 55:252-60
[60] Berry C, Hamilton CA, Brosnan MJ, et al. 2000 Investigation into the sources of superoxide in human blood vessels: angiotensin II increases superoxide production in human internal mammary arteries. Circulation 101:2206-12
[61] Granger DN, Rutili G, McCord JM 1981 Superoxide radicals in feline intestinal ischemia. *Gastroenterology* 81:22-9
[62] Parks DA, Bulkley GB, Granger DN, Hamilton SR, McCord JM 1982 Ischemic injury in the cat small intestine: role of superoxide radicals. *Gastroenterology* 82:9-15
[63] Suematsu M, DeLano FA, Poole D, et al. 1994 Spatial and temporal correlation between leukocyte behavior and cell injury in postischemic rat skeletal muscle microcirculation. *Lab Invest* 70:684-95
[64] Suzuki H, Poole DC, Zweifach BW, Schmid-Schonbein GW 1995 Temporal correlation between maximum tetanic force and cell death in postischemic rat skeletal muscle. *J Clin Invest* 96:2892-7
[65] Jarasch ED, Bruder G, Heid HW 1986 Significance of xanthine oxidase in capillary endothelial cells. *Acta Physiol Scand Suppl* 548:39-46
[66] Suzuki H, DeLano FA, Parks DA, et al. 1998 Xanthine oxidase activity associated with arterial blood pressure in spontaneously hypertensive rats. *Proc Natl Acad Sci U S A* 95:4754-9
[67] Swei A, Lacy F, Delano FA, Parks DA, Schmid-Schonbein GW 1999 A mechanism of oxygen free radical production in the Dahl hypertensive rat. *Microcirculation* 6:179-87
[68] Fleming I 2001 Cytochrome p450 and vascular homeostasis. *Circ Res* 89:753-62
[69] Suzuki H, Zweifach BW, Schmid-Schonbein GW 1995 Dependence of elevated mesenteric arteriolar tone on glucocorticoids in spontaneously hypertensive rats. *Int J Microcirc Clin Exp* 15:309-15
[70] Roman RJ 2002 P-450 metabolites of arachidonic acid in the control of cardiovascular function. *Physiol Rev* 82:131-85
[71] Sacerdoti D, Escalante B, Abraham NG, McGiff JC, Levere RD, Schwartzman ML 1989 Treatment with tin prevents the development of hypertension in spontaneously hypertensive rats. *Science* 243:388-90
[72] Levere RD, Martasek P, Escalante B, Schwartzman ML, Abraham NG 1990 Effect of heme arginate administration on blood pressure in spontaneously hypertensive rats. *J Clin Invest* 86:213-9
[73] Goda N, Suzuki K, Naito M, et al. 1998 Distribution of heme oxygenase isoforms in rat liver. Topographic basis for carbon monoxide-mediated microvascular relaxation. *J Clin Invest* 101:604-12
[74] Morita T, Mitsialis SA, Koike H, Liu Y, Kourembanas S 1997 Carbon monoxide controls the proliferation of hypoxic vascular smooth muscle cells. *J Biol Chem* 272:32804-9
[75] Suematsu M, Goda N, Sano T, et al. 1995 Carbon monoxide: an endogenous modulator of sinusoidal tone in the perfused rat liver. *J Clin Invest* 96:2431-7
[76] Motterlini R, Gonzales A, Foresti R, Clark JE, Green CJ, Winslow RM 1998 Heme oxygenase-1-derived carbon monoxide contributes to the suppression of acute hypertensive responses in vivo. *Circ Res* 83:568-77

[77] Wakabayashi Y, Takamiya R, Mizuki A, et al. 1999 Carbon monoxide overproduced by heme oxygenase-1 causes a reduction of vascular resistance in perfused rat liver. *Am J Physiol* 277:G1088-96
[78] Imai T, Morita T, Shindo T, et al. 2001 Vascular smooth muscle cell-directed overexpression of heme oxygenase-1 elevates blood pressure through attenuation of nitric oxide-induced vasodilation in mice. *Circ Res* 89:55-62
[79] Virdis A, Schiffrin EL 2003 Vascular inflammation: a role in vascular disease in hypertension? *Curr Opin Nephrol Hypertens* 12:181-7
[80] Ross R 1999 Atherosclerosis--an inflammatory disease. *N Engl J Med* 340:115-26
[81] Barnes PJ, Karin M 1997 Nuclear factor-kappaB: a pivotal transcription factor in chronic inflammatory diseases. *N Engl J Med* 336:1066-71
[82] Dzau VJ 2001 Theodore Cooper Lecture: Tissue angiotensin and pathobiology of vascular disease: a unifying hypothesis. *Hypertension* 37:1047-52
[83] Schiffrin EL 2001 Role of endothelin-1 in hypertension and vascular disease. *Am J Hypertens* 14:83S-89S
[84] Chae CU, Lee RT, Rifai N, Ridker PM 2001 Blood pressure and inflammation in apparently healthy men. *Hypertension* 38:399-403
[85] Schieffer B, Schieffer E, Hilfiker-Kleiner D, et al. 2000 Expression of angiotensin II and interleukin 6 in human coronary atherosclerotic plaques: potential implications for inflammation and plaque instability. *Circulation* 101:1372-8
[86] Shekhonin BV, Domogatsky SP, Muzykantov VR, Idelson GL, Rukosuev VS 1985 Distribution of type I, III, IV and V collagen in normal and atherosclerotic human arterial wall: immunomorphological characteristics. *Coll Relat Res* 5:355-68
[87] Schiffrin EL, Lariviere R, Li JS, Sventek P, Touyz RM 1995 Enhanced expression of endothelin-1 gene may cause blood pressure-independent vascular hypertrophy. *J Cardiovasc Pharmacol* 26 Suppl 3:S5-8
[88] Intengan HD, Schiffrin EL 1998 Mechanical properties of mesenteric resistance arteries from Dahl salt-resistant and salt-sensitive rats: role of endothelin-1. *J Hypertens* 16:1907-12
[89] Park JB, Schiffrin EL 2001 ET(A) receptor antagonist prevents blood pressure elevation and vascular remodeling in aldosterone-infused rats. *Hypertension* 37:1444-9
[90] Li JS, Sharifi AM, Schiffrin EL 1997 Effect of AT1 angiotensin-receptor blockade on structure and function of small arteries in SHR. *J Cardiovasc Pharmacol* 30:75-83
[91] Rizzoni D, Porteri E, Guefi D, et al. 2000 Cellular hypertrophy in subcutaneous small arteries of patients with renovascular hypertension. *Hypertension* 35:931-5
[92] Luft FC, Mervaala E, Muller DN, et al. 1999 Hypertension-induced end-organ damage : A new transgenic approach to an old problem. *Hypertension* 33:212-8
[93] Griendling KK, Ushio-Fukai M 2000 Reactive oxygen species as mediators of angiotensin II signaling. *Regul Pept* 91:21-7
[94] Kranzhofer R, Schmidt J, Pfeiffer CA, Hagl S, Libby P, Kubler W 1999 Angiotensin induces inflammatory activation of human vascular smooth muscle cells. *Arterioscler Thromb Vasc Biol* 19:1623-9
[95] Ruiz-Ortega M, Lorenzo O, Ruperez M, Konig S, Wittig B, Egido J 2000 Angiotensin II activates nuclear transcription factor kappaB through AT(1) and AT(2) in vascular smooth muscle cells: molecular mechanisms. *Circ Res* 86:1266-72

[96] Muller DN, Dechend R, Mervaala EM, et al. 2000 NF-kappaB inhibition ameliorates angiotensin II-induced inflammatory damage in rats. *Hypertension* 35:193-201

[97] Tummala PE, Chen XL, Sundell CL, et al. 1999 Angiotensin II induces vascular cell adhesion molecule-1 expression in rat vasculature: A potential link between the renin-angiotensin system and atherosclerosis. *Circulation* 100:1223-9

[98] Pueyo ME, Gonzalez W, Nicoletti A, Savoie F, Arnal JF, Michel JB 2000 Angiotensin II stimulates endothelial vascular cell adhesion molecule-1 via nuclear factor-kappaB activation induced by intracellular oxidative stress. *Arterioscler Thromb Vasc Biol* 20:645-51

[99] Hernandez-Presa M, Bustos C, Ortego M, et al. 1997 Angiotensin-converting enzyme inhibition prevents arterial nuclear factor-kappa B activation, monocyte chemoattractant protein-1 expression, and macrophage infiltration in a rabbit model of early accelerated atherosclerosis. *Circulation* 95:1532-41

[100] Mervaala EM, Muller DN, Park JK, et al. 1999 Monocyte infiltration and adhesion molecules in a rat model of high human renin hypertension. *Hypertension* 33:389-95

[101] Diep QN, El Mabrouk M, Cohn JS, et al. 2002 Structure, endothelial function, cell growth, and inflammation in blood vessels of angiotensin II-infused rats: role of peroxisome proliferator-activated receptor-gamma. *Circulation* 105:2296-302

[102] Muller DN, Mervaala EM, Schmidt F, et al. 2000 Effect of bosentan on NF-kappaB, inflammation, and tissue factor in angiotensin II-induced end-organ damage. *Hypertension* 36:282-90

[103] Parissis JT, Korovesis S, Giazitzoglou E, Kalivas P, Katritsis D 2002 Plasma profiles of peripheral monocyte-related inflammatory markers in patients with arterial hypertension. Correlations with plasma endothelin-1. *Int J Cardiol* 83:13-21

[104] Ammarguellat FZ, Gannon PO, Amiri F, Schiffrin EL 2002 Fibrosis, matrix metalloproteinases, and inflammation in the heart of DOCA-salt hypertensive rats: role of ET(A) receptors. *Hypertension* 39:679-84

[105] Browatzki M, Schmidt J, Kubler W, Kranzhofer R 2000 Endothelin-1 induces interleukin-6 release via activation of the transcription factor NF-kappaB in human vascular smooth muscle cells. *Basic Res Cardiol* 95:98-105

[106] Bund SJ, West KP, Heagerty AM 1991 Effects of protection from pressure on resistance artery morphology and reactivity in spontaneously hypertensive and Wistar-Kyoto rats. *Circ Res* 68:1230-40

[107] Stacy DL, Prewitt RL 1989 Effects of chronic hypertension and its reversal on arteries and arterioles. *Circ Res* 65:869-79

[108] Prewitt RL, Rice DC, Dobrian AD 2002 Adaptation of resistance arteries to increases in pressure. *Microcirculation* 9:295-304

[109] Giancotti FG, Ruoslahti E 1999 Integrin signaling. *Science* 285:1028-32

[110] Wilson E, Sudhir K, Ives HE 1995 Mechanical strain of rat vascular smooth muscle cells is sensed by specific extracellular matrix/integrin interactions. *J Clin Invest* 96:2364-72

[111] Reusch P, Wagdy H, Reusch R, Wilson E, Ives HE 1996 Mechanical strain increases smooth muscle and decreases nonmuscle myosin expression in rat vascular smooth muscle cells. *Circ Res* 79:1046-53

[112] MacKenna DA, Dolfi F, Vuori K, Ruoslahti E 1998 Extracellular signal-regulated kinase and c-Jun NH2-terminal kinase activation by mechanical stretch is integrin-dependent and matrix-specific in rat cardiac fibroblasts. *J Clin Invest* 101:301-10

[113] Schaller MD, Hildebrand JD, Shannon JD, Fox JW, Vines RR, Parsons JT 1994 Autophosphorylation of the focal adhesion kinase, pp125FAK, directs SH2-dependent binding of pp60src. *Mol Cell Biol* 14:1680-8

[114] Schlaepfer DD, Hanks SK, Hunter T, van der Geer P 1994 Integrin-mediated signal transduction linked to Ras pathway by GRB2 binding to focal adhesion kinase. *Nature* 372:786-91

[115] Intengan HD, Thibault G, Li JS, Schiffrin EL 1999 Resistance artery mechanics, structure, and extracellular components in spontaneously hypertensive rats : effects of angiotensin receptor antagonism and converting enzyme inhibition. *Circulation* 100:2267-75

[116] Meininger GA, Lubrano VM, Granger HJ 1984 Hemodynamic and microvascular responses in the hindquarters during the development of renal hypertension in rats. Evidence for the involvement of an autoregulatory component. *Circ Res* 55:609-22

[117] Allen SP, Wade SS, Prewitt RL 1997 Myogenic tone attenuates pressure-induced gene expression in isolated small arteries. *Hypertension* 30:203-8

[118] Jacob MP, Badier-Commander C, Fontaine V, Benazzoug Y, Feldman L, Michel JB 2001 Extracellular matrix remodeling in the vascular wall. *Pathol Biol* (Paris) 49:326-32

[119] Prockop DJ, Kivirikko KI 1995 Collagens: molecular biology, diseases, and potentials for therapy. *Annu Rev Biochem* 64:403-34

[120] van der Rest M, Garrone R 1991 Collagen family of proteins. *Faseb J* 5:2814-23

[121] Mayne R 1986 Collagenous proteins of blood vessels. *Arteriosclerosis* 6:585-93

[122] Thybo NK, Mulvany MJ, Jastrup B, Nielsen H, Aalkjaer C 1996 Some pharmacological and elastic characteristics of isolated subcutaneous small arteries from patients with essential hypertension. *J Hypertens* 14:993-8

[123] Intengan HD, Schiffrin EL 2001 Vascular remodeling in hypertension: roles of apoptosis, inflammation, and fibrosis. *Hypertension* 38:581-7

[124] Ooshima A, Fuller GC, Cardinale GJ, Spector S, Udenfriend S 1974 Increased collagen synthesis in blood vessels of hypertensive rats and its reversal by antihypertensive agents. *Proc Natl Acad Sci U S A* 71:3019-23

[125] Ooshima A, Fuller G, Cardinale G, Spector S, Udenfriend S 1975 Collagen biosynthesis in blood vessels of brain and other tissues of the hypertensive rat. *Science* 190:898-900

[126] Anversa P, Melissari M, Tardini A, Olivetti G 1984 Connective tissue accumulation in the left coronary artery of young SHR. Hypertension 6:526-9

[127] Bezie Y, Lamaziere JM, Laurent S, et al. 1998 Fibronectin expression and aortic wall elastic modulus in spontaneously hypertensive rats. *Arterioscler Thromb Vasc Biol* 18:1027-34

[128] Mizutani K, Ikeda K, Kawai Y, Yamori Y 1999 Biomechanical properties and chemical composition of the aorta in genetic hypertensive rats. *J Hypertens* 17:481-7

[129] Karam H, Heudes D, Gonzales MF, Loffler BM, Clozel M, Clozel JP 1996 Respective role of humoral factors and blood pressure in aortic remodeling of DOCA hypertensive rats. *Am J Hypertens* 9:991-8

[130] Chamiot Clerc P, Renaud JF, Blacher J, et al. 1999 Collagen I and III and mechanical properties of conduit arteries in rats with genetic hypertension. *J Vasc Res* 36:139-46

[131] Kim S, Ohta K, Hamaguchi A, et al. 1995 Angiotensin II type I receptor antagonist inhibits the gene expression of transforming growth factor-beta 1 and extracellular matrix in cardiac and vascular tissues of hypertensive rats. *J Pharmacol Exp Ther* 273:509-15

[132] Sharifi AM, Li JS, Endemann D, Schiffrin EL 1998 Effects of enalapril and amlodipine on small-artery structure and composition, and on endothelial dysfunction in spontaneously hypertensive rats. *J Hypertens* 16:457-66

[133] Intengan HD, Deng LY, Li JS, Schiffrin EL 1999 Mechanics and composition of human subcutaneous resistance arteries in essential hypertension. *Hypertension* 33:569-74

[134] Takasaki I, Takizawa T, Sugimoto K, Gotoh E, Shionoiri H, Ishii M 1994 Effects of hypertension and aging on fibronectin expression in aorta of Dahl salt-sensitive rats. *Am J Physiol* 267:H1523-9

[135] Himeno H, Crawford DC, Hosoi M, Chobanian AV, Brecher P 1994 Angiotensin II alters aortic fibronectin independently of hypertension. *Hypertension* 23:823-6

[136] Ford CM, Li S, Pickering JG 1999 Angiotensin II stimulates collagen synthesis in human vascular smooth muscle cells. Involvement of the AT(1) receptor, transforming growth factor-beta, and tyrosine phosphorylation. *Arterioscler Thromb Vasc Biol* 19:1843-51

[137] Otsuka S, Sugano M, Makino N, Sawada S, Hata T, Niho Y 1998 Interaction of mRNAs for angiotensin II type 1 and type 2 receptors to vascular remodeling in spontaneously hypertensive rats. *Hypertension* 32:467-72

[138] Levy BI, Benessiano J, Henrion D, et al. 1996 Chronic blockade of AT2-subtype receptors prevents the effect of angiotensin II on the rat vascular structure. *J Clin Invest* 98:418-25

[139] Tharaux PL, Chatziantoniou C, Fakhouri F, Dussaule JC 2000 Angiotensin II activates collagen I gene through a mechanism involving the MAP/ER kinase pathway. *Hypertension* 36:330-6

[140] Itoh H, Mukoyama M, Pratt RE, Gibbons GH, Dzau VJ 1993 Multiple autocrine growth factors modulate vascular smooth muscle cell growth response to angiotensin II. *J Clin Invest* 91:2268-74

[141] Schlumberger W, Thie M, Rauterberg J, Robenek H 1991 Collagen synthesis in cultured aortic smooth muscle cells. Modulation by collagen lattice culture, transforming growth factor-beta 1, and epidermal growth factor. *Arterioscler Thromb* 11:1660-6

[142] Boffa JJ, Tharaux PL, Placier S, Ardaillou R, Dussaule JC, Chatziantoniou C 1999 Angiotensin II activates collagen type I gene in the renal vasculature of transgenic mice during inhibition of nitric oxide synthesis: evidence for an endothelin-mediated mechanism. *Circulation* 100:1901-8

[143] Rizvi MA, Katwa L, Spadone DP, Myers PR 1996 The effects of endothelin-1 on collagen type I and type III synthesis in cultured porcine coronary artery vascular smooth muscle cells. *J Mol Cell Cardiol* 28:243-52

[144] Benetos A, Lacolley P, Safar ME 1997 Prevention of aortic fibrosis by spironolactone in spontaneously hypertensive rats. *Arterioscler Thromb Vasc Biol* 17:1152-6

[145] Park JB, Schiffrin EL 2002 Cardiac and vascular fibrosis and hypertrophy in aldosterone-infused rats: role of endothelin-1. *Am J Hypertens* 15:164-9
[146] Reiser K, McCormick RJ, Rucker RB 1992 Enzymatic and nonenzymatic cross-linking of collagen and elastin. *Faseb J* 6:2439-49
[147] Brayden JE, Halpern W, Brann LR 1983 Biochemical and mechanical properties of resistance arteries from normotensive and hypertensive rats. *Hypertension* 5:17-25
[148] Briones AM, Gonzalez JM, Somoza B, et al. 2003 Role of elastin in spontaneously hypertensive rat small mesenteric artery remodelling. *J Physiol* 552:185-95
[149] Tamura K, Chiba E, Yokoyama N, et al. 1999 Renin-angiotensin system and fibronectin gene expression in Dahl Iwai salt-sensitive and salt-resistant rats. *J Hypertens* 17:81-9
[150] Koffi I, Lacolley P, Kirchengaast M, Pomies JP, Laurent S, Benetos A 1998 Prevention of arterial structural alterations with verapamil and trandolapril and consequences for mechanical properties in spontaneously hypertensive rats. *Eur J Pharmacol* 361:51-60
[151] Boumaza S, Arribas SM, Osborne-Pellegrin M, et al. 2001 Fenestrations of the carotid internal elastic lamina and structural adaptation in stroke-prone spontaneously hypertensive rats. *Hypertension* 37:1101-7
[152] Pu Q, Neves MF, Virdis A, Touyz RM, Schiffrin EL 2003 Endothelin antagonism on aldosterone-induced oxidative stress and vascular remodeling. *Hypertension* 42:49-55
[153] Fogerty FJ, Akiyama SK, Yamada KM, Mosher DF 1990 Inhibition of binding of fibronectin to matrix assembly sites by anti-integrin (alpha 5 beta 1) antibodies. *J Cell Biol* 111:699-708
[154] Hahn AW, Kern F, Jonas U, John M, Buhler FR, Resink TJ 1995 Functional aspects of vascular tenascin-C expression. *J Vasc Res* 32:162-74
[155] Gadeau AP, Campan M, Millet D, Candresse T, Desgranges C 1993 Osteopontin overexpression is associated with arterial smooth muscle cell proliferation in vitro. *Arterioscler Thromb* 13:120-5
[156] Liaw L, Almeida M, Hart CE, Schwartz SM, Giachelli CM 1994 Osteopontin promotes vascular cell adhesion and spreading and is chemotactic for smooth muscle cells in vitro. *Circ Res* 74:214-24
[157] Wiener J, Lombardi DM, Su JE, Schwartz SM 1996 Immunohistochemical and molecular characterization of the differential response of the rat mesenteric microvasculature to angiotensin-II infusion. *J Vasc Res* 33:195-208
[158] Shapiro SD, Endicott SK, Province MA, Pierce JA, Campbell EJ 1991 Marked longevity of human lung parenchymal elastic fibers deduced from prevalence of D-aspartate and nuclear weapons-related radiocarbon. *J Clin Invest* 87:1828-34
[159] Werb Z, Banda MJ, McKerrow JH, Sandhaus RA 1982 Elastases and elastin degradation. *J Invest Dermatol* 79 Suppl 1:154s-159s
[160] Robert L 1988 [Proteases of the elastase type]. *Pathol Biol* (Paris) 36:1101-7
[161] Galis ZS, Muszynski M, Sukhova GK, et al. 1994 Cytokine-stimulated human vascular smooth muscle cells synthesize a complement of enzymes required for extracellular matrix digestion. *Circ Res* 75:181-9
[162] Galis ZS, Khatri JJ 2002 Matrix metalloproteinases in vascular remodeling and atherogenesis: the good, the bad, and the ugly. *Circ Res* 90:251-62

[163] Badier-Commander C, Verbeuren T, Lebard C, Michel JB, Jacob MP 2000 Increased TIMP/MMP ratio in varicose veins: a possible explanation for extracellular matrix accumulation. *J Pathol* 192:105-12

[164] Gonzalez W, Fontaine V, Pueyo ME, et al. 2000 Molecular plasticity of vascular wall during N(G)-nitro-L-arginine methyl ester-induced hypertension: modulation of proinflammatory signals. *Hypertension* 36:103-9

[165] Diez J, Panizo A, Gil MJ, Monreal I, Hernandez M, Pardo Mindan J 1996 Serum markers of collagen type I metabolism in spontaneously hypertensive rats: relation to myocardial fibrosis. *Circulation* 93:1026-32

[166] Diez J, Hernandez M 1996 Is the extracellular degradation of collagen type I fibers depressed in spontaneously hypertensive rats with myocardial fibrosis? *Circulation* 94:2998

[167] Diez J, Laviades C, Mayor G, Gil MJ, Monreal I 1995 Increased serum concentrations of procollagen peptides in essential hypertension. Relation to cardiac alterations. *Circulation* 91:1450-6

[168] Laviades C, Varo N, Fernandez J, et al. 1998 Abnormalities of the extracellular degradation of collagen type I in essential hypertension. *Circulation* 98:535-40

[169] Intengan HD, Schiffrin, E.L. 1999 Collagen degradation is diminished in mesenteric arteries of spontaneously hypertensive rats after hypertension is established. *Hypertension* 34:329. Abstract.

[170] Hein M, Fischer J, Kim DK, Hein L, Pratt RE 1996 Vascular smooth muscle cell phenotype influences glycosaminoglycan composition and growth effects of extracellular matrix. *J Vasc Res* 33:433-41

[171] Castro CM, Cruzado MC, Miatello RM, Risler NR 1999 Proteoglycan production by vascular smooth muscle cells from resistance arteries of hypertensive rats. *Hypertension* 34:893-6

[172] Zervoudaki A, Economou E, Stefanadis C, et al. 2003 Plasma levels of active extracellular matrix metalloproteinases 2 and 9 in patients with essential hypertension before and after antihypertensive treatment. *J Hum Hypertens* 17:119-24

[173] Thompson CB 1995 Apoptosis in the pathogenesis and treatment of disease. *Science* 267:1456-62

[174] Hamet P, Richard L, Dam TV, et al. 1995 Apoptosis in target organs of hypertension. *Hypertension* 26:642-8

[175] Diez J, Panizo A, Hernandez M, et al. 1997 Cardiomyocyte apoptosis and cardiac angiotensin-converting enzyme in spontaneously hypertensive rats. *Hypertension* 30:1029-34

[176] Fortuno MA, Ravassa S, Etayo JC, Diez J 1998 Overexpression of Bax protein and enhanced apoptosis in the left ventricle of spontaneously hypertensive rats: effects of AT1 blockade with losartan. *Hypertension* 32:280-6

[177] Rodriguez-Lopez AM, Flores O, Arevalo MA, Lopez-Novoa JM 1998 Glomerular cell proliferation and apoptosis in uninephrectomized spontaneously hypertensive rats. *Kidney Int Suppl* 68:S36-40

[178] Cho A, Courtman DW, Langille BL 1995 Apoptosis (programmed cell death) in arteries of the neonatal lamb. *Circ Res* 76:168-75

[179] Hamet P, deBlois D, Dam TV, et al. 1996 Apoptosis and vascular wall remodeling in hypertension. *Can J Physiol Pharmacol* 74:850-61

[180] Sharifi AM, Schiffrin EL 1997 Apoptosis in aorta of deoxycorticosterone acetate-salt hypertensive rats: effect of endothelin receptor antagonism. *J Hypertens* 15:1441-8
[181] Sharifi AM, Schiffrin EL 1998 Apoptosis in vasculature of spontaneously hypertensive rats: effect of an angiotensin converting enzyme inhibitor and a calcium channel antagonist. *Am J Hypertens* 11:1108-16
[182] Diep QN, Li JS, Schiffrin EL 1999 In vivo study of AT(1) and AT(2) angiotensin receptors in apoptosis in rat blood vessels. *Hypertension* 34:617-24
[183] Devlin AM, Clark JS, Reid JL, Dominiczak AF 2000 DNA synthesis and apoptosis in smooth muscle cells from a model of genetic hypertension. *Hypertension* 36:110-5
[184] Dickhout JG, Lee RM 1999 Apoptosis in the muscular arteries from young spontaneously hypertensive rats. *J Hypertens* 17:1413-9
[185] Rizzoni D, Rodella L, Porteri E, et al. 2000 Time course of apoptosis in small resistance arteries of spontaneously hypertensive rats. *J Hypertens* 18:885-91
[186] Vega F, Panizo A, Pardo-Mindan J, Diez J 1999 Susceptibility to apoptosis measured by MYC, BCL-2, and BAX expression in arterioles and capillaries of adult spontaneously hypertensive rats. *Am J Hypertens* 12:815-20
[187] Irani K 2000 Oxidant signaling in vascular cell growth, death, and survival : a review of the roles of reactive oxygen species in smooth muscle and endothelial cell mitogenic and apoptotic signaling. *Circ Res* 87:179-83
[188] Yamada T, Horiuchi M, Dzau VJ 1996 Angiotensin II type 2 receptor mediates programmed cell death. *Proc Natl Acad Sci U S A* 93:156-60
[189] Cattaruzza M, Dimigen C, Ehrenreich H, Hecker M 2000 Stretch-induced endothelin B receptor-mediated apoptosis in vascular smooth muscle cells. *Faseb J* 14:991-8
[190] Tea BS, Der Sarkissian S, Touyz RM, Hamet P, deBlois D 2000 Proapoptotic and growth-inhibitory role of angiotensin II type 2 receptor in vascular smooth muscle cells of spontaneously hypertensive rats in vivo. *Hypertension* 35:1069-73
[191] deBlois D, Tea BS, Than VD, Tremblay J, Hamet P 1997 Smooth muscle apoptosis during vascular regression in spontaneously hypertensive rats. *Hypertension* 29:340-9
[192] Stead S, Werstiuk ES, Lee RM 2000 Nifedipine induces apoptosis in cultured vascular smooth muscle cells from spontaneously hypertensive rats. *Life Sci* 67:895-906
[193] Leszczynski D, Zhao Y, Luokkamaki M, Foegh ML 1994 Apoptosis of vascular smooth muscle cells. Protein kinase C and oncoprotein Bcl-2 are involved in regulation of apoptosis in non-transformed rat vascular smooth muscle cells. *Am J Pathol* 145:1265-70
[194] Diez J, Panizo A, Hernandez M, Pardo J 1997 Is the regulation of apoptosis altered in smooth muscle cells of adult spontaneously hypertensive rats? *Hypertension* 29:776-80

In: Hypertension: New Research
Editor: Elwood F. Benhagen, pp. 165-177
ISBN: 1-59454-204-X

Chapter VI

MARTORELL'S HYPERTENSIVE LEG ULCERS

John W. Graves
Division of Hypertension
Mayo Clinic and Mayo Foundation

ABSTRACT

The differential diagnosis of lower extremity ulcers is large. Most commonly, lower extremity ulcers are due to vascular disease, both arterial insufficiency and venous disease. Venous ulcers are the most common ulcers of the lower extremity. They are typically on the medial malleolus, at the point of highest venous hydrostatic pressure. Venous ultrasonography usually quickly confirms the presence of clot or venous insufficiency as the etiology of the ulcer. Arterial disease leading to ischemic leg ulcers is primarily from large vessel occlusive disease (atherosclerosis obliterans). The clinical examination and simple testing such as the ankle brachial index (ABI) and transcutaneous oximetry can usually identify ulcers on the basis of large vessel occlusive disease. A reduction in both the ankle brachial index and transcutaneous oximetry is diagnostic of that condition. Ulcers from small vessel (arteriolar) ischemia may also occur. They have a normal ankle brachial index due to normal large vessel perfusion and a reduced transcutaneous oximetry. Small vessel ischemic ulcers may be due to vasculitis, atheroemboli, and smoking (Berger's disease). A unique form of arteriolar ischemic ulcers occurs only in hypertensive patients. First described in the 1940s by Martorell, and by Hines and Farber, these ulcers have a distinct clinical presentation and specific therapy. Several key clinical features define hypertensive leg ulcers. These clinical features include: (1) the location of the ulcers on the medial malleolus, medial to posterior aspect of the thigh, or dorsum of the foot; (2) by their intense pain which is out of proportion of the size of the ulcer; (3) the presence of long-standing poorly controlled hypertension; (4) female predominance; and finally; (5) how refractory these ulcers are to conventional ischemic ulcer therapy.

The pathophysiology of these ulcers is inappropriate vasoconstriction accompanying the structural changes arteriolar hypertrophy of the dermal vessels due to long-standing poorly controlled hypertension. Resolution of these ulcers requires that effective blood pressure control be achieved with vasodilatory antihypertensive therapy to reverse the arteriolar vasoconstriction that is the physiologic hallmark of the hypertensive leg ulcers.

Two cases are presented to illustrate the cardinal features of Martorell's hypertensive leg ulcers including the painful delay in diagnosis and successful therapy common to this condition.

All physicians who deal with lower extremity ischemic vascular disease need to be aware of this entity's unique presentation and therapy to avoid needless suffering by the patient.

INTRODUCTION

First described by Martorell [1] and by Hines and Farber [2], these two cases of hypertensive leg ulcers demonstrate the classic features including: the presence of an extremely painful ulcer in the characteristic position on the anterolateral surface of the lower two thirds of the leg, significant arterial hypertension, absence of large vessel arterial occlusive disease or significant lower extremity venous disease, and lesions that are refractory to the usual topical therapies. There are now 107 cases of Martorell's hypertensive leg ulcers reported in the world's literature, most of them reported in the 1940-1970s [1-22]. Of the 107 cases, 84 are female and 23 male with the first male case reported by Valls-Serra in 1950 [3]. Only three cases in patients of African-American descent have been reported, all females [4]. These ulcers occur over a wide age range with patients as old as age 86 [5] and as young as 41 [6]. The blood pressures in these patients are almost always poorly controlled at presentation and healing of the ulcer does not occur until the blood pressure has been controlled with agents that reverse the arteriolar vasoconstriction found in the skin. The ulcers are classically found on the anterolateral aspect of the lower two thirds of the leg [7]. Pathophysiology of these ischemic skin ulcers represents a perturbation of the changes in the vascular bed that occur in hypertension. Bell and Clausen [23] described at autopsy arteriolosclerosis occurring in multiple organs in hypertensives, and they were the first to describe these changes in dermal vessels. For hypertensive ischemic leg ulcers to occur, the medial hyperplasia and reduction in wall to lumen ratio that is common in long standing poorly treated hypertension [23] must also be accompanied by a local inappropriate increase in vascular resistance as shown by Duncan and Ferris [11]. Successful healing of these painful ulcers was reported first by Orbach [12] using a low sodium rice diet and subsequently by Fogola [13] using antihypertensive medication. Henderson's series of 16 cases [14] revealed that the resolution of the ulcer was dependent not only of achieving blood pressure control but also on the particular antihypertensive agents used to lower blood pressure. He describe four cases where the ulcers did not resolve with reduction in blood pressure but only when the beta blockers used to treat the hypertension were withdrawn. Nikolova [24], in the only randomized trial of treatment of hypertensive ischemic ulcers, further confirmed that blood pressure control and the use of vasodilatory antihypertensive agent to lower blood pressure (nifedipine) was critical to resolution of the ulcers. The latest two cases in the literature [21, 22] are illustrative of the classic features of Martorell's ulcers and suggest that ACE inhibitors and angiotensin receptor blockers may also be effective in reversing dermal vasoconstriction in these patients.

CASES

Case 1

A 67-year-old white female with a history of peripheral arterial occlusive disease was referred for treatment of a non-healing leg ulcer of four months duration. In 1996, she had an aortobifemoral (ABF) bypass graft for claudication. She underwent a left leg femoral-popliteal bypass in July 1997 for non-painful ulcers of the left leg and the ulcers resolved. In August of 1998, she developed right leg claudication, and an arteriogram showed occlusion of the right limb of the ABF graft and a right femoral-femoral graft was done with relief of claudication. Four months prior to coming to the Mayo Clinic she had developed a painful leg ulcer without accompanying claudication. She saw her local doctor who instituted topical wound care and two weeks of oral ciprofloxacin which did not improve the ulcer. She was seen in a wound center in Minneapolis and noninvasive Doppler studies revealed good flow in the right leg graft. Topical therapy with Silvadene and Sorbsan and oral therapy with pentoxifylline and cephalosporin was instituted again without improvement in the ulcer.

On arrival at the Mayo Clinic, she had been taking hypertensive medications for more than five years. She had not measured home blood pressures so her previous degree of blood pressure control was unclear but was suspected to be poor. Medications were verapamil 240 mg per day, simvastatin 5 mg per day, pentoxifylline 400 mg t.i.d., warfarin 5 mg five days per week and 2.5 mg two days per week, ranitidine 150 mg per day, calcium 1500 mg per day, and a multivitamin one daily. Her physical examination revealed a blood pressure of 188/82 mmHg in the left arm sitting and 200/92 mmHg in the right arm sitting. A 2 x 2 cm extremely painful ulceration was observed on the posterolateral aspect of the right leg (Plate 1). The base was covered by fibrinous exudate with some buds of granulation and sharply demarcated margins. There was trace edema of the lower extremities bilaterally. The pulses in the right leg were 2+ femoral and absent distal to the femoral pulse. X-ray of the right foot and ankle was negative for osteomyelitis. Ultrasound revealed the right femoral-femoral bypass graft to be patent with an arterial flow of 52 to 60 cm per second in the right popliteal artery. WBC was 7000, hemoglobin was 14.1 g/dL, fasting glucose was 93 mg/dL, serum creatinine was 1.4 mg/dL, serum protein electrophoresis was normal, and homocysteine level was 14 umol/L (N $<$13 umol/L). The patient was seen at the Wound Center where her Sorbsan was discontinued and saline gauze dressings (which she had used previously without effect), a Rooke boot, and reduced ambulation were prescribed. Enalapril/hydrochlorothiazide 5/12.5 mg once daily was prescribed. No further changes were made in her topical wound therapy, and her leg ulcer dramatically improved over the next seven weeks. At three weeks, the patient returned and her blood pressure was significantly better at 133/58 mmHg. The ulcer was reduced in size to 1.4 x 1.3 cm and was less painful (Plate 2). At five weeks after her initial visit, her blood pressure was 142/70 mmHg. By seven weeks, the blood pressure remained well controlled and the ulcer had 100% epithelialization and the patient was pain-free (Plate 3).

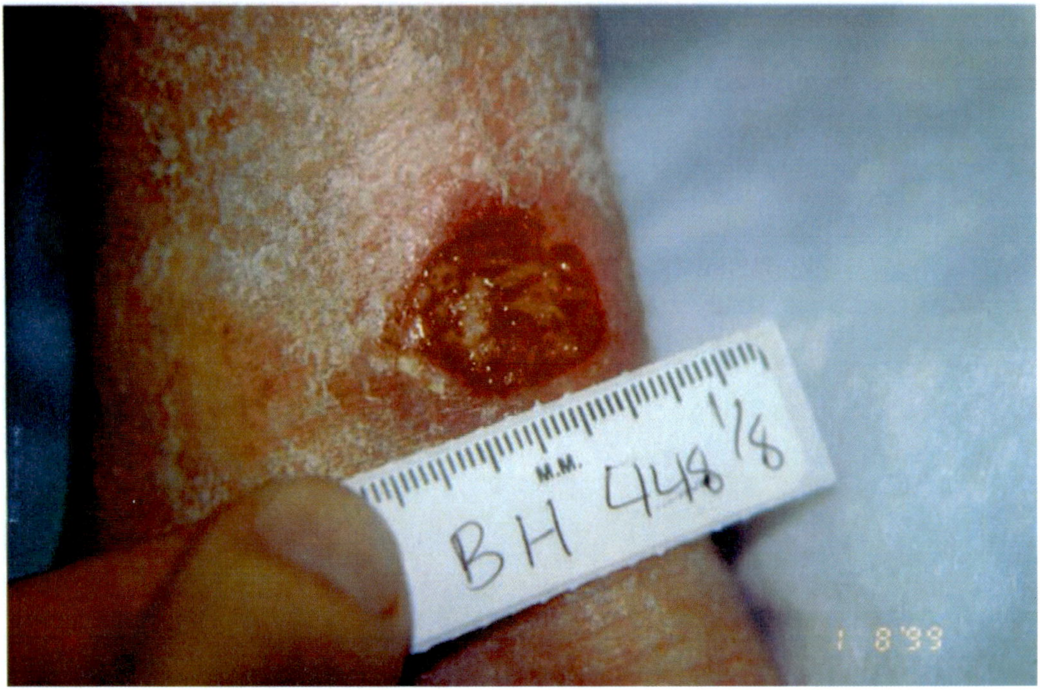

Plate 1

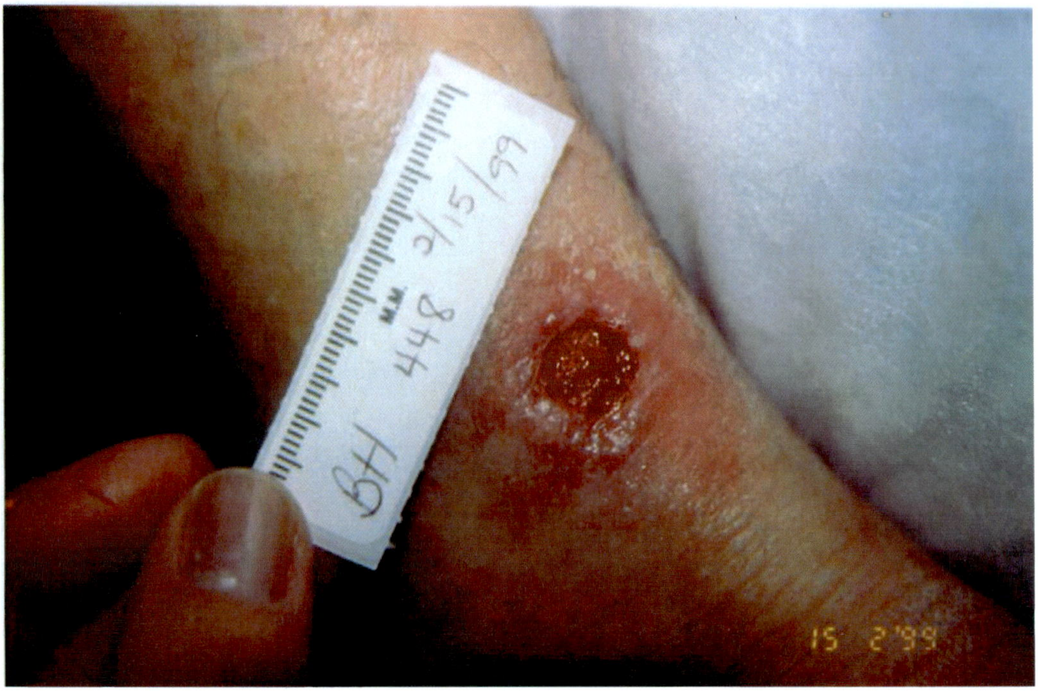

Plate 2

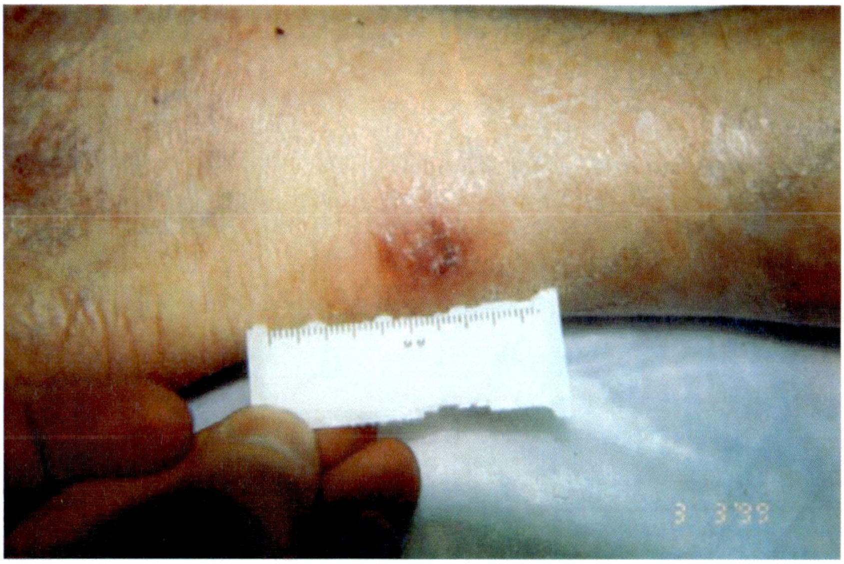

Plate 3

Case 2

A 65-year-old female presented to the Mayo Clinic Rochester for a second opinion concerning chronic non-healing lower extremity ulcers. Eighteen months prior to presentation, she spontaneously developed an ulcer on her right lateral calf that was moderately painful. This ulcer was treated with multiple topical therapies including collagenase, regular DuoDerm dressing changes, bacitracin, and Jobst compression garments without evidence of improved healing. The right lower extremity ulcer was then débrided surgically which seemed to make it worse. Twelve months prior to presentation at the Mayo Clinic, she developed a similar but more painful ulcer on her left lateral calf. This, too, was resistant to topical treatment. She was given an empiric course of oral prednisone for possible vasculitic etiology without improvement—laboratory workup had been negative. Surgical debridement was again recommended, but the patient refused and presented to the Mayo Clinic for a second opinion.

She denied any previous history of lower extremity ulcers, and previous work up for diabetes was unremarkable when her ulcers presented. There was no history of deep venous thrombosis, claudication, or tobacco use. Past medical history was remarkable for poorly controlled hypertension and mild osteoarthritis. Her medications were alpha methyldopa 250 mg three times daily, potassium 10 mEq twice daily, furosemide 20 mg twice daily, indomethacin 25 mg three times daily, and glucosamine chondroitin twice daily.

Her examination revealed a blood pressure of 152/82 mmHg. The remainder of her exam was unremarkable with the exception of her lower extremities. Dorsalis pedis and posterior tibial pulses were easily palpable bilaterally. There was minimal edema. She had bilateral ulcers, 0.5 x 1.5 cm on the right and 2.5 x 3.0 cm on the left (Plate 4). Both ulcers had a surrounding zone of erythema with sharply demarcated borders and minimal granulation tissue. There was no evidence of purulent discharge or infectious odor associated with the ulcers. The ulcers appeared somewhat macerated upon examination due to the occlusive dressings she had been wearing. She was referred to the Hypertension Division and her antihypertensive therapy changed to diltiazem 180 mg, irbesartan 150 mg (lisinopril was stopped due to cough), and a thiazide diuretic. At six weeks, her diltiazem was increased to 240 mg and the irbesartan to 300 mg. Eight weeks after initial presentation, her blood pressures were 122 to 145 systolic and diastolics all less than 83 mmHg and the ulcers had healed. After three years of follow up, the blood pressure is well controlled on the same agents and the ulcers have not recurred.

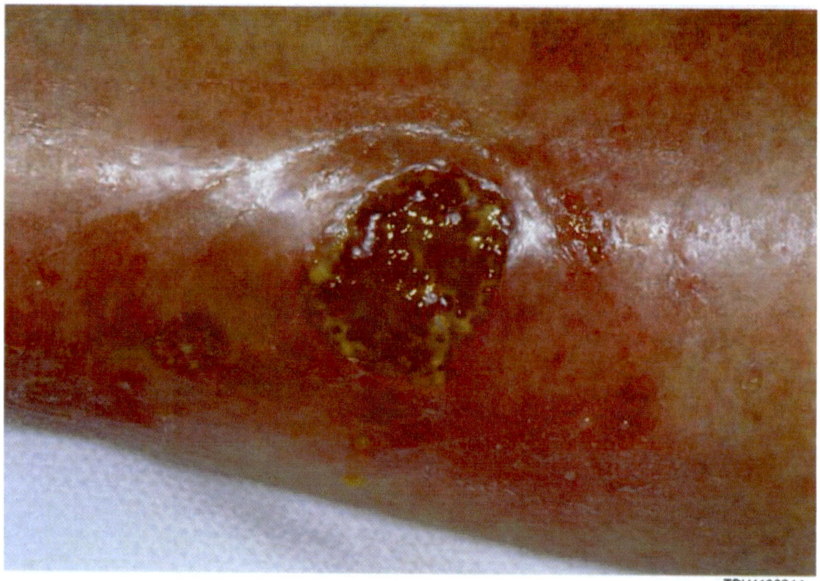

Plate 4

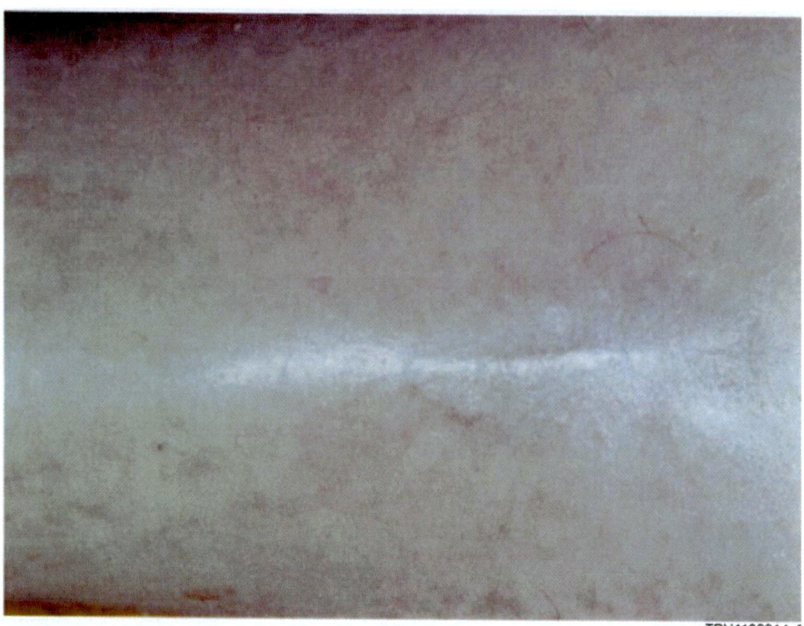

Plate 5

Discussion

Martorell's hypertensive leg ulcers are an uncommon form of lower extremity ulcer. As these two cases demonstrate, early recognition of this rare condition is critical, as these ulcers are very painful and refractory to common topical therapies. First described by Martorell [1] and Hines and Farber [2], these small vessel ischemic ulcers have unique pathophysiology and clinical presentation that allows the astute clinician to differentiate hypertensive leg ulcers from the more common forms of leg ulcers. There are now 107 reported cases of Martorell's hypertensive leg ulcers in the world's literature, most reported before 1970 [1-23]. The majority of reported cases, as seen with the two presented here, are in women (84 female and 23 male cases). The reason for this gender difference is unknown. In addition to a gender difference, there also seems to be a racial difference as only three cases have been reported in African-Americans [4], all of who were female. The mean age at presentation can not be calculated as not all case reports provide the patient's age but the usual age is mid-50s to mid-60s (range: 41 to 86 years). The age of the patients reported in the literature with Martorell's ulcers seems to be on the rise. This is most likely due to the need for long-standing significant hypertension to cause the structural and functional derangements of the dermal vessels. The early cases, where younger patients are reported, are likely influenced by their occurring in the pretreatment era of hypertension.

The largest single series is from Schnier and Sheps [7] at the Mayo Clinic and this consisted of 40 patients (13 male and 27 female, age range 42 to 81 years). They reported 40 cases for Martorell's ulcers occurring at the Mayo Clinic from 1950 to 1961. These cases were seen predominately by consultants in the Peripheral Vascular Department rather than in Dermatology. In only half of their patients could they define an antecedent traumatic event that led to ulcer formation. Two thirds of the patients reported had had hypertension for more than ten years prior to the onset of the ulcer. They reported a marked variability in ulcer size from 1cm to 13 x 27 cm with the average lesion of 3 centimeters. As seen in the two patients presented here, the ulcers had been present for up to 18 months prior to diagnosis. With the topical measures employed at that time and blood pressure reduction, the ulcers healed in an average of four months (range: 2 weeks to one year). They were the first to report the occurrence of Martorell's ischemic ulcer in the patient with concomitant large vessel atherosclerotic disease. In the patients where both were present, the atherosclerotic disease was not felt to be sufficiently severe to cause the ulcers seen. Combined with the location of the ulcers and the disproportionate pain seen, the Martorell's ulcers could be differentiated clinically from ulcers due to large vessel occlusive disease. There was, however, a reduced rate of healing of Martorell's ischemic ulcers in the patients with atherosclerotic disease (10 of 19 healed in patients with atherosclerosis versus 19 of 21 in patients without it).

As in the two cases presented, hypertension is usually poorly controlled and in the earlier reports often severe. In 62 of 107 cases, the mean systolic blood pressure was 204 mmHg (R=120 to 290 mmHg) and diastolic blood pressure 115 mmHg (R=70 to 160 mm Hg).

Our patients demonstrated the distinct character and position of hypertensive ischemic leg ulcers. These lesions are most commonly found on the anterolateral aspects of the lower extremities and often are symmetrical (Figure 1). These ulcers are identified by severe pain disproportionate to their size, refractoriness to topical therapies that are unsuccessful in healing most other forms of ulcers, and their episodic and irregular extension by skin infarction with associated satellite lesions. Painful lower extremity ulcers may occur in association with multiple conditions including large vessel atheromatous occlusive disease, atheroembolic disease, diffuse vasculitis, insect bites, and after pyoderma gangrenosum, to name just a few. Forms of large vessel lower extremity arterial ischemic ulcers typically affect the more distal areas of the foot first and are accompanied by absent lower extremity pulses, dependent rubor, and delayed capillary filling. Appropriate laboratory and radiologic evaluation for these other conditions must be negative before considering the possibility that the painful ulcer may be due to hypertensive ischemic ulcers. Venous ulcers are the most common forms of leg ulcer and are not often confused with hypertensive leg ulcers. They occur on the medical aspect of the leg where venous hydrostatic pressure is the highest, are not usually painful, and have associated chronic edema and stasis skin changes. Finally, neurotrophic ulcers, most commonly from diabetes mellitus, occur at pressure points and are, by definition, painless, making them easy to separate from hypertensive ischemic ulcers.

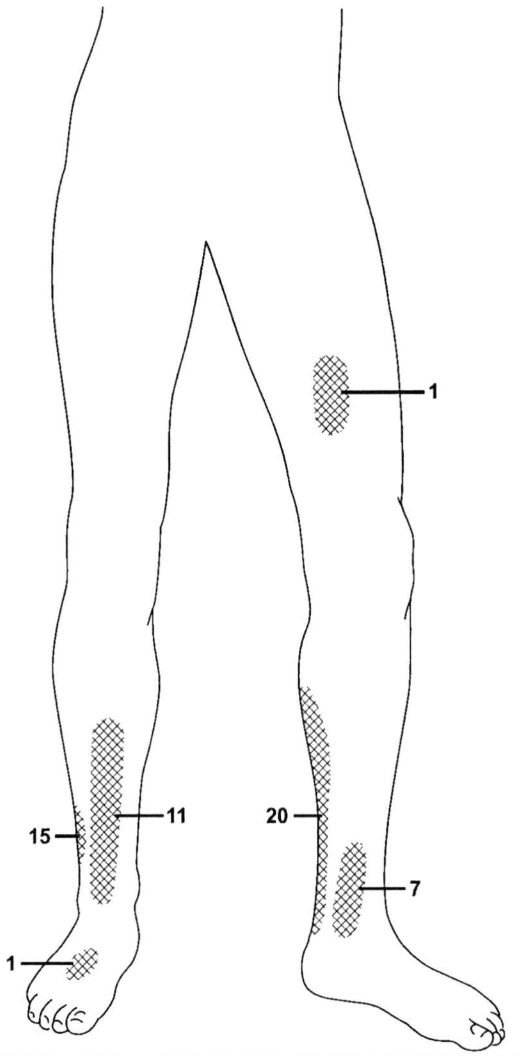

Figure 1

The diagnostic evaluation of lower extremity ulcers is relatively straightforward. First, one must decide whether the painful ulcers are due to large vessel or small vessel occlusive disease. A simple and reliable noninvasive test to determine the presence and importance of large vessel arterial occlusive disease is to obtain lower extremity segmental systolic blood pressure levels and calculate the ankle brachial index (ABI). Dividing the systolic ankle blood pressure for each leg by the highest systolic arm blood pressure does this. The blood pressure level at the ankle should be equal to or slightly higher than that at the arm. Thus, an ABI of 1.0 or more is normal. Transcutaneous oximetry of the skin assesses oxygenation and, thus, the blood flow in the dermal arterioles. Transcutaneous PO2 may be decreased because of large artery occlusive disease and this would be associated with a reduced ankle brachial index of <0.6. The clinical examination would show diminished or absent pulses and loss of dermal hair. On occasion, a contrast aortogram with lower extremity runoff views is required to make the diagnosis of large vessel occlusive disease. In patients with renal insufficiency where intravenous contrast is to be avoided, magnetic resonance arteriograms may yield sufficient information to make the diagnosis of large vessel occlusive disease as the cause of the painful lower extremity ulcers. Where as in arteriolar disease such as Martorell's hypertensive ischemic ulcers, the transcutaneous oximetry would show reduced perfusion and the ankle brachial index would be normal, as would the pulse examination in the lower extremity.

Evaluation of venous ulcerations relies on the use of duplex ultrasonography. Venous ultrasonography is able to document the presence of venous occlusion due to acute or chronic clot formation. It may also show the presence of venous incompetence which leads to further increases in venous hydrostatic pressure and enhances ulcer formation. Contrast venography can also demonstrate these findings but is seldom worth the added risk of contrast administration due to the clinical utility of noninvasive venous Doppler studies. The pathophysiology of hypertensive leg ulcers is a failure of dermal arteriolar vasodilatation in response to the classic arteriolar hypertrophy from long-standing poorly controlled hypertension. The arteriolar hypertrophy in the dermal vessels, first reported by Bell and Clausen [23], was seen less frequently in the skin compared to the arterioles in the brain and kidney. Hines and Farber [2] further characterized the hypertensive changes seen in skin arterioles as thickening of the arteriolar wall and resultant change in the wall to lumen ratio. In their study of 122 subjects, the wall to lumen ration is 1:2.14 in normotensives (N=52) and 1:1.57 in hypertensives (N=70). This wall thickening was a result of hyperplasia of the nuclear elements of the media and hypertrophy of the elastic lamina. Henderson [14] demonstrated these same changes in sixteen consecutive patients with hypertensive ischemic ulcers. Using the same technique to measure the wall to lumen ratio as Hines and Farber, Henderson found that the loss of wall to lumen ration seen in hypertensive ischemic ulcers was not seen in other forms of chronic lower extremity ulcers. These common anatomic changes due to poorly controlled hypertension did not explain the much rarer occurrence of hypertensive leg ulcers.

Duncan and Farris [11] studied skin perfusion in 12 normotensive patients, 8 patients with large vessel peripheral vascular disease, and 6 patients with Martorell's hypertensive ulcers. Significant reductions in skin perfusion were seen in both large vessel vascular disease and hypertensive ischemic leg ulcers but from entirely different mechanisms. In peripheral arterial occlusive disease, skin perfusion was reduced due to proximal reductions in blood flow with local compensatory dermal arteriolar vasodilation. In the patients with hypertensive leg ulcers, large vessel inflow was normal and the reduction is skin perfusion was due to an increase in vascular resistance from the dermal arterioles. This inability to vasodilate in response in dermal arteriolar narrowing may reduce tissue perfusion to such a level that minor skin trauma will result in formation of a significant skin ulcer. This apparent structural and functional alteration of the dermal microvasculature requires further study, and laser dermography may be the tool required to effectively study the function of dermal vessels in hypertension [25, 26].

Catalano and colleagues [27], using the laser Doppler flowmeter technique, showed that the vasoconstrictive properties of the precapillary vessels was impaired in patients with hypertensive when compared to matched normotensive controls. They studied 34 subjects with mild to moderate essential hypertension and compared them to 22 sex- and age-matched healthy subjects. The laser Doppler measurements were performed with the probe at the fingertip at baseline, after an ischemic test, and during mental stress. The essential hypertensives showed a statistically significant lower rest flow compared to controls. During mental stress, the essential hypertensive patients showed a statistically lower mean relative skin blood flow. This data suggests that the vasoconstrictor capacity of precapillary vessels is abnormal in the hypertensives. Sieg-Dobrescu, using the same method, demonstrated that when antihypertensive agents were withdrawn from 18 stable hypertensives the postischemic blood flow responses remained impaired during the six months of the study [28]. This impairment was present regardless of the height of the blood pressure after medication withdrawal. More importantly, the impaired endothelial function, demonstrated by laser Doppler in these hypertensive subjects, preceded the redevelopment of their hypertension after the blood pressure medications had been removed. They were not able to tell from their study design whether these findings were due to hypertension-induced structural, functional vascular abnormalities, or a combination of both. Finally Irving, et al, looked at the skin microvasculature in 105 healthy males. They measured skin vasodilation with laser Doppler fluximetry on the forearm following heating and iontophoresis with acetylcholine. They found that higher systolic blood pressure was associated with impaired maximal dermal blood flow during heating but no impact on the vasodilator response to acetylcholine. Higher fasting glucose did not correlate with microvascular changes with heating or acetylcholine but was associated with lower capillary density and increased capillary blood flow. These significant changes in the dermal microvasculature are associated with early and subtle elevations of the blood pressure and fasting plasma glucose in advance of the subjects crossing the threshold for the diagnosis of hypertension or diabetes [29]. Thus, there are clear changes of structure and function of the dermal microvasculature in the hypertensive subject but as yet, no research using laser Doppler techniques has been reported in Martorell's hypertensive leg ulcers.

Therapy of hypertensive ischemic leg ulcers is dependent on understanding of the underlying dermal microvasculature derangements. Prior to the availability of antihypertensive drugs, multiple topical preparations, including desiccated red blood cells [2], boric acid solutions [2], brilliant green [8, 15), Lassar's paste [12], sulfadiazine powder [2, 15], and topical Varidase (streptokinase-streptodornase) [16], were tried with little success. Skin grafting, when attempted, often met with failure [16, 17]. Other treatments such as cod liver oil [5], typhoid vaccine [5], intra-atrial novocaine [13], and intravenous calcium thionate [5] were tried and failed as well. Recognizing the ischemic basis of these ulcers, lumbar sympathectomy was tried [1, 2, 7, 8, 15, 18, 19]. Since sympathectomy rarely significantly reduced arterial blood pressure, this treatment remained ineffective.

Orbach [12] first described the importance of blood pressure reduction in the healing of Martorell's ischemic ulcers in 1948. He placed a single patient on a rice diet (very low sodium) and the patients blood pressure fell from 260/130 to 160/110, and with the aide of skin grafting, the ulcer healed by the second month of lower blood pressure. Initial reports of antihypertensive drug therapy on hypertensive ulcers were disappointing. Fogola [13], in 1971, used diuretics and other "hypotensive drugs" to little effect in five patients with Martorell's ischemic leg ulcers. Rude [6], in 1983, reported a single case where despite impressive blood pressure reduction (200/120 mmHg to 130/80 mmHg) with a diuretic and methyldopa little improvement in ulcer healing was seen. Henderson's [14] 16 patient series had 9 of 16 with uncontrolled hypertension and 7 with controlled blood pressures. Critically, he noted that in four of the seven patients where good blood pressure control was achieved with beta-blockers, the ulcers healed only after the beta-blockers were stopped. This observation that the type of antihypertensive agent chosen to reduce blood pressure was as or more important, as reducing the blood pressure was further advanced by the only placebo-controlled trial on antihypertensive agents in this condition. Reported by Niklova [24] in 1995, 30 patients with hypertensive ischemic ulcers were randomized to a two-month trial of nifedipine (10 mg three times daily) versus placebo. Significant reductions in the ulcer pain and size occurred in the nifedipine treated patients when compared to placebo. This benefit occurred despite a very modest reduction in systolic blood pressure between the two groups (SBP nifedipine: 165.5±12.2 mmHg versus 170.8±13.1 placebo). Available information demonstrates that healing of Martorell's ischemic ulcers is dependent on reduction in both blood pressure and dermal arteriolar vasoconstriction, as these two cases demonstrate. In addition, these cases supply initial evidence that use of ACE inhibitors [21] and angiotensin receptor blockers [22] may also be effective in counteracting the dermal vasoconstriction seen in hypertensive ischemic ulcers just as they improve capillary hemodynamics in the renal microvasculature.

Conclusion

Martorell's hypertensive ischemic leg ulcers are a unique and under-recognized clinical entity. Failure to correctly diagnose and treat these ulcers results in months of significant pain and potential limb loss due to secondary infection. The clinical presentation of these ulcers is pain disproportionate to ulcer size, position of the ulcers on the antero-lateral surface of the lower extremities, and absence of significant arterial or venous.

Occlusive disease, female predominance, and association with poorly controlled hypertension need to be known to more clinicians. Eighteen of the twenty-three manuscripts on this topic were written from 1945 to 1989. Thus, most clinicians now in practice have not seen or read about this subject. Three of the most commonly used textbooks on hypertension fail to mention ischemic leg ulcers as a consequence of poorly controlled hypertension [30-32]. The pathophysiology of these ulcers means that effective therapy must not only reduce blood pressure to less than 140/90 to decrease the microvascular structural changes that occur due to hypertension, they must counteract the local vasoconstriction as well. These two cases extend the observations of Nikolova about the effectiveness of calcium channel.

Blockers and preliminary data suggesting that ACE inhibitors and angiotensin receptor blockers may also be effective in reversing dermal vasoconstriction. Renewed appreciation of the occurrence of Martorell's hypertensive ischemic ulcers should lead to early diagnosis and effective therapy with resultant relief of pain and debility associated with these ulcers.

REFERENCES

[1] Martorell F. Las ulceros supramaleolares por arteriolitis de las grandes hipertensas. *Acta Inst Policlinico Barcelona*. December 1945;1:6-9.
[2] Hines EA, Farber EM. Ulcer of the leg due to arteriosclerosis and ischemia occurring in the presence of hypertensive disease (hypertensive ischemic ulcers): A preliminary report. *Proceedings of the Staff Meetings of the Mayo Clinic*. 4 September 1946; 21(18):337-346.
[3] Valles-Serra J. Sobre el tratamiento de la ulcera supramaleolar de las grandes hipertensos. *Acta del I. Policlinico*. 1946;9:86.
[4] Farber EM, Schmidt OEL. Hypertensive ischemic leg ulcers. *California Medicine*. 1950;72(1):4-6.
[5] Martorell F. Hypertensive ulcer of the leg. *Angiology*. 1950;1:133-140.
[6] Rude T, Bunkis J, Walton RL. Hypertensive leg ulcers. *The J of Foot Surgery*. 1983;22(2):134-138.
[7] Schnier BR, Sheps SG, Juergens JL. Hypertensive ischemic ulcer: A review of 40 cases. *American J of Cardiology*. 1966;17:560-565.
[8] Monserrat J. Diastolic arterial hypertension and ulcer of the leg--Martorell's syndrome. *Angiology*. 1958;9:226-227.
[9] Farber EM, Hines EA, Montgomery H, Craig WM. The arterioles of the skin in essential hypertension. *J of Investigative Dermatology*. 1947;9:285-298.
[10] Young JR. Differential diagnosis of leg ulcers. *Cardiovascular Clinics*. 1983;13(2):171-93.
[11] Duncan HJ, Faris IB. Martorell's hypertensive ischemic leg ulcers are secondary to an increase in the local vascular resistance. *J of Vascular Surgery*. 1985;2:581-584.
[12] Orbach EJ. Hypertensive ischemic leg ulcer. *Angiology*. 1955;6:153-161.
[13] Fogola N, Pataro EF, Zerbos FC, Acrich MW. Hypertensive ulcer. *J of Cardiovascular Surgery*. September-October 1971;12(5):406-410.
[14] Henderson CA, Highet AS, Lane SA, Hall R. Arterial hypertension causing leg ulcers. *Clinical and Experimental Dermatology*. 1995;20:107-114.
[15] Alonso T. Diastolic arterial hypertension and ulcer of the leg--Martorell's syndrome. *Lancet*. 22 May 1954;266:1059.
[16] Wooling KR. Hypertensive ischemic ulcer. *JAMA*. 18 January 1964;187:196-201.
[17] Palou J. Lumbar sympathectomy in the treatment of hypertensive ischemic leg ulcers of the leg (Martorell's Syndrome). *Circulation*. August 1955;12:239-241.
[18] Mozes M, Salomy M, Jahr J, Adar R. Hypertensive ischemic ulcer of the leg. *J of Cardiovascular Surgery*. 1962;3:201-206.
[19] Gohil P, Young JR, Clarke TH. Hypertensive ischemic ulcers of the leg. *J of American Podiatry Association*. July 1981;71(7):363-367.

[20] Leu HJ. Hypertensive ischemic leg ulcer (Martorell's ulcer): A specific disease entity. *International Angiology*. April-June 1992;11(2):132-136.

[21] Graves JW, Morris JC, Sheps SG. Case Report: Martorell's hypertensive leg ulcer: Case report and concise review of the literature. *Journal of Human Hypertension*. 2001;15:279-283.

[22] Tillman TW, Graves JW. 65 year old woman with painful leg ulcers. *Mayo Clinic Proceedings*. 2002;77:965-968.

[23] Bell ET, Clawson BJ. Primary (essential) hypertension: A study of four hundred and twenty cases. *Archives of Pathology*. June 1928;5(6):939-1001.

[24] Nikolova K. Treatment of hypertensive venous leg ulcers with nifedipine. *Meth Find Exp Clin Pharmacol*. 1995;17(8):545-549.

[25] Fagrell B. Advances in Micro-circulation Network Evaluation: An update. *Int J Microcirculation*. 1995;(suppl 1):34-40.

[26] Goldman L. Future of laser dermatology. *Laser in Surgery and Medicine*. 1998 22:3-8.

[27] Catalano M, Schioppa S, Sampietro G, Contini P Ninno D. Skin blood flow during vasoconstriction and vasodilative stimuli in essential hypertension patients: A laser Doppler flowmetry study. *J Microcirculation*. 1997;17:80-85.

[28] Sieg-0Dobrescu D, Burnier M, Hayoz D, Rudolf Brunner H, Waeber B. The return of increased blood pressure after discontinuation of antihypertensive treatment is associated with an impaired post-ischemic skin blood flow response. *Journal of Hypertension*. 2001;19(8):1387-1392.

[29] Irving RJ, Walker BR, Noon JP, Watt GCM, Webb DJ, Shore AC. Microvascular correlates of blood pressure, plasma glucose, and insulin resistance in health. *Cardiovascular Research*. 2002;53:271-276.

[30] Kaplan NM. In: *Clinical Hypertension,* Sixth Edition. Williams & Wilkins: Baltimore, Maryland, 1994.

[31] The essentials of high blood pressure. In: Izzo JL, Jr. and Black H from The Council on High Blood Pressure Research (Senior Editors). *Hypertension Primer,* Second Edition. American Heart Association 1999.

[32] Clinical Hypertension. In: Robertson JIS (ed). *Handbook of Hypertension,* Vol. 14. Elsevier Science Publishers: Amsterdam, The Netherlands, 1992.

In: Hypertension: New Research
Editor: Elwood F. Benhagen, pp. 179-199
ISBN: 1-59454-204-X

Chapter VII

SEX HORMONES AND BLOOD PRESSURE

***Raghvendra K. Dubey**[*1,2,3] **and Edwin K. Jackson** [1,3,4]*
Center for Clinical Pharmacology,[1] Department of Medicine[3], and Department of Pharmacology[4], University of Pittsburgh School of Medicine, Pittsburgh, PA 15216, USA; and University Hospital Zurich, Department of Obstetrics and Gynecology[2], Clinic for Endocrinology, 8091-Zurich, Switzerland

ABSTRACT

High arterial blood pressure (hypertension) is a major health problem that significantly increases the risk of myocardial infarction, heart failure, stroke, renal disease and peripheral vascular disease. There is increasing evidence that gender influences blood pressure and that sex hormones contribute to the pathophysiology of hypertension. For example, on average premenopausal women have lower arterial blood pressures than either age-matched men or age-matched postmenopausal women, and these findings suggest that ovarian hormones modulate blood pressure. Moreover, in aging males, increases in blood pressure correlate with decreases in androgen levels, and these findings imply that testosterone may also influence blood pressure. However, whether sex hormones are responsible for the observed differences in blood pressure in women versus men and premenopausal versus postmenopausal women remains unclear. The purpose of this book chapter is to discuss the blood pressure modulating actions of female and male sex hormones, and to describe cellular, biochemical and molecular mechanisms by which sex hormones may modulate the cardiovascular effects of hypertension.

Key words: hypertension, estradiol, testosterone, androgens, metabolism, metabolic disorders, methoxyestradiol, hyperplasia, growth factors, anti-mitogenic, smooth muscle cells, mesangial cells, cardiac fibroblasts, endothelial cells.

* Dr. Raghvendra K. Dubey Clinic for Endocrinology Department of Obstetrics and Gynecology University Hospital Zurich Frauenklinikstrasse 10 CH-8051, Zurich Switzerland Phone: 41-1-255-5383 Fax: 41-1-255-4439 E-mail: Raghvendra.Dubey@usz.ch

INTRODUCTION

Gender differences in arterial blood pressure begin in adolescence and are maintained throughout adulthood [1]. In men less than 60 years-of-age, on average systolic and diastolic blood pressures are higher by 6-7 and 3-5 mmHg, respectively, than in age-matched women [2]. However after 60 years-of-age, blood pressure increases in women so that hypertension becomes more or at least as prevalent in women as men [3]. Ovarian hormones may be responsible in part for lower blood pressure in premenopausal women and for the increase in blood pressure in postmenopausal women because gender-related differences in the prevalence of hypertension disappear or cross over after women enter menopause. However, the correlation between reduced testosterone levels and increased blood pressure in older males suggests that testosterone also lowers blood pressure. Like humans, animals also display sex-associated differences in blood pressure [4, 5, 6], and male spontaneously hypertensive rats (SHR), Dahl salt-sensitive rats, deoxycorticosterone acetate-salt hypertensive rats, and New Zealand genetically hypertensive rats have higher blood pressures compared with females. However, contrary to expectations from observations in human beings, in these animal models of high blood pressure, arterial blood pressure is decreased by castration [4, 5, 6], but is not increased by ovariectomy [4, 5, 6]. Thus, although both testicular and ovarian sex hormones appear to affect arterial blood pressure, their role in this regard remains controversial. The purpose of this review is to describe the evidence regarding the possible involvement of female and male sex hormones in regulating blood pressure.

Regulation of Blood Pressure by Estrogens

Evidence from Clinical Observations

The main endogenous estrogen is estradiol, and clinical evidence suggests that endogenous estradiol lowers blood pressure in women. In this regard, multiple cross sectional studies report a significant increase in both systolic and diastolic blood pressure after menopause [4, 7, 8]. For example, a four-fold increase in the incidence of hypertension occurs in postmenopausal women (40% in postmenopausal women versus 10% in premenopausal women) [9]. Moreover, prospective evaluation of blood pressure using conventional and ambulatory methods indicates that the progression from the premenopausal to the postmenopausal state is associated with a 4-5 mm Hg increase in systolic blood pressure [10], and each decade is associated with a 5 mm Hg greater increase in systolic blood pressure in perimenopausal and postmenopausal women than in premenopausal women [10]. Inasmuch as a decrease in the synthesis of endogenous estradiol occurs during menopause, these findings strongly suggest that reductions in estradiol production are causally connected to increases in arterial blood pressure. That endogenous estradiol has a blood pressure lowering effect in women is also supported by the observation that during the menstrual cycle blood pressure is lower in the luteal phase compared with the follicular phase [11]. Finally, during normal pregnancy, blood pressure decreases as estradiol levels increase [12].

Clinical studies with various estrogen replacement therapies provide evidence that estrogens either lower blood pressure or have neutral effect [13-29; Table 1] Studies with exogenous estradiol support the hypothesis that endogenous estradiol lowers blood pressure. In this regard, administration of authentic estradiol generally reduces arterial blood pressure in normotensive, healthy, postmenopausal women (Table 1). For example, two months of treatment with transdermal estradiol (50 μg/day; achieves physiological levels of estradiol) decreases nocturnal, but not day time (office) blood pressure (systolic, diastolic and mean) [13]. Multiple other studies utilizing 24-hour ambulatory blood pressure measurement report blood pressure lowering effects of estradiol given for up to one year [14, 15] (Table 1). Investigators also observe significant decreases in nighttime systolic, diastolic, and mean blood pressure blood pressure in healthy postmenopausal women treated with transdermal estradiol (0.1 mg patches administered twice per week to attain physiologic estradiol levels) alone or in combination with intravaginal progesterone (300 mg) [16]. It is important to note that although exogenous estradiol or estradiol/progestin does not significantly reduce *daytime/office* systolic and diastolic blood pressures, women appear to be more prone to white coat hypertension [30] so nocturnal blood pressure is a more valid measure of the effects of estradiol on blood pressure.

Estradiol also appears to lower blood pressure in hypertensive postmenopausal women (Table 1). For example, results from a randomized, double-blind crossover trial in 30 postmenopausal women with mild hypertension indicate that estradiol (transdermal; delivery rate 100 μg/day) significantly lowers 24-hour ambulatory blood pressure [17]. A significant decrease in blood pressure is also observed in postmenopausal women with mild to moderate hypertension who receive transdermal estradiol [18]. Reports from a prospective study conducted in 34 postmenopausal women with treated hypertension indicate that administration of estradiol plus the progestin norgestrel for 19 weeks lowers 24-hour ambulatory blood pressure [19], and a study in 13 postmenopausal women with concurrent treatment for hypertension suggests that acute administration of transdermal estradiol reduces 24-hour ambulatory day time systolic blood pressure and nocturnal systolic and diastolic blood pressure [20]. However, when ambulatory blood pressure measurements are not employed, blood pressure lowering effects of chronic estradiol administration are generally not detectable [21].

Although endogenous estradiol appears to lower blood pressure, administration of estrogenic preparations that contain little or no estradiol produce inconsistent effects on blood pressure (**Table 1**) (**see review 4 for original citations**). Tibolone (a synthetic estrogen with both androgenic and gestagenic properties), for example, has little effect on blood pressure [31], and the results of the Postmenopausal Estrogen/Progestin Interventions Trial (PEPI) suggest that conjugated equine estrogens, which contain little estradiol, in combination with a variety of progestins do not change blood pressure in normotensive postmenopausal women [32]. Similarly, data from two large randomized hormone replacement trials using conjugated equine estrogens for the primary and secondary prevention of cardiovascular disease also demonstrate no significant effects of these estrogens on blood pressure [33, 34]. However, a prospective study of 160 postmenopausal women taking either conjugated equine estrogens or piperazine estrone sulphate (Ogen) reports development of hypertension in women taking conjugated equine estrogens [35].

Table 1: Effects of estrogens on blood pressure in human beings

Study	Subjects Normotensive (N) / Hypertensive (H)	Treatment	Outcome	Ref
1	62 PMW (42 no HRT; 20 HRT); N	CEE	24 hr. ambulatory BP was decreased	22
2	30 PMW (randomized, double blind crossover; mild H)	Transdermal 17β-E	24 hr. BP was decreased	17
3	29 PMW (15 placebo; 14 treated; N)	Oral 17β-E daily plus dydrogesterone every 3-4 week	Follow-up after 1 year of treatment showed a significant decrease in BP	15
4	16 PMW (mild to moderate H)	Transdermal 17β-estradiol	Ambulatory 24 hr. BP was decreased	18
5	12 surgically PMW (N)	Oral CEE Oral CE plus MPA	Auscultatory BP unchanged after 1 wk Auscultatory BP lowered after 1 wk	23
6	73 PMW (38 oral; 35 transdermal; N)	Oral 17β-E + norethindrone Transdermal 17β-E + norethindrone	24 hr ambulatory BP decreased after 2 and 6 mo 24 hr ambulatory BP decreased after 2, but not 6 mo	24
7	34 PMW (prospective study, 34 PMW with treated H)	Cyclic Estradiol + norgestrel (19 wks)	24 hr ambulatory BP decreased after 19 wks	19
8	60 PMW (20 placebo, 20 CEE, 20 17β-E; CAD) Treatment for 1 year; Transdermal	Oral CEE ± MPA (10d) Transdermal 17β-E ± MPA (10d)	Night time ambulatory BP decreased No significant change in BP	25
9	16 PMW (placebo-controlled, randomized crossover study; N)	17β-E plus cyclic NETA	24hr ambulatory BP decreased and this effect was more pronounced in presence of NETA	26
10	17 PMW (3 month, placebo-controlled, randomized crossover study; N)	Oral CEE Oral CEE plus MPA	24 hr ambulatory BP decreased 24 hr ambulatory BP decreased	27
11	18 PMW (placebo-controlled, randomized crossover study, N)	Transdermal 17β-E for 2 months	24 hr nocturnal, but not day time, BP decreased	13

Table 1: Continued

Study	Subjects Normotensive (N) / Hypertensive (H)	Treatment	Outcome	Ref
12	15 PMW (placebo-controlled, randomized crossover study, N)	Transdermal 17β-E (8wks) ± P (vaginal; 2wks)	24 ambulatory BP (nocturnal & daytime) decreased by 17β-E alone and the effect was enhanced by P	16
13	107 PMW + ERT; 223 PMW –HRT; population based sample; H and N	Oral CEE, 17β-E and other Es oral or transdermal	No change in BP	28
14	PEPI trial-875 PMW; N	CEE ± various progestins	No change in BP	32
15	13 PMW (with ongoing treatment for Hypertension, placebo-controlled double blind, crossover study; H)	Transdermal 17β-E	24 hr ambulatory daytime diastolic BP decreased at 24 hr. and 24 hr ambulatory nocturnal systolic and diastolic BP decreased at 24 hr.	20
16	90 PMW women (oophorectomized, 30-59 yrs.), non-randomized, prospective study; N	Transdermal 17β-E (n=40) Oral ERT (n=50)	24hr. ambulatory nocturnal systolic and daytime as well as night time BP reduced at 3 and 6 months. No change in BP in subjects receiving oral ERT	14
17	20 PMW, double blind, cross over study. (N)	Oral CEE plus oral cyclical MPA	Ambulatory day time diastolic and mean BP reduced and MPA lowered BP dose-dependently in presence of conjugated estrogens.	29
18	16608 PMW, randomized control trial (WHI study)	Oral CEE plus MPA	No change in BP	34
19	2763 PMW, randomized controlled trial, with CHD (HERS trial)	CEE plus MPA	No change in BP	33

PMW, postmenopausal women; N, normotensive; H, hypertensive; ERT, estradiol replacement therapy; HRT, hormone replacement therapy; CEE, conjugated equine estrogens; , 17β-E, , 17β-estradiol; MPA, medroxyprogesterone; NETA, norethisterone acetate. Original references are cited in reference 4. (Reproduced with permission from ref 4)

In contrast to estradiol (lowers blood pressure) and conjugated equine estrogens (little effect on blood pressure), contraceptive estrogens in general elevate blood pressure [reviewed in detail in ref 4]. The risk of hypertension due to oral contraceptives increases with age, duration of use, body mass and progestin potency [4]. Estrogens used in contraceptive pills (e.g., ethinyl estradiol) are chemically different than estradiol and conjugated equine estrogens; moreover, the doses for contraceptive estrogens and estrogens used for hormone replacement therapy vary considerably. Clearly, the blood pressure effects of estrogenic preparations cannot be equated just because the preparations belong to the same pharmacological class.

Evidence from Animal Studies

In various animal models of hypertensive, including SHR, stroke prone SHR (SHRSP), rats with deoxycortisterone acetate-salt induced hypertension, Dahl salt-sensitive rats and rats with pulmonary hypertension estradiol also decreases arterial blood pressure [reviewed in 4, 7, 8, 36]. On the other hand, removal of endogenous estradiol by ovariectomy does not affect the development of hypertension in SHRs [4], a finding which suggests that the blood pressure lowering effects of exogenous estradiol in rats are pharmacological rather than physiological. In contrast to estradiol, the synthetic estrogen ethinyl estradiol increases blood pressure in animals [4], a finding that suggests that the effects of natural and synthetic estrogens differ and may influence different mechanisms of blood pressure regulation.

From an "up close" perspective, the published reports regarding the effects of estrogens on blood pressure appear confusing and inconsistent. However, stepping back and viewing the data from a broader perspective reveals several important trends. Specifically, the available data indicate that the effect of a given estrogen on blood pressure depends on the type of estrogenic preparation, the dose of estrogen and, at least in human beings, how blood pressure is monitored. In this regard, contraceptive estrogens tend to increase blood pressure, conjugated equine estrogens have little effect on blood pressure and authentic estradiol tends to lower blood pressure. Also, the risk of estrogen-induced hypertension is more with high doses compared with low doses. Finally, the blood pressure lowering and antihypertensive actionss of estradiol are best detected by 24-hour ambulatory blood pressure monitoring.

Cellular and Biochemical Mechanisms by which Estadiol Regulates Blood Pressure

Multiple organs and autocrine/paracrine factors are involved in mediating the blood pressure lowering effects of estradiol, and have been reviewed in depth recently [4, 7, 8, 36]. As shown in Table 2, estradiol decreases the synthesis, release or activity of several molecules known to cause vasoconstriction and to increase blood pressure including endothelin-1, angiotensin II, catecholamines, α-adrenergic receptors, angiotensin converting enzyme, renin and the angiotensin type 1 receptor [7, 8]. Moreover, estradiol increases the synthesis, release or activity of additional molecules know to cause vasodilation and to decrease blood pressure including NO, bradykinin, angiotenin 1-7, cAMP, cGMP, prostacyclin, adenosine, vascular endothelial growth factor and K^+ channels [7, 8]. In addition, estradiol protects the endothelium by acting as an anti-oxidant against free radicals and by lowering the levels of homocysteine, Lp(a) and LDL [7, 8]. Estradiol increases insulin sensitivity and insulin like growth factor-1 (IGF-1), thus further generating beneficial effects on the cardiovascular system and blood pressure [7, 8]. Moreover, estradiol inhibits the proliferation of, migration of and extracellular matrix synthesis by vascular smooth muscle cells and cardiac fibroblasts, processes that play a key role in the remodeling of peripheral resistance vessels and the heart, respectively, associated with hypertension (Figure 1) [4, 8]. Taken together the above findings may explain the blood pressure lowering potential of estradiol and the ability of estradiol to provide cardiovascular protection (Table 2).

The kidneys modulate blood pressure, and renal dysfunction is involved in the development and maintenance of hypertension. Single nephron glomerular filteration rate (GFR), glomerular plasma flow, preglomerular resistance, glomerular pressure and renovascular responses to Ang II are quantitatively different in males versus females [4, 8]. In this regard, in male rats compared with female rats, single nephrons GFR and glomerular plasma flow are higher and preglomerular resistance is lower [4]. Because a reduction in preglomerular resistance is associated with increased glomerular injury, particularly if systemic blood pressure is also increased, these gender-based differences in renal hemodynamics may predispose males to more severe progression of glomerulopathies. In addition to favorable effects on renal hemodynaimcs, estradiol also may guard against glomerulosclerosis by inhibiting the proliferation of and extracellular matrix synthesis by mesangial cells and by stimulating endothelial cell proliferation [4, 8]. Finally, estradiol positively influences the synthesis and actions of multiple autocrine/paracrine factors implicated in the etiology of renal disease (Figure 1 and Table 2). Consistent with the aforementioned effects of estradiol, evidence from epidemiological studies, clinical trials and experimental studies using animal models of renal injury indicate that ovarian hormones delay progression of renal disease.

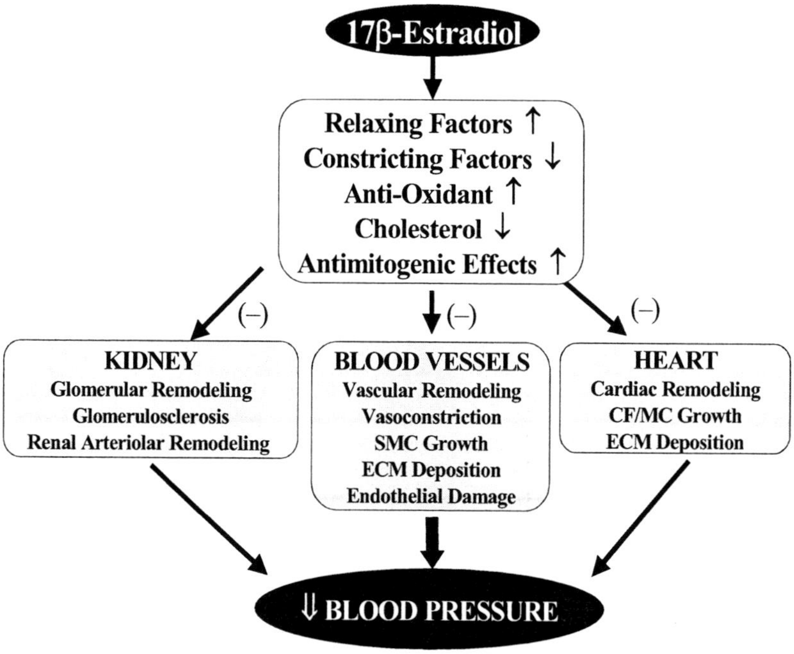

Figure 1. A schematic representation summarizing and comparing the potential mechanisms via which estradiol can influence blood pressure and be associated with preventing hypertension. Smooth muscle cell (SMC); cardiac fibroblast (CF); cardiac myocyte (MC); extracellular matrix synthesis (ECM); inhibition, (); induction (+); increased (↑); decreased (↓); highly increased (⇑); neutral effects (↔).

Table 2. Effects of estradiol and androgens on factors regulating blood pressure directly or indirectly

BLOOD PRESSURE REGULATORY VASOACTIVE FACTORS / ENZYMES / RECEPTORS	INFLUENCE ON BLOOD-PRESSURE	MODULATORY EFFECTS OF ESTRADIOL	MODULATORY EFFECTS OF ANDROGENS
ANGIOTENSIN CONVERTING ENZYME	INCREASES	↓	↑
ANGIOTENSIN II/RENIN RELEASE	INCREASES	↓	↑
ANGIOTENSIN 1-7	LOWERS	↑	?
ANGIOTENSIN TYPE 1 RECEPTORS	INCREASES	↓	↑
BRADYKININ	LOWERS	↑	↑↓
ENDOTHELIN-1	INCREASES	↓	↑
CATECHOLAMINES	INCREASES	↓	↑
α-ADRENERGIC RECEPTORS	INCREASES	↓	↑
NITRIC OXIDE	LOWERS	↑	↑
ADENOSINE	LOWERS	↑	?
VEGF	LOWERS	↑	↓↑
ATRIAL NATURECTIC PEPTIDE (ANP)	LOWERS	↑	↔ or ↓
ANP RECEPTORS	LOWERS	↑	?
NEUROPEPTIDE Y	INCREASES	↓	↑
PROSTACYCLIN	LOWERS	↑	↔ or ↓
20-HETE	INCREASES	↔	↑
ION CHANNEL (Na+, K+, Ca2+) Activity	VARIABLE	↑↑ K+ ; ↔Na+; ↓Ca 2+	↑ K+ ; ↔Na+; ↓Ca 2+
CYCLIC GMP	LOWERS	↑	↑
CYCLIC AMP	LOWERS	↑	↑
INSULIN RESISTANCE	INCREASES	↓	↑
INSULIN SENSITIVITY	DECREASES	↑	↓
IGF-1	INCREASES	↓	↔
HDL-C	POSITIVE	↑	↓
TRIGLYCERIDE	NEGATIVE	↑	↑↓
Lp(a)	NEGATIVE	↓	↓
LDL-C	NEGATIVE	↓	↑↓

↑, INCREASES or INDUCES, ↓, DECREASES or INHIBITS; ↔, NO CHANGE; ?, UNKNOWN

Effects of Estradiol on the Sympathetic Nervous System

The interaction of estradiol with the sympathetic nervous system may also play a role in lowering blood pressure [4]. Studies by Sudhir et al [37] in 12 perimenopausal women randomized to recieve estradiol valerate (n=7) or placebo (n=5) demonstrate that estradiol decreases norepinephrine-induced vasoconstriction and total body norepinephrine spillover. A randomized, crossover, placebo-controlled study in 12 normotensive postmenopausal women demonstrates that transdermal estradiol, but not conjugated equine estrogens, decreases the 24-hour ambulatory blood pressure and sympathetic nerve discharge after eight weeks of treatment [38]. However, a diffenent study demonstrates that in 11 healthy postmenopausal women, conjugated equine estrogens significantly increase sympathetic baroreflex gain [39]. In menopausal women, acute administration of estradiol and progesterone attenuates cardiovascular responses and increases in plasma catecholamines induced by mental stress [40]. Consistent with the hypothesis that estradiol inhibits sympathetic tone is the observation that muscle sympathetic nerve activity as measured by microneurography is lower in women compared with age-matched men [41]. As in human beings, estradiol, but not conjugated estrogens, inhibit the sympathetic nervous system in animal models of hypertension [4]. Thus the totality of the evidence indicates that estradiol, in contrast to conjugated equine estrogens, decreases basal sympathetic tone, an effect that may contribute to the blood pressure lowering effects of estradiol.

Role of Estrogen Receptors and Estradiol Metabolism

There is some evidence that estrogens affect blood pressure via estrogen receptors (ERs). For example, mice lacking ERβ develop sustained systolic and diastolic hypertension [42], and a polymorphism in the ERβ gene is associated with increased systemic blood pressure in Japanese women [43]. Also, estradiol induces the synthesis of potent blood pressure lowering factors like NO via activation of ERα [4, 7, 9].

It is difficult, however, to explain the differential effects of conjugated equine estrogens, contraceptive estrogens and estadiol on blood pressure under the hypothesis that ERs mediate all the blood pressure effects of estrogenic preparations because this hypothesis would predict that all estrogenic compounds would have similar effects on blood pressure. Although many of the biological actions of estradiol are mediated by ERs, recent findings provide evidence that ER-independent mechanisms mediate some of the cardiovascular effects of estradiol. In this regard, endogenous metabolites of estradiol, with little or no affinity for ERs, can affect components of the cardiovascular system, suggesting that estradiol may have cardiovascular actions via its downstream metabolites [44]. Indeed, recent studies from our laboratory provide evidence that the anti-growth effects of estradiol on vascular smooth muscle cells, cardiac fibroblasts and glomerular mesangial cells are mediated by oxidation of estradiol to 2-hydroxyestradiol (mediated by cytochrome P450s), followed by methylation of 2-hydroxyestrdiol to 2-methoxyestradiol (mediated by catechol-O-methyltransferase). Both 2-hydroxyestradiol and 2-methoxyestradiol are major endogenous metabolites of estradiol with little or no, respectively, affinity for ERs [45]. Increased proliferation of these cell types leads to vascular remodeling, left ventricular hypertrophy and glomerulosclerosis, respectively (Figure 1), and these actions of estradiol metabolites may account in part for the ability of estradiol to lower blood pressure and protect the cardiovascular and renal systems from hypertension-induced damage.

Recent studies from our laboratory support the concept that estradiol metabolites mediate in part the blood pressure lowering effects and cardioprotective effects of estradiol. Long-term treatment with 2-hydroxyestradiol decreases body weight, improves vascular endothelial function, decreases nephropathy, exerts anti-diabetic actions and lowers blood pressure and blood cholesterol in male obese ZSF1 rats that exhibit the metabolic syndrome (i.e. hypertension, obesity, diabetes, and hyperlipidemia) and have left ventricular, renal and vascular dysfunction [45]. Also, 2-hydroxyestradiol attenuates puromycin aminonucleoside-induced nephropathy, increases in blood pressure and urinary excretion of albumin [46]. These findings support the hypothesis that the blood pressure lowering effects of estradiol as well as the cardiovascular and renal protective effects of estradiol are in part mediated via endogenous metabolites of estradiol, specifically 2-hydroxyestradiol and 2-methoxyestradiol (Figure 2).

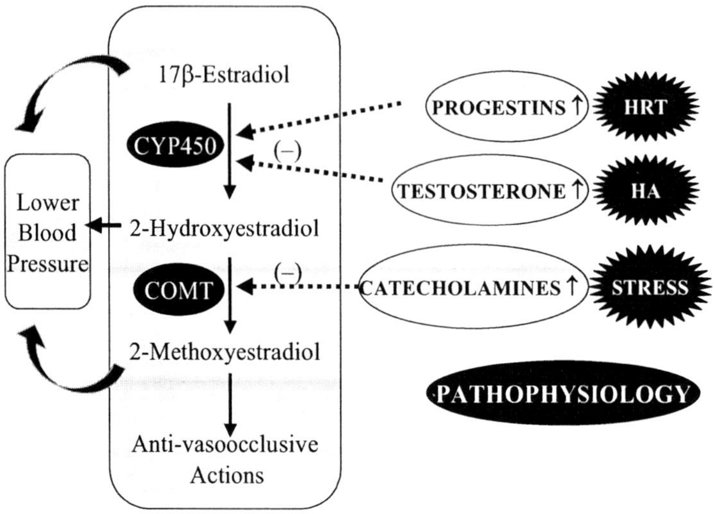

Figure 2. A schematic representation delineating the possible mechanisms via which pathological conditions such as stress, hypertesteronemia (HA), or hormone replacement therapy for postmenopausal disorders can influence endogenous metabolism of estradiol to 2-hydroxyestradiol and 2-methoxyestradiol and abrogate their blood pressure lowering or anti-hypertensive actions. Catechol-O-methyltransferase, COMT; Cytochrome P450, CYP450; Hormone replacement therapy, HRT; inhibition, (–).

The above findings also suggest that endogenous or exogenous factors that interfere with estradiol metabolism may abrogate the cardiovascular protective effects of estradiol. In this context, medroxyprogesterone (a progestin often co-administered with estrogens during hormone replacement therapy) and testosterone inhibit the metabolism of estradiol to 2-hydroxyestradiol [44] and abrogate the effects of estradiol on blood pressure and the cardiovascular system [4]. Also, catecholamines block the antimitogenic effects of estradiol and 2-hydroxyestardiol on vascular smooth muscle cells, cardiac fibroblasts and glomerular mesangial cells by inhibiting catechol-O-methyltransferase and thereby preventing the conversion of 2-hydroxyestradiol to 2-methoxyestradiol [47, 48]. Additionally, life style factor, such as dietary habits (for example consumption of dietary factors, such as resveratrol, that inhibit cytochrome P450s) and stress (leading to increased catecholamine release which inhibits catechol-O-methyltransferase), can also alter the metabolism of estradiol to 2-hydroyestradiol and 2-methoxyestradiol [44]. Based on these observations, we hypothesize that endogenous metabolism of estradiol to 2-hydroxyestradiol and 2-methoxyestradiol may play a very important role in defining the blood pressure lowering effects of estradiol. In this context and as hypothesized in **Figure 2,** several factors may abrogate the beneficial effects of estradiol on blood pressure by inhibiting the conversion of estradiol to 2-hydroxyestradiol and 2-methoxyestradiol including: 1) increased testosterone levels in pathophysiological conditions such as polycystic ovarian syndrome, pregnancy-induced hypertension and during hormone therapy for female-to-male transsexuals; 2) administration of progestins during hormone replacement therapy in postmenopausal women; and 3) increased catecholamine levels during stress. In summary, either genetic or acquired abnormalities in the metabolism of estradiol to 2-hydroxyestradiol and 2-methoxyestadiol may play a critical role in defining the cardioprotective and blood pressure lowering effects of estradiol.

Regulation of Blood Pressure by Progestins

Animal studies demonstrate that acute administration of progesterone does not alter mean arterial blood pressure [4]. In contrast, chronic exposure to progesterone tends to decrease blood pressure. For example, progression of pregnancy is associated with an increase in progesterone and a decrease in blood pressure [4]. Also, in men and postmenopausal women with mild to moderate hypertension, oral administration of progesterone significantly lowers blood pressure [49]. However, in normotensive postclimacteric women, oral progesterone does not affect blood pressure [50]. Sequential administration of the non-androgenic progestogen medroxyprogesterone acetate (MPA) or the androgenic progestogen norethisterone acetate (NETA) either does not alter or enhances the blood pressure lowering effects of estrogens. For example, one study reports that in 53 postmenopausal women treated for 4 weeks with conjugated equine estrogens (0.625 mg daily), sequentially treatment with either 2.5, 5 and 10 mg of MPA during the last 14 days causes a dose-dependent decrease in daytime ambulatory diastolic and mean arterial blood pressure [51]. Similarly, the progestin NETA significantly enhances the blood pressure lowering effects of estradiol in a placebo-controlled randomized crossover study in 16 normotensive postmenopausal women [4]. In summary, acute administration of progestins has little if any affect on blood pressure, whereas chronic administration of progestins tends to lower blood pressure.

Regulation of Blood Pressure by Androgens

Evidence from Clinical Observations

Some clinical findings support the concept that androgens lower blood pressure and protect the cardiovascular system. For example, testosterone and androstenedione levels tend to be lower in hypertensive men, and circulating testosterone levels in men with coronary artery disease or myocardial infarction are either unchanged or decreased (for details and original references see 4, 52, 53). These observations suggest that decreased, rather than increased, androgen levels are associated with hypertension, myocardial infarction and coronary artery disease. It is likely, however, that the lower testosterone level in unhealthy men is a result rather than a cause of cardiovascular disease. In this regard, myocardial infarction, surgery, head trauma, burns, hypoxia, sleep deprivation and psychological stressors reduce testosterone levels [4]. Therefore, it is possible that the reduced levels of testosterone in men with hypertension and cardiovascular disease is merely a consequence of the underlying disease.

Most clinical findings support the concept that androgens increase blood pressure and the risk of cardiovascular disease. For example, the low prevalence of coronary disease among men with hypotestosteronemia plus hyperestrogenemia favors the hypothesis that androgens increase, rather than decrease, the risk of cardiovascular disease [4, 52, 53]. Also, the fact that women suffering from hypertestosteronemia have an increased risk of coronary artery disease and myocardial infarction supports the concept that testosterone is a risk factor for cardiovascular disease and hypertension [4]. Moreover, androgen levels and blood pressure are increased in women with polycystic ovarian syndrome (PCOS) and pregnancy-induced hypertension (PIH) [4, 52, 53], and men with testosterone deficiency following orchiectomy have a slightly lower mortality from heart disease [4, 52, 53]. Data from several small clinical studies [54-69] provide evidence that testosterone and androgens have either adverse or neutral effects on blood pressure (**Table 3**). The blood pressure elevating effects of testosterone/androgens in women with hypertestosteronemia (PCOS, PIH, anovulation, or male-to-female transsexuals) may be due to testosterone blocking the blood pressure lowering effects of estradiol. As shown in **Figure 2,** testosterone and androgens can inhibit the conversion of estradiol to 2-hydroxyestradiol, a major estradiol metabolite which lowers blood pressure [45, 46].

Abuse of synthetic derivatives of testosterone (for example some anabolic steroids) is associated with hypertension, ventricular remodeling, myocardial ischemia and sudden cardiac death [4]. In this regard, a double blind placebo-controlled study in 21 men demonstrates that treatment with testosterone enanthate (3.5 mg/kg bwt) for 12 weeks significantly increases systolic blood pressure by 10 mm Hg [70]. In contrast, administration of testosterone to 20 male subjects (mean age 70.6±6.2 years) to achieve physiologic and superphysiologic serum testosterone concentrations does not increase blood pressure [68], and testosterone undecanoate (120 mg/day for 5 days) does not affect blood pressure [62]. Apparently, the effects of andogens on the cardiovascular system are modulated by age, duration of treatment and exercise.

Evidence from Animal Studies

Animal studies indicate that testosterone increases blood pressure. For example, compared with females, blood pressure is significantly higher in male SHR, Dahl salt-sensitive rats, deoxycorticosterone acetate-salt hypertensive rats and New Zealand genetically hypertensive rats [4, 5, 6], and castration at 3 to 5 weeks-of-age attenuates the development of hypertension in SHR and Dahl salt-sensitive rats [4-6]. Also, administration of testosterone increases blood pressure in ovariectomized normotensive female rats, castrated normotensive male rats [4, 5, 6], ovariectomized female SHRs and normotensive, uninephrectomized female rats [4, 5, 6]. Importantly, neonatal androgen imprinting determines the gender dimorphic pattern of blood pressure. In this regard, a single dose of testosterone administered to newborn females increases their blood pressure to male levels at maturity [52]. There is also evidence for Y chromosome locus producing gender-selective hypertension mediated by testosterone and androgen receptors [52].

Cellular and Biochemical Mechanisms by which Androgens Regulate Blood Pressure

Testosterone/andrognes may elevate blood pressure and damage blood vessels via a number of mechanisms (**Figure 3**). In this regard, testosterone/androgens modulate the synthesis of multiple vasoactive factors that regulate blood pressure (**Table 2**). Testosterone increases plasma levels of homocysteine, and homocysteine damages vascular and glomerular endothelial cells, which may contribute to the development of atherosclerosis and glomerulosclerosis [4]. Unlike estradiol which decreases endothelin-1 release, testosterone increases endothelin-1 levels in subjects undergoing a sex change, and this may be a humoral mechanism by which testosterone elevates blood pressure [4]. In male SHR, increased levels of catecholamines are associated with high blood pressure [4, 5, 6], and castration reduces catecholamine levels to those observed in normotensive controls [4], suggesting that testosterone can augment catecholamine synthesis [4]. Indeed, testosterone stimulates tyrosine hydroxylase, the rate limiting enzyme for catecholamine synthesis [4, 7, 8].

Androgens also induce the synthesis of 20-HETE, a potent vasoconstricting and blood pressure elevating factor [72]. Thus, testosterone may elevate blood pressure and contribute to the pathogenesis of cardiovascular disease by altering a number of humoral factors, including homocysteine, endothelin-1 and catecholamines.

Table 3: Effects of androgens on blood pressure in human beings

Study	Subjects Normal (N); Diabetic (D); Obese (O); Male (M); Female (F) No treatment (NT) ; Treated (T); Placebo (P);	Treatment Days (D); intramuscular (IM); intravenous (IV); Percutaneous gel (PG)	Outcome	Ref
1	48 Middle aged men; D (type-II); 24 NT; 24 T; Open Label sStudy	TU (120mg/day) for 3 months	No adverse effects or no change in BP	54
2	8 men; N; age 44±3; randomized, double blind crossover study	Oral A (200mg/day) for 28 days with 28 day washout period.	No significant change in BP	55
3	37 transexuals (17 F to M); 16-36 years; prospective intervention study	TE (250mg/2wk IM) for 12 months	No significant change in BP	56
4	36 hypogonadal men; 37±12 years; 19 treated with T; 20 eugonadal M served as controls	TEN (250mg/2wk IM) for 3 months	No change or adverse effects on BP	57
5	32 M with provocable myocardial ischemia; age 69±6.4; randomized controlled trial (16 placebo and 18 treated)	T(2 doses, IV) for acute effects	No significant change in BP	58
6	18 healthy M; age 51-55; randomized double blind unicentric controlled trial (6 placebo; 6 T treated; 6 DHT treated);	T (125 mg/d) and DHT (25mg/d) via percutaneous gels for 3 months.	No significant change in BP	59
7	21 Hypogonadal men (7 in study 1 and 14 in study II)	TU, 1000mg in tea seed oil (study 1) or in castor ol (study II), IM for acute T.	No significant change in BP	60
8	12 F to M transexuals; 12 healthy F (controls); cross sectional and non-randomized	Treated with long term high dose androgen therapy (200 to 800 mg T depot implants and TE as IM) for at least 2-months.	No significant change in BP	61

Table 3: Effects of androgens on blood pressure in human beings

Study	Subjects	Treatment	Outcome	Ref
9	23 eugonadal men with osteoporosis (age 34-73); open, prospective therapeutic trial.	TE (250 mg / fortnightly IM) for 6 months	Favorable changes in diastolic BP (-4.7 mm Hg; p<.01)	62
10	30 healthy obese M; age 40 ; randomized, double blind, placebo controlled clinical trial (Groups: placebo, TEN, anabolic steroids)	TEN orally; anabolic steroids (oral oxandralone or parenteral nandrolone decaoate) for 9 months	No significant change in BP	63
11	23 middle aged Obese Men; Randomized placebo controlled trial	Testosterone treatment for 8 months	Diastolic BP decreased with T treatment	64
12	11 obese middle aged men.	Testosterone (500 mg as single IV or 40mgx4 orally) for 6 weeks.	No signficant change in BP	65
13	Middle aged obese men; exploratory study with three groups	Groups: T 250 or 500mg IM for 6 weeks; TU oral for 6 weeks; T and DHT transdermal for 3 months	No significant change in BP	66
14	The Helsinki Heart Study. Randomized controlled trial; nested case control design; 62 subjects; 97 controls on placebo		Increased DHEAS levels associated with increased Systolic and Diastolic BP	67
15	20 men; age 70.6±6.2; studied at three occasions after receiving placebo or T to achieve physiologic T or supraphysiologic T; randomized trial	Physiologic T (bolus plus continuous IV to increase T levels by 2 and 6 times, respectively); duration 28 minutes	No significant change in BP	68
16	9 hypogonadal men; age 35±4; receiving T replacement therapy	Treated with T (800mg / month depot) for 2-4 weeks. Subjects served as their own control; measurements made at trough and peak levels	No significant change in BP	69

T, testosterone; TU, testosterone undecanoate ; TE, testosterone ester; TEN, testosterone enanthate; A, androstenedione; DHT, dihydrotestosterone; DHEAS, dehydroepiandrosterone sulfate;

Androgens may also cause hypertension by inducing renal injury [4, 5, 6]. Compared with females, ageing males exhibit decreased glomerular filtration rate and develop glomerular injury, glomerulosclerosis, proteinuria and increased blood pressure [4, 5, 6]. Castration early in life decreases renal injury and attenuates the development of hypertension. Conversely, administration of testosterone to castrated animals increases blood pressure to levels similar to those found in intact males [5, 6]. Together, these observations indicate that testosterone adversely affects renal function, eventually leading to hypertension.

An important question is whether the effects of testosterone on blood pressure are androgen-receptor mediated. In this regard, flutamide, an androgen receptor antagonist, lowers blood pressure in male SHRs to levels found in female or castrated male SHRs [6]. These findings suggest that the effects of androgens on blood pressure are mediated by androgen receptors. In support of this concept, androgen-receptor blockade suppresses sodium-induced increases in blood pressure in Wistar-Kyoto rats and SHR [5, 6].

Disruption of the CYP4A14 gene causes hypertension that is more severe in males, and male CYP4A14 (-/-) mice have increased levels of plasma androgens, kidney CYP4A12 expression, and the prohypertensive arachidonic acid metabolite 20-HETE. Castration normalizes blood pressure in CYP 4A14 (-/-) mice, decreases CYP4A12 expression and reduces 20-HETE formation, and the effects of castration are reversed by androgen replacement. These data support the hypothesis that androgens may increase blood pressure by up-regulating the production of 20-HETE.

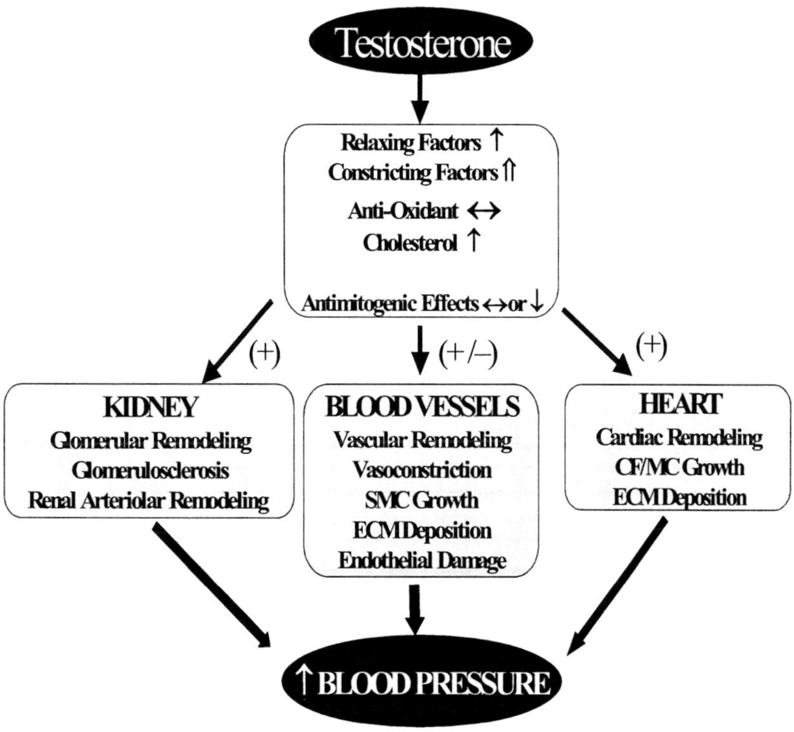

Figure 3: A schematic representation summarizing and comparing the potential mechanisms via which testosterone can influence blood pressure and be associated with inducing hypertension. Smooth muscle cell (SMC); cardiac fibroblast (CF); cardiac myocyte (MC); extracellular matrix synthesis (ECM); inhibition, (–); induction (+); increased (↑); decreased (↓); highly increased (⇑); neutral effects (↔).

Androgens may increase blood pressure by several other mechanisms including shifting the pressure-natriuresis relationship to the right to increase sodium retention and by increasing plasma renin activity [4, 5]. In addition, in contrast to estradiol, androgens induce insulin resistance [73, 74], increase insulin like growth factor-1 levels, decrease HDL-C and increase neuropeptide Y levels, catecholamine levels and the expression of α-adrenergic receptors (Table 2).

CONCLUSION

Men and postmenopausal women are relatively more susceptible to hypertension and its sequelae compared to premenopausal women. There is now strong evidence, based on animal studies, that estradiol is an antihypertensive sex hormone, whereas testosterone is a pro-hypertensive sex hormone. Estradiol and testosterone affect blood pressure via multiple mechanisms involving direct effects on vascular, renal and cardiac cells and indirect effects mediated by humoral factors. Current evidence does not allow a conclusion regarding the role for progesterone in the regulation of arterial blood pressure. Additional research is badly needed to provide clear answers to important questions regarding the role of sex hormones in hypertension and cardiovascular disease. Two important questions in need of answers are: 1) Do estradiol metabolites mediate any beneficial effects of sex hormones on the cardiovascular system and blood pressure? 2) How does estradiol/progesterone compare to conjugated equine estrogens/synthetic progestins with regard to long-term effects on blood pressure and cardiovascular disease in a large cohort of hypertensive postmenopausal women? The answers to these and other important related questions may be long in coming.

ACKNOWLEDGEMENTS

This work was supported by grants from the Swiss National Science Foundation (Dr. R.K.Dubey; 32-54172.98), and the National Institutes of Health (Dr. E.Jackson, HL69846).

FOOT NOTE: Due to page limitations we could not cite all the original and highly valued scientific work of several authors and would like to extend our sincere apologies. We have made every attempt to cite review articles from where the original citations can be obtained.

REFERENCES

[1] Yong LC, Kuller LH, Rutan G, et al.: Longitudinal study of blood pressure changes and determinants from adolescence to middle age. The Dormont High School Follow-Up Study, 1957–1963 to 1989–1990. *Am J Epidemiol* 1993; 138: 973–983.

[2] Burt Vl, Whelton P, Rocella EJ, et al. Prevalence of hypertension in the US adult population: results of the Third National Health and Nutrition Examination Survey, 1988–1991. *Hypertension* 1995; 25: 305–313.

[3] Stamler J, Stamler R, Riedlinger WF, et al.: Hypertension screening of 1 million Americans. Community Hypertension Evaluation Clinic (CHEC) Program, 1973–1975. *JAMA*. 1976; 235: 2299–2306.

[4] Dubey RK, Oparil S, Imthurn B, et al.: Sex hormones and hypertension. *Cardiovascular Research* 2002; 53: 688-708. [This article provides an in-depth review of the cellular and biochemical mechanisms by which estrogens and androgens can influence the cardiovascular system. It reviews the evidence for the effects of sex hormones on blood pressure from both clinical and animal studies.]

[5] Reckelhoff JF, Granger JP. Role of androgens in mediating hypertension and renal injury. *Clin Expt Pharmacol Physiol* 1999; 26: 127-131. [In-depth review providing evidence linking androgens to hypertension.]

[6] Reckelhoff JF, Zhang H, Srivastava K, et al.: Gender differences in hypertension in spontaneously hypertensive rats: role of androgens and androgen receptor. *Hypertension* 1999; 34: 920–923.

[7] Mendelsohn ME, Karas RH: The protective effects of estrogen on the cardiovascular system. *N Engl J Med* 1999; 340: 1801-1811. [Extensive and in-depth review on the protective effects of estrogens on the cardiovascular system and the mechanisms involved.]

[8] Dubey RK, Jackson EK.: Estrogen-induced cardiorenal protection: potential cellular, biochemical, and molecular mechanisms. *Am J Physiol Renal Physiol* 2001; 280: F365-F388. [Extensive and in-depth review on the protective effects of estrogens on the cardiorenal system and the cellular, biochemical and molecular mechanisms involved.]

[9] Staessen J, Bulpitt CJ, Fagard R, et al.: The influence of menopause on blood pressure. *J Hum Hypertens* 1989; 3: 427–433.

[10] Staessen JA, Ginnochio G, Thijs L,et al.: Conventional and ambulatory blood pressure and menopause in a prospective population study. *J Hum Hypertens* 1997; 11: 507-514.

[11] Chapman AB, Zamudio S, Woodmansee W, et al. Systemic and renal hemodynamic changes in the luteal phase of the menstrual cycle mimic early pregnancy. *Am J Physiol* 1997; 273: F777–F782.

[12] Siamopoulos KC, Papanikolaou S, Elisaf M, et al.: Ambulatory blood pressure monitoring in normotensive pregnant women. *J Hum Hypertens* 1996; 10 (suppl 3): S51-S54.

[13] Cagnacci A, Rovati L, Annalisa Z, et al.: Physiological doses of estradiol decrease nocturnal blood pressure in normotensive postmenopausal women. *Am J Physiol Heart Circ Physiol.* 1999; 276: H1355-H1360.

[14] Akkad AA, Halligan AWF, Abrams K,et al.: Differing responses in blood pressure over 24 hours in normotensive women receiving oral or transdermal estrogen replacement therapy. *Obstet Gynecol* 1997; 89: 97–103.

[15] van Ittersum FJ, van Baal WM, Kenemans P, et al.: Ambulatory –not office—blood pressure decline during hormone relacement therapy in healthy postmenopausal women. *Am J Hypertens* 1998; 11: 1147-1152.

[16] Seely EW, Walsh BW, Gerhard MD, et al.: Estradiol with or without progesterone and ambulatory blood pressure in postmenopausal women. *Hypertension* 1999; 33: 1190-1194.

[17] Mercuro G, Zoncu S, Piano D, et al.: Estradiol-17β reduces blood pressure and restores the normal amplitude of the circadian blood pressure rhythm in postmenopausal hypertension. *Am J Hypertens* 1998; 11: 909-13.
[18] Mercuro G, Zoncu S, Pilia I, et al.: Effects of acute administration of transdermal estrogen on postmenopausal women with systemic hypertension. *Am J Cardiol* 1997; 80: 652-655.
[19] Szekacs B, Najo Z, Acs N, et al.: Hormone replacement therapy reduces mean 24-hour blood pressure and its variability in postmenopausal women with treated hypertension. *Menopause* 2000; 7: 31-35.
[20] Manhem K, Ahlm H, Milsom I, et al.: Transdermal oestrogen reduces daytime blood pressure in hypertensive women. *J Hum Hypertens* 1.998; 12:323-327.
[21] Lip GYH, Beevers M, Churchill D, et al.: Hormone replacement therapy and blood pressure in hypertensive women. *J Hum Hypertens* 1994; 8: 491–494.
[22] Butkevich A, Abraham C, Phillips RA. Hormone replacement therapy and 24-hour blood pressure profile of postmenopausal women. *Am J Hypertens* 2000; 13: 1039-1041.
[23] Regensteiner JG, Hiatt WR, Byyny RL et al. Short-term effects of estrogen and progestin on blood pressure of normotensive post-menopausal women. *J Clin Pharmacol* 1991; 31: 543-548.
[24] Cacciatore B, Paakkari I, Hasselblatt R et al. Randomized comparison between o rally and transdermally administered replacement therapy regimens of long-term effects on 24-hour ambulatory blood pressure in postmenopausal women. *Am J Obstet Gynecol* 2001; 184: 904-909.
[25] Pripp U, Hall G, Csemiczky G et al. A randomized trial on effects of hormone replacement therapy on ambulatory blood pressure and lipoprotein levels in women with coronary artery disease. *J Hypertens* 1999; 17:1379-1386.
[26] Sorensen MB, Rasmussen V, Jensen G, Ottesen B. Temporal changes in clinic and ambulatory blood pressure during cyclic post-menopausal hormone replacement therapy. *J Hypertens* 2000; 18: 1387-1391.
[27] Manwaring P, Morfis L, Diamond T, Howes LG. Effects of hormone replacement therapy on ambulatory blood pressure responses in normotensive women. *Blood Press* 2000; 9: 22-27.
[28] Schunkert H, Danser AHJ, Hense H-W et al. Effects of estrogen replacement therapy on the renin-angiotensin system in post-menopausal women. *Circulation* 1997; 95:39-45.
[29] DeMeersam R, Zion AS, Giardina EGV et al. Estrogen replacement, vascular distensitibility, and blood pressure in postmenopausal women. *Am J Physiol* 1998; 274: H1539-H1544.
[30] Meyers MG, Reeves RA. White coat effect in treated hypertensive patients: sex differences. *J Hum Hypertens* 1995; 9: 729-773.
[31] Lloyd G, McGing E, Cooper A, et al.: A randomized placebo controlled trial of the effects of tibolone on blood pressure and lipids in hypertensive women. *J Hum Hypertens* 2000; 14: 99-104.
[32] PEPI Trial Writing Group: Effects of estrogen or estrogen/progestin regimens on heart disease risk factors in postmenopausal women. The postmenopausal estrogen/protestin interventions (PEPI) trial. *JAMA.* 1995; 3:199–208.

[33] Hulley S, Grady D, Bush T, et al.: Randomized trial of estrogen plus progestin for secondary prevention of coronary heart disease in postmenopausal women: Heart and estrogen/progestin replacement study (HERS) research group. *JAMA* 1998; 280: 605-613.

[34] Rossouw JE, Anderson GL, Prentice RL, et al.: Writing Group for the Women's Health Initiative Investigators. Risks and benefits of estrogen plus progestin in healthy postmenopausal women: principal results from the Women's Health Initiative randomized controlled trial. *JAMA*. 2002 17; 288: 321-33.

[35] Wren BG, Routledge DA. Blood pressure changes. Oestrogens in climacteric women. *Med J Aust* 1981; 2: 528–531.

[36] Reckelhoff JF: Gender differences in the regulation of blood pressure. *Hypertension* 2001; 37: 1199-1208.

[37] Sudhir K, Esler M, Jennings G, et al.: Estrogen supplementation decreases norepinephrine-induced vasoconstriction and total body norepinephrine spillover in perimenopausal women. *Hypertension* 1997; 30:1538-1543.

[38] Vongpatanasin W, Tuncel M, Mansour Y. Transdermal estrogen replacement therapy decreases sympathetic activity in postmenopausal women. *Circulation* 2001; 103: 2903-2908.

[39] Hunt BE, Taylor JA, Hamner JW, et al.: Estrogen replacement therapy improves baroreflex regulation of vascular sympathetic outflow in postmenopausal women. *Circulation* 2001; 103: 2909-2914.

[40] Del Rio G, Velardo A, Menozzi R, et al.: Acute estradiol and progesterone administration reduced cardiovascular and catecholamine responses to mental stress in menopausal women. *Neuroendocrinology* 1998; 67: 269-274.

[41] Ng VA, Callister R, Johnson DG, et al.: Age and gender influence muscle sympathetic nerve activity at rest in healthy humans. *Hypertension* 1993; 21: 498-503.

[42] Zhu Y, Bian Z, Lu P, et al.: Abnormal vascular function and hypertension in mice deficient in estrogen receptor β. *Science* 2002; 295: 505-508. [Provides evidence that estrogen receptor β regulates the blood pressure lowering effects of estradiol.]

[43] Ogawa S, Emi M, Shiraki M, et al.; Association of estrogen receptor beta (ESR2) gene polymorphism with blood pressure. *J Hum Genet* 2000; 45: 327-330.

[44] Dubey RK, Jackson EK: Cardiovascular protective effects of 17β-estradiol metabolites. *J Appl Physiol* 2001; 91: 1868-1883. [In depth review highlighting the role of estradiol metabolites as biologically active molecules which can regulate cardiovascular and renal function and influence blood pressure.]

[45] Tofovic S, Dubey RK, Jackson EK.: 2-Hydroxyestradiol attenuates the development of obesity, the metabolic syndrome, and vascular and renal dysfunction in obese ZSF1 rats. *J Pharmacol Expt. Therap* 2001; 299: 973-977. [Study showing the blood pressure lowering and vasoprotective effects of estradiol metabolites.]

[46] Tofovic SP, Dubey RK, Salah EM, et al.: 2-Hydroxyestradiol attenuates renal disease in chronic puromycin aminonucleoside nephropathy. *J Am Soc Nephrol* 2002; 13: 2737-2747.

[47] Zacharia LC, Jackson EK, Gillespie DG, et al.: Catecholamines abrogate antimitogenic effects of 2-hydroxyestradiol on human aortic vascular smooth muscle cells. *Arterioscler Thromb Vasc Biol 2001;* 21: 1745-1750.

[48] Dubey RK, Zacharia LC, Gillespie DG, et al.: Catecholamines block the anti-mitogenic effect of estradiol on human glomerular mesangial cells. *Hypertension* 2003; 42:349-355. [Study demonstrating that catecholamines can block the antimitogenic effects of estradiol by inhibiting its metabolism to 2-methoxyestradiol.]

[49] Rylance PB, Brincat M, Lafferty K, et al.: Natural progesterone and antihypertensive action. *Br Med J* 1985; 5: 13-14.

[50] Tapanainem J, Kauppila A, Metsa-Ketela T, et al.: Prostanoids and catecholamines after oral administration of natural progesterone. *Gynecol Endocrinol* 1989; 3: 135-142.

[51] Harvey PJ, Molloy D, Upton J, et al.: Dose response effect of cyclical medroxyprogesterone on blood pressure in postmenopausal women. *J Hum Hypertens* 2001; 15: 313-321.

[52] Liu PY, Death AK, Handelsman DJ: Androgens and cardiovascular disease. *Endocrine Reviews* 2003; 24: 313-340. [An extensive review providing in-depth review on the association between androgens and cardiovascular disease.]

[53] Wu FCW, von Eckardstein A. Androgens and coronary artery disease. *Endocrine Reviews* 2003; 24: 183-217. [An extensive review providing in-depth review on the association between androgens and coronary artery disease. Highlights the effects on lipids, cholesterol and insulin sensitivity.]

[54] Boyanov MA, Boneva Z, Christov VG: Testosterone supplementation in men with type 2 diabetes, visceral obesity and partial androgen deficiency. *Aging Male* 2003; 6: 1-7.

[55] Beckham SG, Earnest CP: Four weeks of androstenedione supplementation diminishes the treatment response in middle aged men. *Br J Sports Med* 2003; 37: 212-218.

[56] Elbers JM, Giltay EJ, Teerlink T, et al.: Effects of sex steroids on components of the insulin resistance syndrome in transsexual subjects. *Clin Endocrinol (Oxd)* 2003; 58: 562-571.

[57] Zitzmann M, Brune M, Nieschlag E. Vascular reactivity in hypogonadal men is reduced by androgen substitution. *J Clin Endocrinol Metab* 2002; 87: 5030-5037.

[58] Thompson PD, Ahlberg AW, Moyna NM, et al.: Effect of intravenous testosterone on myocardial ischemia in men with coronary artery disease. *Am Heart J* 2002; 143: 249-256.

[59] Simon D, Charles M-A, Lahlou N, et al.: Androgen therapy improves insulin sensitivity and decreases leptin level in healthy adult men with low plasma total testosterone. *Diabetes Care* 2001; 24: 2149-2151.

[60] Behre HM, Abshagen K, Oettel M, et al.: Intramuscular injection of testosterone undecanoate for the treatment of male hypogonadism: phase 1 studies. *Eur J Endocrinol* 1999; 140: 414-419.

[61] McCredie RJ, McCrohon JA, Turner L, et al.: Vascular reactivity is impaired in genetic females taking high-dose androgens. *J Am Coll Cardiol* 1998; 32: 1331-1335.

[62] Anderson FH, Francis RM, Faulkner K. Androgen supplementation in eugonadal men with osteoporosis : effects of 6 months of treatment on bone mineral density and cardiovascular risk factors. *Bone* 1996; 18: 171-177.

[63] Lovejoy JC, Bray GA, Greeson CS, et al.: Oral anabolic steroid treatment, but not parenteral androgen treatment, decreases abdominal fat in obese, older men. *Int J Obes Relat Metab Disord* 1995; 19: 614-624.

[64] Marin P, Holmang S, Jonsson L, et al.: The effects of testosterone on body composition and metabolism in middle aged men. *Int J Obes Relat Metab Disord* 1992; 16: 991-997.

[65] Rebuffe-Scrive M, Marin P, Bjorntorp P: Effect of testosterone on abdominal adipose tissue in men. *Int J Obes* 1991; 15: 791-795.

[66] Marin P, Krotkiewski M, Bjorntorp P. Androgen treatment of middle-aged, obese men: effects on metabolism, muscle and adipose tissue. *Eur J Med* 1992; 1: 329-336.

[67] Hautanen A, Manttari M, Manninen V, et al.: Adrenal androgens and testosterone as coronary risk factors the Helsinki Heart Study. *Atherosclerosis* 1994; 105: 191-200.

[68] White CM, Ferraro-Borgida MJ, Moyna NM, et al.: The effect of pharmacokinetically guided acute intravenous testosterone administration on electrocardiographic and blood pressure variables. *J Clin Pharmacol* 1999; 39: 1038-1043.

[69] Sader MA, Griffiths KA, Skilton MR, et al.: Physiological testosterone replacement and arterial endothelial function in men. *Clin Endocrinol (Oxf)* 2003; 59: 62-67.

[70] Giorgi A, Weatherby RP, Murphy PW. Muscular strength, body composition and health responses to the use of testosterone enanthate: a double blind study. *J Sci Med Sport.* 1999; 2: 341-355.

[71] Whitworth JA, Scoggins BA, Andrews J, et al.: Haemodynamic and metabolic effects of short term administration of synthetic sex steroids in humans. *Clin Exp Hypertens.* 1992; 14: 905-922.

[72] Nakagawa K, Marji JS, Schwartzman ML, et al.: The androgen-mediated induction of the kidney arachidonate hydroxylase is associated with the development of hypertension. *Am J Physiol Regul Integr Comp Physiol 2003*; 284: R1055-R1062.

[73] Galipeau DM, Yao L, McNeill JH: Relationship among hyperinsulinemia, insulin resistance and hypertension is dependent on sex. *Am J Physiol Heart Circ Physiol.* 2002; 283: H562-H567.

[74] Suzuki M, Kanazawa A, Hasegawa M, et al.: A close association between insulin resistance and dehydroepiandrosterone sulfate in subjects with essential hypertension. *Endocr J* 1999; 46: 521-528.

In: Hypertension: New Research
Editor: Elwood F. Benhagen, pp. 201-238
ISBN: 1-59454-204-X

Chapter VIII

IMMUNOSUPPRESSIVE DRUGS DURING PREGNANCY: HYPERTENSION FOR MOTHER AND CHILD?

Anne Prévot[1] *and Jean-Pierre Guignard*
Department of Pediatrics, Nephrology Unit,
Centre Hospitalier Universitaire Vaudois,
CH 1011, Lausanne, Switzerland.

ABSTRACT

The number of pregnant women receiving immunosuppressants in the context of anti-rejection therapy or autoimmune diseases is constantly increasing and over 80% of these pregnancies result in surviving infants. Yet, all immunosuppressive drugs cross the placental barrier, raising questions about the long-term outcome of the children exposed *in utero*.

Although there is no higher risk of congenital anomalies, an increased incidence of prematurity (from 14 to 83%, as compared to 5-15% in the general population), intrauterine growth retardation (IUGR) and generally low birthweight (19 to 67% of neonates, as compared to 5-13% in the general population in developed countries) has been reported, along with maternal hypertension (71% with cyclosporine A vs 31.5%) and preeclampsia.

Neonatal complications include adrenal insufficiency associated with corticosteroids; immunological disturbances with azathioprine and cyclosporine; hyperkalemia with tacrolimus. However, the most frequent complications are those associated with prematurity, IUGR and low birthweight, mostly respiratory tract diseases and neurological affections such as periventricular leukomalacia and intraventricular hemorrhage.

Experimental as well as epidemiological studies have shown that low birthweight is also a predisposing factor for metabolic abnormalities such as atherosclerosis,

[1] Present address: Department of Medicine - Division of Physiology, Rue du Musée 5 - CH 1700 Fribourg, Switzerland. prevotanne@hotmail.com

cardiovascular diseases, renal disease, non-insulin diabetes, hypertension, obesity or the metabolic syndrome. Indeed, the human fetus adapts to undernutrition by redistribution of blood flow, but also by metabolic and endocrine changes in the production of fetal and placental growth hormones. These adaptations may all lead to a programming of the fetus with lifelong effects. The long-term follow-up of infants exposed to immunosuppressants *in utero* is still limited, but experimental studies raise the question whether there could be an increased incidence at adult age of some pathologies including renal insufficiency and hypertension.

Key Words: Autoimmune diseases; Barker hypothesis; cyclosporine; fetal programming; hypertension; immunosuppressive drugs; infant, newborn; intrauterine growth retardation; nephrogenesis; pregnancy; prematurity; prenatal exposure delayed effects; transplantation.

INTRODUCTION

The number of pregnancies under immunosuppressive drugs is constantly increasing, either in the context of organ/tissue transplants, or autoimmune diseases including systemic lupus erythematosus, rheumatoid arthritis, psoriasis or dermatomyositis [Armenti 2002b, Bermas 95, Ramsey-Goldman 97]. Despite the maternal and fetal risks of these pregnancies, 57% (lung transplant) to 94% (kidney transplant) result in surviving infants [Armenti 2002b, Davison 97]. Therefore, the possibility that immunosuppressed women of childbearing age might become pregnant should be considered [Prévot 2002a].

The drugs given to pregnant women include corticosteroids, purine metabolism inhibitors (azathioprine, mycophenolate mofetil), calcineurin inhibitors (cyclosporine, tacrolimus), the cell-growth inhibitor sirolimus, or monoclonal antibodies (basiliximab, daclizumab) [Armenti 98]. In addition to these drugs, alkylating agents (cyclophosphamide, chlorambucil) and methotrexate have been used to achieve immunosuppression, mostly in immune-mediated diseases [Bermas 95, Ramsey-Goldman 97].

All immunosuppressive drugs and their metabolites cross the placental barrier [Armenti 98, Bermas 95, Ramsey-Goldman 97]. To date, case reports and registries have not observed a specific pattern or an increase in the incidence of malformations. Nonetheless, pregnancy in immunosuppressed patients carries an increased risk of prematurity, intrauterine growth retardation (IUGR) and more generally low birthweight (<2500 g), in addition to maternal complications including hypertension and preeclampsia [Armenti 98, 2002b].

Experimental as well as epidemiological studies have shown that low birthweight could be a predisposing factor for metabolic abnormalities such as hypertension, cardiovascular diseases, atherosclerosis, renal diseases, non-insulin diabetes, obesity or the metabolic syndrome [Barker 98, Holemans 2003]. Moreover, experimental studies raise the question whether *in utero* exposure to cyclosporine could result *per se* in an increased incidence at adult age of pathologies including renal insufficiency and hypertension [Tendron 2003].

A- THE IMMUNOSUPPRESSED MOTHER

Transplantation and Fertility

Fertility, which is markedly reduced by chronic heart, hepatic, or renal failure, is usually restored between one and 12 months post-transplantation [Hou 99]. Therefore, the incidence of unplanned post-transplant pregnancies can be as high as 60%. Contraception should thus be considered in order to wait for both stable graft function and immunosuppressive regimen. Whatever the organ, most teams recommend a delay of 15 to 24 months post-transplantation to avoid the frequent rejection episodes occurring in the first year [Davison 76, 84, 91].

Effect of Pregnancy on Graft Function

A rejection episode during pregnancy occurs in 0% (kidney) to 31% (lung) in the data of the latest report of the US National Transplantation Pregnancy Registry (1324 pregnancies, 1358 children) [Armenti 2002b]. The incidence of graft loss within two years of delivery varies from 0% (heart) to 23% (lung) [Armenti 2002b].

Pregnancy in kidney recipients is considered to be safe and can only be considered as a risk factor for graft loss when serum creatinine levels are ≥1.5 mg/dl (133 μmol/l) before conception [EBPG 2002]. Ten to 15% of women present a deterioration of their renal function during pregnancy and graft loss after delivery is reported in 2 to 20% of these women [Armenti 2002b, Davison 85b, Hou 99, 2003]. Moreover, if chronic rejection is present prior to pregnancy, these patients have a greater risk of pregnancy-related graft loss [Armenti 98, 2002b].

In heart and liver transplantation, pregnancy is generally well tolerated and does not appear to increase the incidence of rejection [Chevalier 96]. However, in liver recipients seropositive for the hepatitis B virus, cytomegalovirus and above all hepatitis C virus, deterioration of liver function can occur during pregnancy [Armenti 98, Radomski 95]. Significantly lower gestational age and birthweight are noted among offspring of recipients with acute rejection episodes when compared with those of mothers without rejection during pregnancy [Armenti 2002b]. The above-mentioned risks justify a careful follow-up of graft function during pregnancy and after delivery, whatever the transplanted organ.

Hypertension in Pregnancy

The hypertensive disorders of pregnancy affect about 10% of all gestations and are a major cause of maternal, fetal and neonatal morbidity and mortality in the USA and worldwide. They can be classified into four separate entities [August 95, Barron 95, Roberts 2003].

1- Preeclampsia is a pregnancy-specific syndrome that usually occurs after the 20th week of gestation, and most often near term. Preeclampsia is a complication in approximately 5-10% of all pregnancies and causes 50-70% of cases of hypertension in pregnancy.

Preeclampsia is defined as *de novo* appearance of hypertension (Systolic Blood Pressure ≥140 mm Hg, Diastolic Blood Pressure ≥90 mm Hg, or increases in systolic and diastolic levels by 30 and 15 mm Hg, respectively), associated with new-onset proteinuria (≥300 mg per 24 hours) [Barron 95]. Edema can also be present but this sign is nonspecific, as it is present in many pregnant non-eclamptic women.

Preeclampsia occurs only in the presence of a placenta. Although the exact etiology of preeclampsia remains unknown, placental dysfunction may initiate the generalized vasoconstriction, ischemia, and thrombosis that eventually damage maternal organs and can result in placental infarction and fetal death. Risk factors for preeclampsia include extremes of maternal age, primigravida, multigravida exposed to a new partner, i.e. new paternal antigen (immunologic basis), multiple gestations, molar pregnancy, preexisting hypertension, diabetes mellitus, renal disease, preexisting connective tissue disease, vascular disease, as well as a prior history of preeclampsia or eclampsia [August 95, Roberts 2003].

Preeclampsia is the second leading cause of maternal mortality, constituting 12-18% of pregnancy-related maternal deaths. Preeclampsia is also associated with high perinatal morbidity and mortality rates, as a result of iatrogenic prematurity [Paruk 2000]. Indeed, maternal death is largely preventable by delivery to prevent disease progression. Therefore, about 15% of preterm births are indicated early deliveries for preeclampsia [August 95, Roberts 2003].

Preeclampsia vanishes rapidly after delivery; however, hypertension can persist for a few weeks, often in women with severe early-onset disease [August 95].

2- Eclampsia occurs when severe preeclampsia is complicated by seizures and/or coma, which are thought to be secondary to hypertensive encephalopathy. It can occur either after mid-pregnancy, during delivery, or during the first 48 hours postpartum. There is also a rare and transient variant called late postpartum eclampsia, where convulsions can occur between 48 hrs and 10 days after delivery.

Little is known of the pathophysiology of this disorder. The incidence of eclampsia varies from 0.05% to 0.2% of all deliveries, and it causes the termination of 1 in 1000 pregnancies [August 95, Paruk 2000]. The fetal and maternal morbidity and mortality rates are high, especially in developing countries. Maternal mortality results mostly from intracranial hemorrhage or pulmonary oedema [August 95, Paruk 2000, Walker 2000].

Nearly 10% of women with severe preeclampsia and 30-50% of women with eclampsia are affected by the hemolysis, elevated liver enzymes, and low platelet count (HELLP) syndrome, although the exact relationship between the HELLP syndrome and preeclampsia is unknown. Women with preeclampsia with this syndrome develop hemolysis, rapid deterioration of the coagulation parameters, hepatocellular necrosis and liver dysfunction. The mortality rate is therefore further increased and prompt termination of the pregnancy is mandatory. One third of women with preeclampsia also develop disseminated intravascular coagulation [August 95, Roberts 2003].

3- Gestational hypertension is defined as *de novo* isolated hypertension arising after mid-pregnancy. In many cases, the course is relatively benign and blood pressure normalizes after delivery, at which time the diagnosis is therefore changed to *transient hypertension of pregnancy*.

4- Chronic hypertension refers to an elevated blood pressure in the mother that predated the onset of the pregnancy. If unknown before, it can be assumed when high blood pressure is detected before mid-pregnancy, but can also be diagnosed in retrospect when hypertension fails to normalize 12 weeks after delivery. There is little consensus on how to treat this condition, which is a cause of concern as these women are at increased risk of surimposed preeclampsia (15 to 25% risk) [Walker 2000], preterm delivery, fetal growth restriction, abruptio placentae, congestive heart failure and acute renal failure. The outcome for mother and infant is then worse than with *de novo* preeclampsia [Roberts 2003].

Preexisting chronic hypertension complicates up to 5% of non-immunosuppressed pregnancies and is associated with an increased risk of preterm labor, uteroplacental insufficiency, placental detachment, and low birthweight [Barron 95, Lindheimer 2001].

Incidence of Hypertension in Immunosuppressed Pregnancies

The prevalence of post-transplant arterial hypertension is high, especially in kidney patients where it is considered that between 50 and 80% of patients with otherwise well-functioning grafts exhibit arterial hypertension [Armenti 2002b, EBPG 2002]. The etiologies include pre-transplant hypertension, chronic allograft nephropathy, renal artery stenosis and immunosuppressive therapy (mainly steroids, cyclosporine and tacrolimus). Because of the adverse effects of hypertension on the renal allograft, hypertension in kidney patients should be treated as to maintain blood pressure around 125/75 mm Hg [Hou 2003]. However, it appears that maternal drug-treated hypertension is a significant pre-pregnancy factor that increases the risk of low birthweight, especially in patients treated with cyclosporine [Armenti 2002b, Mimran 95].

Table 1 shows the incidence of hypertension and preeclampsia episodes during pregnancy in transplant recipients, as reported in the US National Transplantation Pregnancy Registry [Armenti 2002b]. Isolated hypertension occurs in 25% (liver/tacrolimus) to 78% (pancreas/kidney) of transplant patients, while preeclampsia occurs in 11% (heart) to 36% (pancreas/kidney) [Armenti 2002b, EBPG 2002]. The incidence of preeclampsia is 4-fold higher in renal transplant women than in uncomplicated pregnancies [Hou 99].

Table 1. Immunosuppressants and incidence of hypertension and preeclampsia

Organ/Immunosuppressant	Hypertension (%)	Preeclampsia (%)
Kidney		
CsA-Sandimmune®	63	29
CsA-Neoral®	72	30
Tacrolimus	53	32
Kidney		
Multiple gestation (twins or triplets)	77	29
Liver		
CsA-Sandimmune®	40	25
CsA-Neoral®	39	32
Tacrolimus	25	15
Pancreas/kidney	78	36
Heart	48	11
Lung	50	13

Adapted from [Armenti 2002b]

CsA: cyclosporine A.

Management of Hypertension during Pregnancy

Because preeclampsia develops in about 30% of pregnant transplant patients, especially those with prior arterial hypertension, blood pressure, renal function, proteinuria and weight should be monitored every 2-4 weeks, with even more attention during the third trimester. The diagnosis of preeclampsia may be difficult to make in a woman with preexisting renal disease, arterial hypertension or chronic rejection, and an allograft biopsy could thus be required to ensure the diagnosis.

Although delivery is the only definitive treatment for preeclampsia [Barron 95, Khedun 97], adequate treatment of hypertension is essential for the mother and the fetus [Afifi 2003]. Indeed, the leading cause of maternal death from preeclampsia/eclampsia is cerebral hemorrhage, at least in part the consequence of severe hypertension. The goal of treatment is thus to achieve blood pressure levels at which the risk of hypertension-induced cerebral hemorrhage is low, while maintaining sufficient uteroplacental blood flow to avoid fetal compromise.

Antihypertensive agents should be those tolerated during pregnancy [see Afifi 2003, Khedun 97 for extensive review]. Calcium channel blockers, angiotensin-converting enzyme inhibitors (ACEIs), diuretics and beta-blockers are the main drugs used for pharmacologic treatment in posttransplant hypertension [Demme 2001]. However, ACE inhibitors are strictly contra-indicated during pregnancy [EBPG 2002], as they have been associated with oligohydramnios, persistent neonatal anuria, pulmonary hypoplasia and neonatal death by respiratory failure [Guignard 81, 88, Hanssens 91]. Angiotensin II receptor antagonists are also contra-indicated [EBPG 2002]: sartans have been associated with neonatal acute renal failure [Piétrement 2003, Prévot 2002b], as well as fetal or neonatal deaths, all presenting with severe oligohydramnios and enlarged kidneys [Briggs 2001, Martinovic 2001, Saji 2001].

Alpha-methyldopa is usually the first choice to treat chronic hypertension [Barron 95]. It is effective and does not induce any deleterious effect for the fetus [Cockburn 82]. Clonidine and calcium channel blockers could be used as second line. A metaanalysis by Papatsonis *et al.* showed that the use of nifedipine for tocolysis in comparison to betamimetics was associated with increased prolongation of pregnancy resulting in significantly fewer admissions of newborns in intensive care, as well as a lower incidence of respiratory distress syndrome [Papatsonis 2001].

In the case of hypertensive emergencies, a metaanalysis by Magee *et al.* indicated that hydralazine was associated with more low Apgar scores at one minute and a trend towards an increase in stillbirths as compared with other antihypertensives [Magee 2003]. However, hydralazine was associated with less neonatal bradycardia than labetalol. Nifedipine or parenteral labetalol seemed to be reasonable alternatives to hydralazine [Barron 95, Magee 2003].

Interaction between Antihypertensive and Immunosuppressive Drugs

Pharmacokinetic interactions have been reported between some antihypertensive and immunosuppressive drugs, resulting mainly in an increase in the plasma levels of immunosuppressants [Akhlaghi 2001, Fourtounas 2002, Imani 99, Jones 2002, Mimran 95, Ocran 99]. Therefore, blood concentrations should be closely monitored in the mother, so as not to expose the fetus to an even increased risk of exposure *in utero*.

Fetal Monitoring

Frequent fetal testing is indicated when the mother is treated for hypertension, whether isolated or in the context of preeclampsia. However, there is no real consensus on the frequency of the tests, which usually depends on the severity of the maternal disease, the gestational age at diagnosis, and subsequent fetal growth findings [Khedun 97, Sibai 2003]. Most authorities in the USA recommend daily fetal movement/kick counts, a decreased fetal kick count being a reliable parameter of a compromised fetus. Ultrasound estimation of fetal weight as well as amniotic fluid quantity should be performed at diagnosis and subsequently every 3 to 4 weeks if growth is normal, weekly if intrauterine growth restriction and/or oligohydramnios should happen, or even daily if preeclampsia is severe and gestational age is less than 32 weeks [Khedun 97, Sibai 2003]. In any case, delivery should be performed if there is evidence of fetal distress.

B- The Immunosuppressed Fetus and Child

Prematurity - IUGR - Low Birthweight (<2500 g)

Perinatal mortality (stillbirth and neonatal death <30 days) occurs in 0 to 14% of children from transplant patients [Armenti 98, 2002b, Bar 97].

The incidence of prematurity varies from 14 to 83% in immunosuppressed pregnancies, as compared to 5-15% in the general population. In the USA, prematurity affected 12% of all births for all races in 2002, with around 11% for whites and hispanics, and 17.5% for blacks [Martin 2003].

Low birthweight occurs in 19 to 67% of neonates from immunosuppressed mothers, as compared to 5-13% in the general population in developed countries [Meyberg 2000, Villar 82] (See Table 2 for details). In the US, low birthweight affected 7.8% of all births in 2002, with around 7% for whites and hispanics, and 13.3% for blacks [Martin 2003].

As a result, morbidity is increased, with an average hospitalization time in the neonatal intensive care unit of 35.2 ± 16.2 days in the study of Bar *et al.* reporting results from renal transplant patients [Bar 97, Meyberg 2000].

The maternal comorbid factors with a significant relationship to outcome are:

- post-transplantation time: when <24 months, prematurity rate is 92%; when >24 months, 40% [Picaud 91].
- for kidney recipients: serum creatinine before conception ≥1.5 mg/dl (133 μmol/l), rising creatinine and/or graft dysfunction as well as hypertension during pregnancy significantly decrease the birthweight of the offspring [Armenti 95].

Table 2: Immunosuppressive drugs and incidence of prematurity, low birthweight (LBW) and intra-uterine growth retardation (IUGR)

Immunosuppressant	Prematurity (%)	IUGR or LBW <2500 g (%)	Reference
Corticoids	No increased incidence of prematurity	- Significant decrease of BW with prednisone *in utero* as compared to control offspring	[Armenti 98, Ramsey-Goldman 97]
Azathioprine	40 to 52	19 to 40 (IUGR)	[Bermas 95, Pabelick 91, Ramsey-Goldman 97]
Mycophenolate Mofetil	88 (8 children)	75 (LBW)	[Armenti 2002b]
Cyclosporine A	44.5 to 83	44.3 (LBW) - 56 (IUGR)	[Lamarque 97, Lo Giudice 2000, Pabelick 91]
Heart - Liver - Kidney	37.5 – 38.7 - 52	37.5 – 32.3 – 49.6 (LBW)	
Sandimmune® - kidney			[Radomski 95]
Neoral® - kidney	52	45 (LBW)	[Armenti 2002b]
Neoral® - liver	54	51 (LBW)	[Armenti 2002b]
	27	35 (LBW)	[Armenti 2002b]
Tacrolimus	59	5 (IUGR)	[Ramsey-Goldman 97]
Tacrolimus - Liver	38 to 54	0 (IUGR) – 28 (LBW)	[Armenti 2002b, Jain 97]
Tacrolimus - Kidney	56	58 (LBW)	[Armenti 2002b]
Double or triple immunosuppression	14 to 65	7.7 (very LBW<1000g) to 49.6 (LBW) - 7.7 to 33 (IUGR)	[Armenti 95, Bar 97, Gaughan 96, Haugen 94, Picaud 91, Rieu 97, Touraine 97]
Pancreas-kidney	74	59 (LBW)	[Armenti 2002b]
Heart	33	33 (LBW)	[Armenti 2002b]
Lung	63	63 (LBW)	[Armenti 2002b]
Multiple gestations in kidney recipients (14 pregnancies, 32 outcomes, livebirths 88%)	92	93	[Armenti 2002b]

The most frequent complications related to prematurity are respiratory tract diseases [Kainz 2000], with a high incidence of bronchopulmonary dysplasia, a condition with a mortality rate near 30% [Salle 89], as well as apnea of prematurity, isolated or associated with bradycardia, cyanosis, anemia, jaundice and infections [Salle 89]. Neurologically, the most frequent complications are periventricular leukomalacia and intraventricular hemorrhage, the incidence of which is more elevated when birthweight is lower and the infant is more immature [Salle 89]. The immediate complications of IUGR are hypothermia, hypoglycemia, blood hyperviscosity, hypocalcemia and hydroelectrolytic disorders, associated with respiratory and/or vital diseases related to the acute fetal failure, such as intraventricular hemorrhage often associated with *in utero* acquired leukomalacias [Relier 89].

Epidemiological data indicate that a low birthweight is associated with a higher incidence at adult age of hypertension, type 2 diabetes, chronic renal failure and cardiovascular diseases. Blood pressure is inversely correlated with birthweight, either from extra-renal (elevated plasma cortisol levels, resistance to insulin, decreased Na^+/K^+-ATPase activity), or intrinsic reasons (decreased nephron number hypothesis, gene programming) [Lackland 2000, 2003, Manalich 2000].

These aspects will be further developed in section C called "fetal programming of adult hypertension".

Immunosuppressive Treatment

The immunosuppressive treatment is usually maintained at pre-pregnancy levels, with adjustments according to standard parameters such as cyclosporine A (CsA) trough levels or 2 hours post-dose monitoring (C2) [Armenti 2000].

Follow-up is not long enough to determine whether there is a higher incidence of childhood cancers or sterility in the offspring. Chromosomal studies from children of kidney transplant recipients treated with conventional therapy or CsA showed normal caryotypes or shortly reversible chromatid breaks (5 to 32 months after birth), with no increase in the incidence of congenital malformations [Chevalier 96, Picaud 91]. However, chromosome aberrations have been described in somatic cells of infants exposed to azathioprine (AZA) *in utero* and the repercussion on germline cells remains to be studied [Picaud 91]. Indeed, of the surviving female offspring of mice treated with low doses of 6-mercaptopurine during pregnancy, despite normal body weight and general appearance, many were either sterile, or had smaller litters and more dead fetuses as compared to offspring of mothers that had not received the drug [Picaud 91]. This underscores the need for long-term follow-up of the children of women receiving immunosuppressants.

1- Corticosteroids

Prednisone and prednisolone cross the placental barrier. However, they are metabolized by a placental 11-hydroxygenase and the fetus is thus exposed only to approximately 10% of the maternal dose [Beitins 72]. When glucocorticoids are needed to treat fetal conditions such as immature lungs, dexamethasone and betamethasone are preferred because they are less well metabolized by the placenta and greater doses are available to the fetus. Prednisone should thus be used to treat the mother, even more since it has been demonstrated that high doses of dexamethasone given to pregnant rats affect nephrogenesis of the offspring leading to substantial nephron deficits [Merlet-Bénichou 99].

The use of corticoids prior to pregnancy does not seem to impair fertility or increase the incidence of spontaneous abortions. However, there may be a higher incidence of pregnancy-specific complications such as premature rupture of the membranes, gestational diabetes and hypertension [Janssen 2000]. An increased incidence of cleft lip and palate has been reported in animals but not demonstrated in humans [Bermas 95]. In 468 cortisone-exposed, non-transplant gravidas, an overall fetal malformation rate of 3.5% was noted, which is no greater than the general population [Armenti 2002a].

Adrenal insufficiency (rapidly recovering after stimulation with synthetic corticotropin [Huynh 94]) and thymic hypoplasia have been occasionally described in the newborn, but their incidence is reduced if the dose is maintained below 15 mg/d. Even if they appear healthy, neonates born to these mothers should thus be carefully monitored for evidence of adrenal insufficiency.

Acute rejection episodes are mainly treated with an increase of the amount of immunosuppression, usually with corticoids, therefore increasing the potential for drug toxicity as well as infections such as cytomegalovirus [Armenti 98]. Therefore, children exposed to a maternal acute rejection episode *in utero* should also be closely followed for any immunological problem.

2- Azathioprine - 6-Mercaptopurine

Azathioprine (AZA) and its active metabolite 6-mercaptopurine (6-MP) are inhibitors of purine metabolism that decrease natural killer cell activity, antibody production, antibody-dependent cellular cytotoxicity and cellular immune responses, such as interleukin-2 secretion [Ramsey-Goldman 97]. AZA crosses the placenta (64 to 93% are found in fetal blood) and 6-MP has been found in cord blood [Armenti 98]. However, 6-MP must be metabolized by the enzyme inosinate pyrophosphorylase to obtain components that act on DNA in dividing cells. Yet this enzyme lacks in the immature fetal liver, so that the majority of the drug is in the form of the inactive metabolite thiouric acid and the fetus should theoretically be relatively protected from the effects of AZA [Hou 99, Huynh 94]. Nonetheless, AZA presents with teratogenicity in animal studies, with a high incidence of embryonic resorption and fetal anomalies [Davison 85a, Janssen 2000]. AZA does not seem to be teratogenic in humans, even if there were isolated case reports of fetal malformations, including craniosynostosis, hypoplasia of the frontal lobe and ventriculomegaly [Bermas 95]. In a population-based cohort study, Norgard *et al.* studied the outcome of 19 pregnancies exposed to AZA or 6-MP for a short duration or during the entire pregnancy. They found an increase in the incidence of preterm birth (30%), low birthweight (30%), malformations (22%) and perinatal mortality (11%), as compared to non-exposed controls (5.5, 4.4, 3.7 and 0.6%, respectively) [Norgard 2003]. However, the number of pregnancies considered is very small as compared to controls (19 versus 19418), and it is thus not possible to conclude definitely on the human teratogenicity. There seems to be no effect of AZA on fertility and no reported increase in abortion rate [Janssen 2000].

6-Mercaptopurine is teratogenic in animals and has long-term effects on germline cells of exposed offspring. Fertility problems affect the female offspring of mice whose mothers have been given low dosages of 6-MP [Armenti 98]. However, there is no information on fertility in humans [Bermas 95].

Azathioprine is most frequently associated with a dose-dependent myelosuppression in the fetus. Cases of lymphopenia and thrombocytopenia and one case of neonatal lethal pancytopenia have been reported [Bermas 95]. Leucopenia seems avoidable if the maternal white blood cell count is maintained over 7.5 G/l. Even if the lymphocytes count is normal, the CD4+/CD8+ ratio of the offspring is usually higher when the mother is immunosuppressed. Koslowska-Boszko *et al.* [Koslowska-Boszko 97] report a high incidence of newborns exposed to prednisone, AZA or CsA *in utero* presenting with a diminished proportion of CD4+ (11/13) and CD8+-positive T cells (7/13) at 1st day of life. In only 2/6 and 1/5 cases, the levels of CD4+ and CD8+, respectively, were normal on the 30th day, suggesting a slow recovery. These neonates were clinically asymptomatic in 12/13 cases, but the immunomonitoring of children exposed to AZA is recommended [Koslowska-Boszko 97]. Other reported adverse effects include decreased thymic shadow, anemia, reduced immunoglobulin levels, infections and sepsis, or chromosomal abnormalities that may persist for up to one year, as well as sequelae from preterm delivery and IUGR [Armenti 98, Davison 85a].

3- Mycophenolate Mofetil (MMF)

MMF is a prodrug metabolized by hepatic ester hydrolysis into its active metabolite, mycophenolic acid, which has antiproliferative effects by inhibition of *de novo* purine synthesis on which lymphocytes are dependent [Armenti 98]. Animal studies have raised the possibility of an increased risk of malformations in newborns of females treated with MMF during pregnancy. The latest report of the National Transplantation Pregnancy Registry found two cases of structural malformations in 8 newborns from MMF-treated mothers (immunosuppressive regimens including MMF associated to prednisone and tacrolimus or cyclosporine-Neoral®) [Armenti 2002b]. The malformations included hypoplastic nails and shortened fifth fingers in an otherwise healthy child developing well after 5 years of follow-up, as well as a child with cleft lip and palate and an ear deformity. Interestingly enough, this child was not only submitted to MMF, tacrolimus and prednisone at conception, but a biopsy-proven acute rejection was documented in the mother who was subsequently treated with steroids, Thymoglobulin® and sirolimus [Armenti 2002b]. Therefore, it is difficult to conclude on a specific role of MMF in this setting. Of these eight children, 7/8 (88%) were premature and 6/8 (75%) had a birthweight below 2500 g [Armenti 2002b].

4- Calcineurine Inhibitors

Calcineurine inhibitors block the helper T cell's signal transduction mechanism by inhibiting calcineurin, a rate-limiting phosphatase required to activate the promoters needed for transcription of the cytokine genes essential for T cell activation and proliferation. The most prominent of these cytokines is interleukin-2 [Armenti 98]. As CsA only affects lymphocytes without depressing bone marrow or leucocyte counts, it is associated with a lower risk of infection than corticosteroids or AZA [Armenti 2002a].

Cyclosporine

Cyclosporine passively crosses the placental blood barrier. No teratogenic effect has been reported in animals and in humans. In 629 pregnancies under CsA, Lamarque *et al.* reported 9.7% of fetal losses and 3% of malformations, which is in the range of the general population [Lamarque 97].

Hypertension is significantly more frequent with CsA than under conventional therapy (71 vs 31.5%) [Rieu 97].

Globally, the incidence of neonatal complications is lower than with other immunosuppressive drugs. A few reports suggest hematological disorders: the T cell counts are either increased or decreased with a CD4+/CD8+ ratio always higher than normal, even after 24 months of follow-up [Baarsma 93]. However, there is no clinical sign of immunosuppression, no increased incidence of infections, either opportunistic or chronic and a normal IgG-antibody response to vaccination [Baarsma 93, Di Paolo 2000, Pilarski 94]. B cell numbers are always in the normal range.

Nephrotoxicity is a feature commonly seen with calcineurin inhibitors [Jain 97, Lamarque 97, Prévot 2000]. CsA being nephrotoxic for the mother, the question of an effect on the renal function of the fetus can be asked. However, studies reporting the nephrologic follow-up of children exposed to CsA *in utero* are scarce (See Table 3 for details) and no study on tacrolimus is available. Data with CsA are reassuring but the maximal follow-up is only 6.9 years [Lo Giudice 2000], which is insufficient. Blood pressure in the study by Lo Giudice *et al.* was normal in 8/12 children and slightly elevated in 4/12, who were only 1.37 to 1.88 years old [Lo Giudice 2000]. Moreover, the methods of measurement have only been briefly described and thus do not allow us to conclude on the real blood pressure status of these children. Although the data show that renal function and integrity are normal in these children, these preliminary results need to be confirmed and further evaluation of renal function parameters as well as blood pressure is required.

Table 3: Renal function and blood pressure of children exposed to cyclosporin (CsA) *in utero*

Mothers	Children			Reference
	n	Duration of follow-up in months (range)	Renal function and blood pressure	
Renal transplantation CsA last trimester: 320 ng/l (109-511)	26	39 (6-72)	Glomerular function: normal urea and creatinine; no hematuria, no proteinuria. Tubular function: normal amino-acids chromatography; normal plasma chloride, phosphate and bicarbonate; no proteinuria.	[Shaheen 93]
Renal transplantation CsA at delivery: 103±30 ng/ml (63-153)	6	28 (16-54)	Normal inulin and PAH clearances; filtration fraction and uric acid clearance slightly elevated.	[Saïd 96]
Transplantation 7 kidneys (1 regraft), 1 pancreas-kidney, 1 liver, 1 heart Mean trough blood CsA during pregnancy: 234±115 g/l (121-511)	12	31 (12-83)	Normal inulin-PAH clearances and filtration fraction. Renal ultrasound within normal ranges (kidney size); normal tubular function; no proteinuria. Blood pressure was normal in 8/12 children and slightly elevated in 4/12.	[Lo Giudice 2000]

Tacrolimus

Tacrolimus is a macrolide antibiotic that acts in a way similar to CsA, i.e. by inhibiting calcineurin [Armenti 98]. Common adverse effects include nephrotoxicity, hypertension, neurotoxicity and diabetes mellitus. When compared with cyclosporin, a lower incidence of hypertension has been highlighted as potentially beneficial in pregnancy management, as well as a lower incidence of hyperlipidemia; however, incidence of diabetes seems to be increased [Armenti 2002a].

Tacrolimus crosses the placenta but maternal and fetal toxicities appear to be dose-dependent. In mice, high dosages of tacrolimus (1.28 mg/kg/d) caused resorption of all fetuses without any obvious detrimental effects on maternal health, whereas in a pharmacological dosage group (0.16 mg/kg/d), the fetuses that survived did not appear to be different from control animals [Armenti 98].

An increased incidence of transient neonatal hyperkalemia (from 30 to 70%), as well as mild reversible renal impairment (anuria for 36 hours) have been reported with tacrolimus [Armenti 98, Hou 99, Kainz 2000]. A study reported a possible adverse effect of tacrolimus on fetal cardiac muscle in twins from a renal transplant recipient [Vyas 99]. The first twin died on day three of life from thrombotic dilated cardiomyopathy. The second twin also had dilated heart chambers with mild tricuspid insufficiency persisting at discharge at two months of age, as well as transient neonatal renal failure. All viral and bacterial cultures were persistently negative, ruling out viral myocarditis, and there was no family history of heart disease. Moreover, experimental data demonstrated a clear relationship between tacrolimus and myocarditis with necrosis, as well as widespread vasculitis of the cardiac muscle of rabbits, baboons and dogs [Vyas 99].

Two studies report a normal outcome in children submitted to tacrolimus *in utero*, but the follow-up is only 3 and 39 months (10 to 76) postpartum, respectively [Jain 97, Midtvedt 97].

5- Sirolimus (Rapamycin)

Sirolimus is a macrolide antibiotic with a different mechanism of action than tacrolimus. It has no effect on calcineurin activity but inhibits cytokine-driven T cell activation and proliferation, thus preventing the progression from the G_1 to the S-phase of the cell cycle at least two steps later in the activation/proliferation cascade in the cell than the calcineurin-dependent steps. In combination with CsA and prednisone, sirolimus provides enhanced immunosuppression and reduced acute rejection episodes.

The most common side effects of sirolimus include hypercholesterolemia/ triglyceridemia, anemia, thrombocytopenia, lymphocele, abdominal pain, diarrhea, arthralgia, hypokalemia, elevated lactate deshydrogenase and acne. In addition, abnormal healing following surgery has been reported.

No mutagenesis was found [Wyeth]. Carcinogenesis studies in mice and rats showed an increase in the incidence of lymphoma, hepatocellular adenoma and leukemia [Wyeth]. However, it is well known that the incidence of neoplasia can increase as a result of chronic use of immunosuppressive drugs. Therefore, this increase might not be attributable to sirolimus.

Reproductive studies have shown a decrease in male fertility [Wyeth]. A decrease in the number of spermatozoids as well as a decrease in testicle weight and/or histological lesions have been described in rats and monkeys [Wyeth].

Embryotoxicity in rat studies is characterized by increased fetal mortality and decreased fetal weight associated with delayed ossification of skeletal structures. No teratogenesis was noted. However, when sirolimus was administered in combination with CsA to pregnant animals, there was an increased fetal mortality, increased numbers of resorptions and decreased numbers of live fetuses, suggesting an increased toxicity in conjunction with calcineurin inhibition [Armenti 2002a]. Yet, there were no effects on rabbit development at a maternally toxic dosage. This might be reassuring as rabbits are a model closer to humans than rats; indeed, rabbit placentation is hemochorial as in human subjects, therefore allowing closer contact between maternal and fetal circulations [Thibault 91]. Nonetheless, definitive clinical pregnancy outcome data are not yet available. Therefore, sirolimus being a cell-growth inhibitor it is recommended that effective contraception must be initiated before sirolimus therapy, continued during therapy and for the 12 weeks following discontinuation of sirolimus.

6- Monoclonal Antibodies

Muromonab CD3 Orthoclone (OKT®3)

OKT®3 is a murine immunoglobulin G_{2A} that binds to the CD3 antigen on human T cells, blocking the function of helper T cells by subsequently causing CD3+ cells to disappear from peripheral circulation.

OKT®3 is used for both induction (duration of treatment = ten to fourteen days) and antirejection regimens. OKT®3 crosses the placenta but data are sparse: two studies reported seven pregnancies with OKT®3 with five surviving infants who were developing normally after a short follow-up [Hou 99]. No animal study on reproduction has been reported.

Basiliximab and Daclizumab

Basiliximab and daclizumab are immunoglobulins (IgG_1) which specifically antagonize the action of interleukine 2 at its membrane CD25 receptor, thus causing inhibition of IL-2-dependent T lymphocyte proliferation in response to antigen recognition. They are both used in the early postoperative period for induction and to prevent acute rejection, in association with cyclosporine and corticoids [Armenti 98].

No maternal toxicity, embryotoxicity or teratogenicity has been reported in the Cynomolgus monkey when basiliximab was used during organogenesis [Armenti 2002a]. No mutagenic potential was observed *in vitro*. However, IgG is known to cross the human placenta and no human study being available, basiliximab is thus contra-indicated during pregnancy and breastfeeding. A delay of eight weeks after the second dose is recommended before conception.

No animal or human study is available for daclizumab either. As for basiliximab, it is thus recommended to take contraception for at least four months after the last dose and to avoid breastfeeding.

7- Chlorambucil and Cyclophosphamide

Chlorambucil and cyclophosphamide are mutagenic and carcinogenic alkylating agents used to achieve immunosuppression in a variety of immune-mediated diseases [Janssen 2000, Ramsey-Goldman 97]. They prevent cell replication, reducing B and T cell numbers by cross-linking strands of DNA [Ramsey-Goldman 97].

Chlorambucil is three times more teratogenic than cyclophosphamide [Bermas 95]. Moreover, it has a selective effect on renal development by retarding both tubular and glomerular growth, and may cause renal and ureteral hypoplasia. In humans the major toxicity appears to be renal agenesis [Bermas 95]. Cyclophosphamide crosses the placenta and accumulates in amniotic fluid at dose levels of 25% of that observed in maternal blood [Bermas 95]. It produces severe growth retardation and congenital abnormalities (risk ranging between 16 and 22%) such as exophtalmos, cleft palate and skeletal abnormalities in animals.

Human data are scarce and usually reassuring for cyclophosphamide. However a worrying case described a male twin exposed *in utero* to cyclophosphamide who developed thyroid papillary cancer at age 11 years and neuroblastoma at 14, while the other twin was not affected [Bermas 95]. Moreover, cyclophosphamide causes infertility when taken daily in women as well as in men: permanent ovarian failure occurs in over 70% of patients with amenorrhea within a year, and azoospermia or oligospermia have been reported [Bermas 95, Janssen 2000]. These data question the long-term effects on fertility of *in utero* exposure. Alkylating agents should thus be avoided during pregnancy and genetic counseling after exposure should be offered, especially during the first trimester.

8- Methotrexate

Methotrexate (MTX) is a folic acid antagonist that impairs dihydrofolate reductase and thus interferes with the biosynthesis of purines [Ramsey-Goldman 97]. MTX is used in the treatment of psoriasis, rheumatoid arthritis and other rheumatic diseases [Chakravarty 2003, Janssen 2000, Ramsey-Goldman 97]. The spontaneous abortion rate is very high with MTX (44%), with no long-term effects on fertility in women. MTX is thus used in obstetrics for termination of early or ectopic pregnancies. MTX also induces reversible oligospermia in men. Therefore, discontinuation of the drug at least three months prior to conception is recommended [Bermas 95, Janssen 2000]. Although some pregnancies have been carried out successfully with MTX [Chakravarty 2003, Janssen 2000, Ramsey-Goldman 97], it is teratogenic and embryotoxic at high or therapeutic doses in mice and humans (88% embryolethality, craniofacial and limb defects, central nervous system abnormalities including anencephaly, hydrocephaly and meningomyelocele) [Chakravarty 2003, Chapa 2003, Ramsey-Goldman 97]. A recent case report by Nguyen *et al.* showed multiple anomalies in a fetus exposed only for 2 days at 3.5 weeks postconception. The pregnancy was terminated at 20 weeks and fetopsy revealed craniofacial, axial skeletal, cardiopulmonary and gastrointestinal abnormalities [Nguyen 2002]. In case of exposure, folate should be supplemented to avoid neural tube defects [Janssen 2000]. Myelosuppression has been reported in two cases. Low-dose MTX has also been proven to result in normal full-term children [Chakravarty 2003, Janssen 2000, Ramsey-Goldman 97]. However, as MTX may be retained in human tissue for up to 8 months after exposure, it is recommended that a reliable form of contraception should be used when using MTX [Nguyen 2002].

C- Fetal Programming of Adult Hypertension

In fetal life, tissues and organs go through critical periods of development which may coincide with periods of rapid cell division and differentiation [Widdowson 75]. These are periods when the tissue/organ is particularly sensitive to any stimulus or insult that might disturb its normal course of development, i.e. the tissue/organ shows great plasticity to environmental stimuli, with possible lifelong effects. Among these stimuli are fetal undernutrition, either via maternal malnutrition or placental insufficiency, as well as *in utero* exposure to drugs.

Fetal Programming: a Multifactorial Process

Depending on the time of exposure during pregnancy, differences appear in the long-term effects of prenatal exposure to various stresses. Therefore, a unique common mechanism has not been found yet, and will probably never be. Regardless of the time of exposure, the mechanisms underlying fetal programming are probably multifactorial (see figure 1). We will try in the following to briefly review some of the available data on this wide topic.

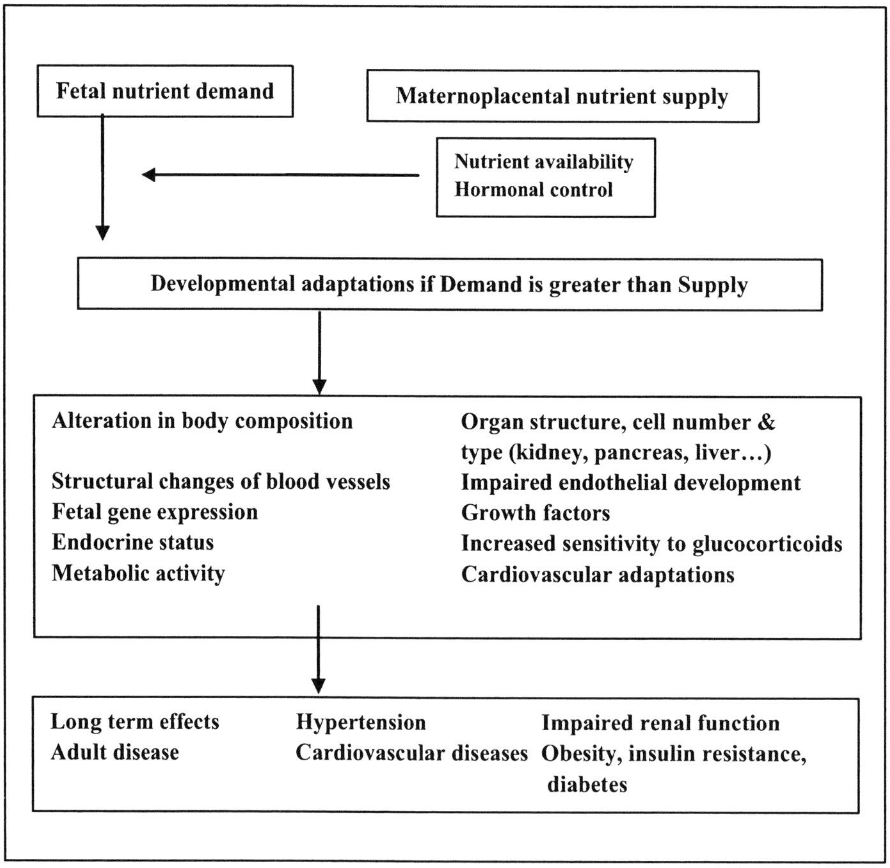

Figure 1: Possible mechanisms of fetal programming of adult diseases.

Low Birthweight and the Fetal Programming Hypothesis

The fetal programming hypothesis, also known now as the Barker hypothesis, states that fetal undernutrition during gestation, which leads to impaired fetal growth, can program adult chronic diseases such as hypertension, renal disease, coronary heart disease, atherosclerosis, stroke, non-insulin dependent type II diabetes, obesity or the metabolic syndrome X, by inducing permanent changes in blood pressure, organ morphology, cholesterol metabolism, insulin response to glucose, and a wide range of other metabolic, endocrine and immune functions [Barker 98, 2002, Baum 2003, Forsen 2000, Godfrey 2000, Holemans 2003, Kohen-Avramoglu 2003, Robinson 2002]. Possible associations with liver diseases such as hepatitis, non-alcoholic fatty liver disease, cirrhosis, hepatoblastoma, or hepatocellular carcinoma can be added to these pathologies [Donma 2003]. Although there are still controversial areas, there is at present sufficient scientific evidence for fetal programming to be regarded as an additional risk factor for chronic disease in interaction with genetic and lifestyle risk factors.

Noteworthy that the sole measure of birthweight is not the best representative of intrauterine growth. It does not allow the thin or stunted baby to be distinguished from the short one, or the disproportionate as a result of "brain-sparing" redistribution of blood flow. The addition of birth length, head circumference and ponderal index (birthweight/length^3) would better reflect different fetal growth patterns that may have different long-term consequences, and should therefore be added in registries. However, most records used so far for epidemiological studies did not include measurements of body size at birth other than weight and we will therefore only focus on the relation between low birthweight and hypertension.

Numerous epidemiological studies have shown that low birthweight is associated with persisting raised blood pressure in all age groups in childhood and adult life, in men and women, in developed as well as developing countries [Law 93, Barker 98]. The relation is not found in adolescence, probably because the tracking of blood pressure is perturbed by the adolescent growth spurt and it is not confounded by socio-economic conditions at birth or in adult life. Because it is found in people who were thin, short, or proportionately small babies, high blood pressure at adult age seems to be associated with interference with fetal growth at any stage of gestation. From these studies, it appears that an increase in birthweight of 1 kg is associated with a decrease in systolic blood pressure at adult age by around 2 to 5 mm Hg [Barker 98, Huxley 2000]. This might not seem to be clinically relevant for individuals, yet an epidemiological study by Rose suggested that lowering systolic blood pressure in a population by 10 mm Hg could result in a 30% reduction in the total attributable mortality of this population [Rose 85].

Maternal Undernutrition

Low birthweight induced by fetal undernutrition is linked to maternal nutrition. In Jamaican women, weight and thinness of the offspring at birth appeared to be related to indices of pre-pregnancy maternal nutritional status, such as height, weight and body mass index (BMI) [Thame 97]. In 10-year-old Jamaican children, blood pressure was related to maternal hemoglobin and triceps skinfold thickness in pregnancy [Godfrey 96]. British men in their forties were found to have higher blood pressure when their mothers had consumed a high-carbohydrate low-protein diet during pregnancy [Campbell 96].

In animals, the most common models of fetal undernutrition are achieved either through uterine artery ligation, or by giving low-protein diet to the pregnant mother. These models result in fetal growth retardation and increases in blood pressure at adult age [Langley-Evans 2001, 2003]. However, differences in the magnitude of long-term effects seemed to be related to different diet compositions. Therefore, it appears that the main nutritional programming influence on the fetus is rather the overall balance of nutrients than low protein per se. Indeed, Langley-Evans *et al.* demonstrated that the effects of the low-protein diet on blood pressure could be replicated by alterations to the fat source [Langley-Evans 96].

Finally, blood pressure of the mothers during and after pregnancy also correlates with the blood pressure of the offspring. However, the associations between body size and proportions at birth and later blood pressure are independent of the blood pressures of the mothers.

Role of the Placenta

Epidemiological and experimental studies have demonstrated that maternal undernutrition during pregnancy is also associated with abnormal placental growth. It is now widely acknowledged that alterations in placental growth and vascular resistance, altered nutrient and hormone metabolism in the placenta, and changes in nutrient transfer and partitioning between mother, placenta and fetus all have important effects on the fetal adaptations associated to programming.

Of note that associations between placental weight and adult disease are not consistent. Some of these associations are U-shaped, suggesting that both low and high placental weight/birthweight ratio (placental ratio) may be associated with fetal programming. It is the case for blood pressure, where small and large placental weights have been reported to be associated with the development of adult hypertension [Godfrey 2002]. In most studies however, the placental ratio is predictive of blood pressure and there is an increase in systolic as well as diastolic blood pressure with increasing placental weight [Barker 98, Godfrey 2002]. It appears from a study in sheep that enlargement occurs only in ewes that were well nourished before pregnancy [McCrabb 91, Symonds 2003]. A possible explanation could be that placental enlargement is an adaptive response to extract more nutrients from the mother that occurs only when these nutrients are available.

Proposed mechanisms for programming through placental modifications include mainly alterations in fetal body composition, as well as changes in fetal endocrinology and metabolism. For example in rats, reduced placental activity of the enzyme 11-beta-hydroxysteroid dehydrogenase type-2, leading to increased fetal exposure to maternal glucocorticoids, is associated with increased blood pressure in the offspring during adult life [Edwards 93].

Fetal Exposure to Excess Maternal Glucocorticoids

During normal fetal development, circulating fetal concentrations of glucocorticoids are very low relative to maternal concentrations. Separation of the fetal circulation from maternal glucocorticoids is achieved through the activity of placental 11-beta-hydroxysteroid dehydrogenase type-2 (11-beta-HSD-2), an enzyme that inactivates maternal cortisol (humans) or corticosterone (rats) before they reach the fetus. This ensures normal development of the fetal hypothalamic-pituitary-adrenal (HPA) axis, and a correct developmental pattern of gene expression. An excess may occur either from fetoplacental stress or from deficiency in the normal placental enzyme barrier. Such a deficiency can be produced experimentally in rats by undernutrition. Indeed, protein restriction has been associated with reductions of the activity level of placental 11-beta-HSD-2, therefore resulting in higher than normal exposure of the fetus to maternal glucocorticoids [Edwards 93, Lindsay 96]. Lowered activity levels or downregulation of 11-beta-HSD-2 have been associated with low birthweight and raised blood pressure in the rat [Bertram 2001]. Metyrapone, an inhibitor of maternal glucocorticoid synthesis, prevented the rise in blood pressure induced by maternal low-protein diet, whereas corticosterone replacement of metyrapone-treated pregnant rats restored the hypertensive effect of the diet. Moreover, the dependence to glucocorticoids seems to extend beyond the fetal period, as adrenalectomy in four-week-old rats exposed to low-protein diet *in utero* restored blood pressure levels comparable to controls. Again, corticosterone replacement reversed the effect of adrenalectomy [Langley-Evans 2001]. Furthermore, administration of dexamethasone, which is a poor substrate for 11-beta-HSD-2 and crosses the placenta freely, to pregnant rats on a normal diet induces low birthweight and hypertension in the offspring. Treatment with carbexolone, an inhibitor of 11-beta-HSD-2, has similar effects. It thus appears that programmed hypertension depends, at least partly, on maternal glucocorticoid production.

The mechanism of this programming remains unclear. In the fetus, maternal glucocorticoid excess may suppress the development of the fetal adrenal glands by inhibiting adrenocorticotropic hormone (ACTH) secretion and thus reducing adrenal growth and steroidogenesis, leading to the suppression of the HPA axis in adulthood [Ashton 2000]. In humans, an inverse relation between birthweight and excretion of cortisol metabolites has been reported in children as well as adult men and women. In men, timed fasting plasma cortisol concentrations fell progressively from 408 to 309 nmol/L when birthweight increased from below 2500 g to over 4310 g, a trend independent of age and BMI [Phillips 98, 2001]. Likely, low birthweight was associated with increased cortisol responsiveness to synthetic adrenocorticotrophic hormone administration, a finding strongly suggestive of increased HPA activity [Phillips 2001]. Moreover, evidence from people without pituitary or adrenal disease shows that elevated plasma cortisol concentrations in morning samples are associated with high blood pressure [Phillips 98, 2000]. Therefore, increased activity of the HPA axis may link low birthweight with raised blood pressure.

In humans, decreased 11-beta-HSD-2 expression may also enhance glucocorticoids availability to both glucocorticoid receptor and mineralocorticoid receptor. This would be likely to induce a state of apparent mineralocorticoid excess similar to that observed in patients with congenital or acquired deficiency of 11-beta-HSD-2 activity, conditions which are accompanied by hypertension [Bertram 2001].

Of interest is also the fact that reduced 11-beta-HSD-2 expression has been reported in placentas of women with preeclampsia and pregnancy-induced hypertension [Quinkler 2003]. The etiology of this inhibition is still unknown, but it reinforces the need for close follow-up of the offspring.

Reduced Nephron Number

One of the mechanisms that are now widely recognized as a possible etiology of elevated blood pressure at adult age in small children is a reduction in the number of nephrons. Widdowson and McCance were among the first to show that brief periods of undernutrition may permanently reduce the number of cells in organs [Widdowson 74, 75]. Among these organs, it seems that the kidney is particularly vulnerable [Moritz 2003]. Studies of growth-retarded infants have shown that the kidneys were disproportionately more affected relative to the other organs [Konje 96].

The total nephron number is fixed, characteristic of a species and among species proportional to body size (average in humans: 1 million per kidney; range: 330'000 to 2 millions per kidney). In humans, about 60% nephrons develop during the 3rd trimester and nephrogenesis is completed by the 36th week of amenorrhea. Nephron number in humans is entirely determined by prenatal factors, since no new nephrons are added after birth [Merlet-Bénichou 99]. Nephrogenesis can thus be modulated by several factors during pregnancy, including IUGR or exposure to maternal drugs [Lelièvre-Pégorier 2000, Merlet-Bénichou 94, 99]. Animal and human studies have established that fetal growth retardation from various etiologies leads to small fetal kidneys, with strong correlation coefficients between birthweight and the number of glomeruli ranging from 0.77 to 0.87 [Hughson 2003, Mackenzie 96, Manalich 2000, Merlet-Bénichou 99, Silver 2003]. A clinical study of infants who died from non-renal causes showed that the infants with a birthweight between the 5th and 10th percentile had 30% less nephrons on average than did infants whose birthweight was above the 10th percentile [Merlet-Bénichou 99].

A reduction of the renal mass causes morphologic and functional compensatory adaptation of the remnant nephrons, which become hyperfiltrating. Therefore, renal function is usually well maintained at first. Yet, hyperfiltration has been associated with the development of renal insufficiency and hypertension. Animal studies have provided evidence that nephron reduction acquired in the perinatal period is eventually related to a higher incidence of focal glomerulosclerosis associated with proteinuria, tubular atrophy, macrophage infiltration, interstitial fibrosis, and decreased glomerular filtration rate at adult age [Brenner 82, Chevalier 2000, Lucas 2000, Merlet-Bénichou 99]. In humans, oligomeganephronic renal hypoplasia, in which the nephron number is always below 300'000 by kidney, inevitably progresses to end-stage renal failure in childhood or adolescence (mean age at onset: 6 years) [Broyer 97, Rostand 2003]. Moreover, even if renal function still appeared normal, Regazzoni *et al.* have shown in adults uninephrectomized during childhood (before 16) that the renal reserve capacity significantly decreased over the years [Regazzoni 98]. These results indicate a vulnerability of the remaining single kidney that could raise the possibility of future renal functional impairment.

As for hypertension, kidneys with a lower nephron number undergo hyperfiltration, which will lead to a progressive deterioration and further loss of nephrons. Single nephron pressure and efferent vascular resistance will further increase to maintain function and will eventually translate into elevated systemic blood pressure. Indeed, Brenner *et al.* showed that the number of nephrons is inversely correlated to the risk of developing hypertension at adult age in the rat. Spontaneously hypertensive rats had 10 to 25% less nephrons compared to normotensive animals [Brenner 88]. Surgical reduction in the number of nephrons from birth also leads to increased blood pressure in adult rats [Ingelfinger 2002]. Mackenzie *et al.* [Mackenzie 96] later postulated that a congenital or acquired nephron deficit could be the explanation for the increased risk of hypertension in later life in low birthweight infants. Post-mortem analysis of the number of glomeruli in white adults with primary hypertension and/or left ventricular hypertrophy showed that the number of glomeruli was significantly lower in these patients, as compared to normotensive controls [Keller 2003]. Moreover, the mean glomerular volume was significantly higher and morphological abnormalities were only found in the hypertensive patients. Unfortunately, the birthweights of these patients were not reported.

A recent study by the team of Brenner demonstrated that supplementation of kidney mass by isograft transplantation in nephrectomized rats significantly decreased systolic blood pressure by about 35 mm Hg. Glomerular hyperfiltration was also reduced in the remnant kidneys, as well as proteinuria and glomerulosclerosis, as compared to sham-operated rats [Ots 04]. The authors thus concluded that a reduced renal mass *per se* is a major independent factor in the development and maintenance of hypertension, which can be reversed in their model by supplementing renal mass.

Finally, neither IUGR nor congenital oligonephronia are sufficient to induce hypertension. Because placental blood flow is reduced, IUGR is associated with low fetal vitamin A levels. Retinoids are known to be potent nephron mass regulators, which can modulate the nephron number at birth in a dose-dependent manner. This suggests that fetal vitamin A homeostasis may play a critical role in the association between size at birth and blood pressure later in life [Merlet-Bénichou 99, Gilbert 2002]. Vitamin C status of the mother has also been implied.

The Renin-Angiotensin System

Components of the renin-angiotensin system (RAS) are key elements of blood pressure control, as well as being involved in normal kidney development and functioning, in particular the maintenance of glomerular filtration rate [Moritz 2003, Prévot 2002b]. Animals lacking genes of the RAS develop markedly abnormal kidneys and may develop hypertension [Ingelfinger 2002].

Maternal dietary protein restriction during pregnancy in the rat causes suppression of the intrarenal RAS during the period of nephrogenesis. Reduced renal renin gene expression, reduced renin immunostaining in the kidney and reduced renal tissue AII levels were present in the offspring [Woods 2000]. As a result, adult male offspring had approximately 25% fewer nephrons and showed an increase of mean arterial pressure by about 10 mm Hg, as compared to controls [Woods 98]. The pharmacological suppression of the RAS with perinatal administration of losartan also resulted in a 42% reduction in the number of nephrons per kidney, associated with reduced renal function and hypertension in adulthood [Tufro-McReddie 95]. Conversely, there is evidence that the fetal RAS is activated during IUGR. In the rat, renin and angiotensin converting activities were elevated in animals exposed to a low-protein diet *in utero*. A two-weeks administration of the ACE inhibitor captopril lowered blood pressure in both neonates and young adults to levels comparable to those observed in control rats [Sherman 98]. Again, it appears that the composition and time of administration of the maternal diet are essential.

Taken together, the data suggest that either inhibition or overexpression of the RAS, resulting in too much or too little intrarenal AII activity, may equally be involved in programming the development of the kidney and further hypertension.

Gene Programming

It has been demonstrated that low birthweight and programmed hypertension are associated with altered expression of numerous genes [Bertram 2001, Lindsay 96, Manning 2002, Quinkler 2003, Sharkey 2001]. We will only mention a few with particular interest for hypertension.

Maternal protein restriction in the rat resulted in upregulation at both the mRNA and the protein levels of two sodium transporters (BSC1 and TSC) of the thick ascending limb and the distal convoluted tubule [Manning 2002]. It is likely that this upregulation is associated with increased Na reabsorption in these two segments. Thus, enhanced Na transport would be a part of the pathogenesis of hypertension by leading to an expansion of extracellular volume. Interestingly enough, upregulation was detected before the development of hypertension and there was no downregulation after hypertension was established. Yet, physiologic downregulation of TSC has been shown to be part of the pressure-natriuresis response designed to correct hypertension by increasing renal Na excretion. Impaired regulation of Na transport would therefore participate in the development as well as maintenance of prenatally-programmed hypertension.

Of interest is also the finding that overexpression of human insulin-like growth factor (IGF) binding protein-1 in the mouse resulted in a significant reduction in the nephron number [Doublier 2001]. Exogenously added IGF-II, but not IGF-I, was effective in stimulating nephrogenesis *in vitro*. In addition, Vickers *et al.* showed in a rat model of programmed hypertension that treatment with either IGF-I or growth hormone (GH) at adult age significantly reduced systolic blood pressure [Vickers 2001, 2002]. This suggests that reduced amounts of circulating growth factors as a result of fetal programming could impair kidney development and participate in blood pressure regulation.

Finally, while most genes are expressed from both parental loci, some called "imprinted genes" are only expressed from either the maternal or the paternal allele [see Young 2001 for review]. Because they are functionally haploid, imprinted genes are particularly vulnerable to being inactivated or overexpressed. Many act mainly during fetal development, making them plausible candidates for programming. It has been well established from animal experiments that nutrition can affect imprinted genes. Among these are the gene of the potent fetal growth factor, insulin-like growth factor II (*Igf2* gene, paternally expressed in most fetal tissues) and the *H19* gene. Disruptions at imprinted gene loci have been demonstrated to significantly affect allometric growth and development of organs, including kidneys, liver and heart. The *H19* gene is activated in human atherosclerotic plaques, suggesting a role in both atherosclerosis and hypertension. Brain development is also regulated by imprinted genes. Therefore, effects on the hypothalamus or pituitary may have direct implications on hypertension through endocrine disruption. Finally, alterations in the DNA methylation components of imprinted genes seem to be stably inherited and could thus have further effects in the next generations [Reik 2001].

Childhood Catch-Up Growth

Blood pressure in childhood predicts the likelihood of developing hypertension in adult life. In children the rise of blood pressure with age is closely related to growth. Moreover, body mass at adult age is also important as the highest pressures are found in people who were small at birth and later became overweight as adults. Therefore, some authors have proposed that hypertension could be a disorder of growth. However, it appears that it is rather that postnatal catch-up growth plays an important role in amplifying changes established *in utero* [Law 2002].

Experimental results in rats exposed to fetal undernutrition showed hyperphagia at all ages [Vickers 2000]. ANOVA revealed significant interaction between programming and diet during the post-pubertal and adult age, suggesting fetal programming of hyperphagia. Moreover, these findings were correlated with the development of increased systolic blood pressure, suggesting amplification of the metabolic and cardiovascular abnormalities by hypercaloric nutrition [Vickers 2000].

In humans, Moore *et al.* demonstrated amplification of the relationship between birthweight and blood pressure over the period from 8 to 20 years, due at least in part to greater rises in blood pressure with age among individuals who were of low birthweight [Moore 99]. In a systematic review of the literature, Huxley *et al.* examined sixteen studies reporting on the role of skeletal or non-skeletal catch-up growth [Huxley 2000]. Twelve studies reported a positive association between the prevalence of hypertension and height in adulthood, the relative change in weight from birth to current or adult BMI. This supports the suggestion that small-for-gestational-age infants who exhibit catch-up growth postnatally are at increased risk of high blood pressure. However, it is difficult to determine whether this postnatal catch-up growth predicts blood pressure independently of prenatal growth as the measures of postnatal growth usually incorporate birthweight in their calculations. Moreover, the heterogeneity of measures may have represented different biological processes to assess adult height and weight, as for example accelerated early childhood growth or fat accumulation in adolescence and adult life.

Immunosuppressive Drugs and Fetal Programming

We have previously seen that *in utero* exposure to immunosuppressive drugs increases the incidence of low birthweight, which is by itself a risk factor for developing hypertension. However, it has been demonstrated that some drugs could play a specific role in fetal programming. As far as we know, experimental evidence for immunosuppressants is only available for dexamethasone and cyclosporine [Celsi 98, Martins 2003, Merlet-Bénichou 99, Tendron 2003]. However, as the mode of action of most immunosuppressive drugs is through inhibition of cell growth, it would be of great interest to consider this aspect for the other drugs.

Prenatal exposure to dexamethasone in rats led to low birthweight and oligonephronia [Celsi 98, Martins 2003, Merlet-Bénichou 99]. It appears that the magnitude of the decreased nephron number was an important factor for later development of adult disease. Indeed, in one study, dexamethasone did not elicit any change in blood pressure or renal function despite mild oligonephronia [Martins 2003], whereas in the other the rats showed a lower glomerular filtration rate, higher albuminuria, increased sodium retention, and a significantly higher blood pressure [Celsi 98]. In the latter study, treatment with hydrocortisone resulted in normal fetal development and adult blood pressure [Celsi 98]. Moreover, in sheep, only two days of exposure to high levels of dexamethasone (mean age at exposure 27 days, gestation length 150 days) resulted in normal birthweight but hypertensive offspring at 3-4 months of age, suggesting that the programming of hypertension could, at least in this study, be dissociated from intrauterine growth retardation [Dodic 2003, Moritz 2003]. Taken together, these results thus suggest a specific action of dexamethasone on fetal programming (see "Fetal exposure to maternal glucocorticoids" for more).

In vitro, CsA altered nephrogenesis in rat metanephric organ culture, leading to a dose-dependent nephron deficit reaching 50% of control values [Merlet-Bénichou 99]. *In vivo*, administration of a therapeutic dose of CsA to pregnant rabbits led to a significant nephron deficit of 25 to 33% in the offspring exposed from day 14 to day 18 or day 20 to day 24 of gestation, respectively (gestation time 31 days, nephrogenesis starts on embryonic day 11. Therefore the first treatment coincides with the onset of metanephros formation, and the second one with the beginning of nephron filtration) [Tendron 2000, 2003]. Histological study showed that the nephron deficit was localized in the deep and superficial cortex, indicating that disturbance of the early steps of renal organogenesis can also impair the following generations of nephrons. Despite the reduced nephron mass and the presence of histopathological findings (including tubular vacuolization, foci of interstitial fibrosis, and enlarged juxtamedullary nephrons), creatinine levels were normal in one-month old rabbits, suggesting normal renal function. However, preliminary data in adult rabbits born to CsA-treated mothers indicated that mean blood pressure was significantly increased in these animals as compared to age-matched controls. Moreover, CsA-exposed rabbits exhibited a significant reduction in glomerular filtration rate, as measured with the gold standard method, i.e. inulin clearance. A significant increase in renal vascular resistance, as well as established proteinuria were also noted [Tendron 2003]. Again, the oligonephronia seen with exposure from day 14 to 18 was present without low birthweight suggesting that, like dexamethasone, CsA per se may have an impact on fetal programming.

Antihypertensive Drugs and Fetal Programming

Bayliss *et al.* showed that the beta-blocker atenolol taken at the time of conception and/or during the first trimester of pregnancy was associated with low birthweight, independently of the development of preeclampsia [Bayliss 2002]. The use of atenolol in the second trimester did not induce any reduction in birthweight. Other antihypertensives were not found to be associated with low birthweight [Bayliss 2002].

Experimental studies in newborn rats and rabbits showed that ACE inhibition with enalapril or specific angiotensin II type 1 (AT_1) receptor blockade with losartan resulted in abnormalities in renal function [Prévot 2002b] and morphology, including fewer and thicker afferent arterioles, reduced glomerular size and number, tubular dilatation and papillary atrophy, associated with hypertension in adulthood [Guron 99, Tufro-McReddie 95, Woods 98]. This was seen when enalapril was administered from the 3rd to the 13th postnatal day, but not later. This early postnatal time span coincides with the completion of nephrogenesis and a period of marked tubular growth and differentiation, thus suggesting a pivotal role for angiotensin II in the regulation of nephrovascular development. Moreover, renal AT_1 receptor expression was increased in rats exposed *in utero* to a maternal low-protein diet [Sahajpal 2003]. These rats had fewer glomeruli, an increase in mean arterial blood pressure and elevated renal vascular resistance at 4 weeks of age. When challenged with angiotensin II, these rats also showed a greater reduction in glomerular filtration rate than did control rats, suggesting an increased sensitivity to angiotensin II [Sahajpal 2003]. These results suggest a contribution of angiotensin II, directly or via the increased AT_1 receptor expression, to the elevated blood pressure in this model.

However, we have seen that ACE inhibitors and angiotensin II receptor antagonists are strictly contra-indicated during pregnancy. Therefore, this should not be an additional risk factor for immunosuppressed pregnancies. Although data are scarce, they again emphasize the need for careful follow-up of the offspring.

Programming of the Next Generations?

The female offspring of rabbit mothers with secondary renal hypertension (2-kidney, 1-wrapped Page hypertension) had increased blood pressure as adults [Denton 2003]. Interestingly, blood pressure in male offspring was unaffected, suggesting either that males were protected, or that females were more susceptible to the intrauterine environment. Other studies have clearly shown gender-based differences in the adult response to adverse prenatal events. However, in a rat model of pharmacologically-induced maternal hypertension, no significant difference was found in the blood pressure of the pups, even after high-salt diet challenge [Gomez-Sanchez 99]. These conflicting results suggest the implications of several different maternal factors as well as different mechanisms of hypertension programming in the fetus. In the first described study, the mothers were not only hypertensive but also had reduced weight gain, elevated plasma renin activity, and renal impairment [Denton 2003].

In a human study, Klebanoff *et al.* reported that women who were small for gestational age at birth were found to be at increased risk of developing hypertension during pregnancy (11.3 versus 7.2%; adjusted odds ratio 1.8; 95% confidence interval 1.1-2.8). The risk could not be explained by the presence of hypertensive disorders during their mother's pregnancies [Klebanoff 99]. These results may have implications beyond pregnancy since hypertension arising during pregnancy is a marker for increased risk of developing chronic hypertension years later [Klebanoff 99]. Unfortunately, there was no report of the outcome of the pregnancies and we therefore do not know if there was an increase in the incidence of low birthweight and IUGR in the second generation. Of note that the same was found for preterm women who experienced increased blood pressure at adult age (mean 26±1.9 years) [Kistner 2000].

In a follow-up study in men and women whose parents' birthweight was known, Barker *et al.* reported blood pressure measurements at 18-40 years of age. Systolic and diastolic blood pressures fell with increasing mother's birthweight and head circumference. Systolic blood pressure fell by 2.4 mm Hg for each pound increase in mother's birthweight and by 4.0 mm Hg for each one inch increase in head circumference. Moreover, these results were independent of the mother's current blood pressure and no sex difference was present [Barker 2000].

It thus appears from these animal and human studies that, if the growth of a female fetus is constrained or the female fetus is exposed *in utero* to the hypertension of the mother, persisting changes appear in her physiology, metabolism, and probably also genetic background, which could lead to reduced fetal growth and raised blood pressure in the next generation [Barker 2000].

We may therefore be in the presence of a vicious cycle of hypertension/low birthweight-induced hypertension/low birthweight. Epidemiological studies are still mandatory to confirm this phenomenon. However, until further data are available, public health policies improving the nutrition of pregnant women and subsequent fetal growth in one generation may contribute to preventing chronic diseases in succeeding generations as well, in addition to enhancing health and survival of mothers and children.

D- BREASTFEEDING

Breastfeeding and Immunosuppressive Drugs

Most immunosuppressants are transferred into breast milk, therefore raising the question of further exposure of the newborn child to the drugs taken by the mother.

Prednisone and prednisolone are considered safe in breastfeeding mothers since less than 10% of the active drug is secreted into breast milk [Bermas 95] and no adverse effects have been reported [Janssen 2000].

Two clinical studies report CsA blood concentrations in seven breastfed infants below the detection limit of 30 μg/l and in one infant lower than 3 μg/l, despite maternal trough levels ranging from 55 to 260 μg/l. The CsA concentrations measured in breast milk suggest that a baby taking 150 ml of milk per kg weight every day would receive less than 300 μg of CsA per day, i.e. less than 0.1 mg/kg, which is under a 60th of the dose of the mother, weight for weight [Nyberg 98, Thiru 97]. Rats exposed to CsA *in utero* and breastfed by untreated mothers showed no decrease in the frequency of anomalies (i.e. temporary defects in the development of hematopoietic organs, such as the thymus, the liver and the spleen). On the other hand, rats not exposed to CsA *in utero* and breastfed by CsA-treated mothers showed similar features to control animals. These results indicate an intrauterine effect of the drug but no effect when CsA is present in breast milk [Rezzani 97].

Azathioprine and 6-mercaptopurine are transferred into breast milk at low levels [Ramsey-Goldman 97].

Jain *et al.* [Jain 97] published a report of the measurement of tacrolimus concentrations in colostrum, which differs in protein content from mature milk. Despite very low concentrations, the mothers were counseled to abstain from breastfeeding [Jain 97]. However, in a recent report French *et al.* described the first account of tacrolimus measurement in human milk following maternal dosing in which the mother decided to carry on breastfeeding while taking the medication [French 2003]. The liver-transplant mother took tacrolimus throughout pregnancy with a stable graft function. Tacrolimus analysis was performed by tandem-mass spectrometry, which is considered a very sensitive and specific method. The average exposure of the exclusively breastfed infant was estimated to be 0.06% of the mother's weight-adjusted dose and the highest concentration in milk (0.57 ng/mL) was observed 1 hour after the dose. At 2.5 months of age, the infant was developing well both physically and neurologically. Chest ultrasound revealed a normally developed thymus [French 2003]. These results therefore suggest that tacrolimus may be compatible with breastfeeding.

It is not known whether sirolimus is excreted in human milk. However, sirolimus is excreted in small quantities in the milk of breastfeeding rats. Therefore, until further studies and considering that sirolimus is a cell-growth inhibitor, breastfeeding should be contra-indicated with this product.

Breastfeeding confers a better immune response to various infectious agents, promotes maturation of the gastrointestinal mucosal barrier, and was claimed to reduce the risk of atopic manifestations, autoimmune disorders and the incidence of admission to hospital [Nyberg 98, Thiru 97]. Furthermore, being breastfed is associated with significantly better intellectual development and the benefits of breastfeeding are considered even more pronounced in low and very low birthweight infants [Horwood 2001].

Data are mandatory for other immunosuppressive agents. However, it seems reasonable to say that, except for alkylating agents, methotrexate and sirolimus which are strictly contraindicated, the benefits of antibacterial and antiviral properties of human milk are higher than the risk of absorbing a small quantity of immunosuppressants [Armenti 98]. Therefore, mothers who still have the desire to breastfeed their baby after being carefully informed of the potential risks should be allowed to do so, with their children closely monitored for any potential adverse effect.

Breastfeeding and Antihypertensive Drugs

We will only briefly review the more commonly used.

The American Academy of Pediatrics considers hydrochlorothiazide and chlorthalidone compatible for breastfeeding. Beta-blockers such as atenolol, metoprolol or acebutolol appear to be concentrated in milk, and clinical signs of beta-blockade were reported in newborns [Barron 95, Boutroy 86]. However, it is not the case for propanolol, which could then be used [Barron 95].

A case report of the measurement of hydralazine showed that the estimated dose per milk feed (i.e. 75 ml) would not exceed 0.013 mg. Therefore, it appears that breastfeeding would not result in a clinically relevant concentration in the infant [Liedholm 82]. Nifedipine is excreted in milk, but only less than 5% of the maternal dose is ingested by the infant. Likewise, captopril and enalapril are excreted in very small quantities. A case report on the measurement of the calcium channel blocker verapamil and norverapamil showed that concentrations in milk were 60% and 16% of the maternal plasma concentration, respectively [Anderson 87]. Therefore, the child received less than 0.01% of the maternal dose and neither verapamil nor norverapamil could be detected in the plasma of the child (detection limit 1 ng/ml). Thus, calcium channel blockers do not seem to be a contraindication to breastfeeding.

Clonidine concentrations in milk were roughly twice that in maternal serum; in the newborn serum the concentrations were about half those of the mothers. However, there was no sign of any adverse effect in the newborns [Hartikainen-Sorri 87].

Finally, the available data indicate that ACE inhibitors, methyldopa, beta-blockers with high protein binding, and calcium channel blockers appear to be safe for a nursing mother, as milk to plasma ratios were low [Beardmore 2002]. However, given the scarcity of data available, mainly being case reports, breastfed infants of mothers treated for hypertension should be closely monitored for adverse effects.

Is There a Prevention of Programmed Hypertension by Breastfeeding?

Singhal *et al.* showed that consumption of breast milk compared to formula in infancy resulted in a significant decrease in diastolic as well as mean blood pressure in 13-16 years-old children by 3 and 4 mm Hg, respectively [Singhal 2001]. In addition, there was a negative dose-response relation between total breast milk consumption and teenage blood pressure within the breast milk-fed group. These findings are consistent with the hypothesis that high blood pressure in later life, at least partly, has early nutritional origins. Moreover, they provide supportive evidence for a potential long-term beneficial effect of breastfeeding. However, the time of breastfeeding also seems to be a crucial point. Leeson *et al.* reported that breastfeeding for more than 3 months decreased the distensibility of the brachial artery in young healthy adults, thereby increasing their theoretical risk of further developing hypertension [Leeson 2001]. Epidemiological studies suggest that serum cholesterol concentrations are also programmed by infant feeding. Men who were breastfed for more than one year had raised low density lipoprotein concentrations associated with increased mortality from coronary heart disease [Fall 92]. Studies of baboons suggest that these effects could be mediated through thyroxine in breast milk and resetting of the infants' hypothalamic-pituitary-thyroid axis [Mott 96]. It is interesting to add that breastfed small for gestational age infants showed greater gains in weight and occipitofrontal head circumference by 18 months than did formula-fed infants. However, as we already mentioned, postnatal catch-up growth can also be an additional risk factor for hypertension by amplifying changes established *in utero* [Barker 98, Fewtrell 2001].

Conclusion

Immunosuppressive treatment should not be a contra-indication to pregnancy. Short-term results of *in utero* exposure in humans are reassuring. However, animal studies raise the possibility of a reduction in the number of nephrons in the exposed offspring, associated with a decrease in renal function as well as an increase in blood pressure.

Therefore, epidemiological studies are mandatory and the long-term follow-up of children exposed to immunosuppressive agents *in utero* should be organized by a multidisciplinary team that should always take the perinatal context into account.

References

Afifi Y, Churchill D. Pharmacological treatment of hypertension in pregnancy. *Curr Pharm Des 2003;9:1745-1753.*

Akhlaghi F, Keogh AM, McLachlan AJ, Kaan A. Pharmacokinetics of cyclosporine in heart transplant recipients receiving metabolic inhibitors. *J Heart Lung Transplant 2001;20:431-438.*

Anderson P, Bondesson U, Mattiasson I, Johansson BW. Verapamil and norverapamil in plasma and breast milk during breast feeding. *Eur J Clin Pharmacol 1987;31:625-627.*

Armenti VT, Ahlswede KM, Ahlswede BA, Cater JR, Jarrell BE, Moritz MJ, Burke JF. Variables affecting birthweight and graft survival in 197 pregnancies in cyclosporine-treated female kidney transplant recipients. *Transplantation 1995;59:476-479.*

Armenti VT, Moritz MJ, Cardonick EH, Davison JM. Immunosuppression in Pregnancy. Choices for infant and maternal health. *Drugs 2002(a);62:2361-2375.*

Armenti VT, Moritz MJ, Davison JM. Drug safety issues in pregnancy following transplantation and immunosuppression. Effects and outcomes. *Drug Saf 1998;19:219-232.*

Armenti VT, Moritz MJ, Radomski JS, Davison JM. Pregnancy and transplantation. *Graft 2000;3:59-63.*

Armenti VT, Radomski JS, Moritz MJ, Gaughan WJ, Philips LZ, McGrory CH, Coscia LA. Report from the National Transplantation Pregnancy Registry (NTPR): outcomes of pregnancy after transplantation. *Clin Transpl 2002(b);121-130.*

Ashton N. Perinatal development and adult blood pressure. *Braz J Med Biol Res 2000;33:731-740.*

August P, Lindheimer MD. Pathophysiology of preeclampsia. *In: Laragh JH, Brenner BM, eds. Hypertension: Pathophysiology, Diagnosis and Management. Second Edition. Raven Press, Ltd., New York, 1995:2407-2426.*

Baarsma R, Kamps WA. Immunological responses in an infant after cyclosporine A exposure during pregnancy. *Eur J Pediatr 1993;152:476-477.*

Bar J, Fisch B, Wittenberg C, Gelerenter I, Boner G, Hod M. Prednisone dosage and pregnancy outcome in renal allograft recipients. *Nephrol Dial Transplant 1997;12:760-763.*

Barker DJ, Shiell AW, Barker ME, Law CM. Growth *in utero* and blood pressure levels in the next generation. *J Hypertens 2000;18:843-846.*

Barker DJP, Gluckman PD, Godfrey KM, Harding JE, Owens JA, Robinson JS. Fetal nutrition and cardiovascular disease in adult life. *Lancet 1993;341:938-941.*

Barker DJP. Fetal programming of coronary heart disease. *Trends Endocrinol Metab 2002;13:364-368.*

Barker DJP. *In utero* programming of chronic disease. *Clin Sci (Lond) 1998;95:115-128.*

Barker DJP. Mothers, babies and disease in later life. *London: BMJ Publishing Group, 1994.*

Barron WM, Lindheimer MD. Management of hypertension during pregnancy. *In: Laragh JH, Brenner BM, eds. Hypertension: Pathophysiology, Diagnosis and Management. Second Edition. Raven Press, Ltd., New York, 1995:2427-2450.*

Baum M, Ortiz L, Quan A. Fetal origins of cardiovascular disease. Curr *Opin Pediatr 2003;15:166-170.*

Bayliss H, Churchill D, Beevers M, Beevers DG. Anti-hypertensive drugs in pregnancy and fetal growth: evidence for "pharmacological programming" in the first trimester? *Hypertens Pregnancy 2002;21:161-174.*

Beardmore KS, Morris JM, Gallery ED. Excretion of antihypertensive medication into human breast milk: a systematic review. *Hypertens Pregnancy. 2002;21:85-95.*

Beitins IZ, Bayard F, Ances IG, Kowarski A, Migeon CJ. The transplacental passage of prednisone and prednisolone in pregnancy near term. *J Pediatr 1972;81:936-945.*

Bermas BL, Hill JA. Effects of immunosuppressive drugs during pregnancy. *Arthritis Rheum 1995;38:1722-1732.*

Bertram C, Trowern AR, Copin N, Jackson AA, Whorwood CB. The maternal diet during pregnancy programs altered expression of the glucocorticoid receptor and type 2 11beta-hydroxysteroid dehydrogenase: potential molecular mechanisms underlying the programming of hypertension *in utero*. *Endocrinology 2001;142:2841-2853.*

Boutroy MJ, Bianchetti G, Dubruc C, Vert P, Morselli PL. To nurse when receiving acebutolol: is it dangerous for the neonate? *Eur J Clin Pharmacol 1986;30:737-739.*

Brenner BM, Garcia DL, Anderson S. Glomeruli and blood pressure. Less of one, more of the other? *Am J Hypertens 1988;1:335-347.*

Brenner BM, Meyer TW, Hotstetter TH. Dietary protein intake and the progressive nature of kidney disease: the role of hemodynamically mediated glomerular injury in the pathogenesis of progressive glomerular sclerosis in aging, renal ablation and intrinsic renal disease. *N Engl J Med 1982;307:652-659.*

Briggs GG, Nageotte MP. Fatal fetal outcome with the combined use of valsartan and atenolol. *Ann Pharmacother 2001;35:859-861.*

Broyer M, Soto B, Gagnadoux MF, Adi M, Rica C, Gubler MC. Oligomeganephronic renal hypoplasia. *Adv Nephrol Necker Hosp 1997;26:47-63.*

Campbell DM, Hall MH, Barker DJ, Cross J, Shiell AW, Godfrey KM. Diet in pregnancy and the offspring's blood pressure 40 years later. *Br J Obstet Gynaecol 1996;103:273-280.*

Celsi G, Kistner A, Aizman R, Eklof AC, Ceccatelli S, de Santiago A, Jacobson SH. Prenatal dexamethasone causes oligonephronia, sodium retention, and higher blood pressure in the offspring. *Pediatr Res 1998;44:317-322.*

Chakravarty EF, Sanchez-Yamamoto D, Bush TM. The use of disease modifying antirheumatic drugs in women with rheumatoid arthritis of childbearing age: a survey of practice patterns and pregnancy outcomes. *J Rheumatol 2003;30:241-246.*

Chapa JB, Hibbard JU, Weber EM, Abramowicz JS, Verp MS. Prenatal diagnosis of methotrexate embryopathy. *Obstet Gynecol 2003;101:1104-1107.*

Chevalier P, Poinsignon Y, Guillemain R, Amrein C, Farge D. Grossesse après greffes d'organe. *Presse Med 1996;25:1643-1648.*

Chevalier RL, Thornhill BA, Chang AY. Unilateral ureteral obstruction in neonatal rats leads to renal insufficiency in adulthood. *Kidney Int 2000;58:1987-1995.*

Cockburn J, Moar VA, Ounsted M, Redman CW. Final report of study on hypertension during pregnancy: the effects of specific treatment on the growth and development of the children. *Lancet 1982;1:647-649.*

Davison JM, Dellagrammatikas H, Parkin JM. Maternal azathioprine therapy and depressed haemopoiesis in the babies of renal allograft patients. *Br J Obstet Gynaecol 1985(a);92:233-239.*

Davison JM, Lind T, Uldall PR. Planned pregnancy in a renal transplant recipient. *Br J Obstet Gynaecol 1976;83:518-527.*

Davison JM, Lindheimer MD. Pregnancy in women with renal allografts. *Semin Nephrol 1984;4:240-251.*

Davison JM, Milne JEC. Pregnancy and renal transplantation. *Br J Urol 1997;80[Suppl 1]:29-32.*

Davison JM. Dialysis, transplantation, and pregnancy. *Am J Kidney Dis 1991;17:127-132.*

Davison JM. The effect of pregnancy on kidney function in renal allograft recipients. *Kidney Int 1985(b);27:74-79.*

Demme RA. Hypertension in the kidney transplant patient. *Graft 2001;4:248-255.*

Denton KM, Flower RL, Stevenson KM, Anderson WP. Adult rabbit offspring of mothers with secondary hypertension have increased blood pressure. *Hypertension 2003;41:634-639.*

Di Paolo S, Schena A, Morrone LF, Manfredi G, Stallone G, Derosa C, Procino A, Schena FP. Immunological evaluation during the first year of life of infants born to cyclosporine-treated female kidney recipients. *Transplantation 2000;69:2049-2054.*

Dodic M, Moritz K, Wintour EM. Prenatal exposure to glucocorticoids and adult disease. *Arch Physiol Biochem 2003;111:61-69.*

Donma MM, Donma O. Low birth weight: a possible risk factor also for liver diseases in adult life? *Med Hypotheses 2003;61:435-438.*

Doublier S, Amri K, Seurin D, Moreau E, Merlet-Bénichou C, Striker GE, Gilbert T. Overexpression of human insulin-like growth factor binding protein-1 in the mouse leads to nephron deficit. *Pediatr Res 2001;49:660-666.*

EBPG Expert Group on Renal Transplantation. European best practice guidelines for renal transplantation. IV.10 Pregnancy in renal transplant recipients. *Nephrol Dial Transplant 2002;17:50-55.*

Edwards CRW, Benediktsson R, Lindsay RS, Seckl JR. Dysfunction of placental glucocorticoid barrier: link between fetal environment and adult hypertension? *Lancet 1993;341:355-357.*

Fall CHD, Barker DJP, Osmond C, Winter PD, Clark PMS, Hales CN. Relation of infant feeding to adult serum cholesterol concentration and death from ischaemic heart disease. *BMJ 1992;304:801-805.*

Fewtrell MS, Morley R, Abbott RA, Singhal A, Stephenson T, MacFadyen UM, Clements H, Lucas A. Catch-up growth in small-for-gestational-age term infants: a randomized trial. *Am J Clin Nutr 2001;74:516-523.*

Forsen T, Eriksson J, Tuomilehto J, Reunanen A, Osmond C, Barker D. The fetal and childhood growth of persons who develop type 2 diabetes. *Ann Intern Med 2000;133:176-182.*

Fourtounas C, Kopelias I, Kiriaki D, Agroyannis B. Increased cyclosporine blood levels after nisoldipine administration in a renal transplant recipient. *Transpl Int 2002;15:586-588. Epub 2002 Sep 27.*

French AE, Soldin SJ, Soldin OP, Koren G. Milk transfer and neonatal safety of Tacrolimus. *Ann Pharmacother 2003;37:815-818.*

Gaughan WJ, Moritz MJ, Radomski JS, Burke Jr JF, Armenti VT. National transplantation pregnancy registry: report on outcomes in cyclosporine-treated female kidney transplant recipients with an interval from transplant to pregnancy of greater than five years. *Am J Kidney Dis 1996;28:266-269.*

Gilbert T. Vitamin A and kidney development. *Nephrol Dial Transplant 2002;17 Suppl 9:78-80.*

Godfrey K, Robinson S, Barker DJ, Osmond C, Cox V. Maternal nutrition in early and late pregnancy in relation to placental and fetal growth. *BMJ 1996;312:410-414.*

Godfrey KM, Barker DJP. Fetal nutrition and adult disease. *Am J Clin Nutr 2000;71:1344S-1352S.*

Godfrey KM. The role of the placenta in fetal programming-a review. *Placenta 2002;23 Suppl A:S20-S27.*

Gomez-Sanchez EP, Gomez-Sanchez CE. Maternal hypertension and progeny blood pressure: role of aldosterone and 11beta-HSD. *Hypertension 1999;33:1369-1373.*

Guignard JP, Burgener F, Calame A. Persistent anuria in a neonate: a side effect of captopril? *Int J Pediatr Nephrol 1981;2:133.*

Guignard JP, Gouyon JB. Adverse effects of drugs on the immature kidney. *Biol Neonate 1988;53:243-252.*

Guron G, Marcussen N, Nilsson A, Sundelin B, Friberg P. Postnatal time frame for renal vulnerability to enalapril in rats. *J Am Soc Nephrol 1999;10:1550-1560.*

Hanssens M, Keirse MJ, Vankelecom F, Van Assche FA. Fetal and neonatal effects of treatment with angiotensin-converting enzyme inhibitors in pregnancy. *Obstet Gynecol 1991;78:128-135.*

Hartikainen-Sorri AL, Heikkinen JE, Koivisto M. Pharmacokinetics of clonidine during pregnancy and nursing. *Obstet Gynecol 1987;69:598-600.*

Haugen G, Fauchald P, Sodal G, Leivestad T, Moe N. Pregnancy outcome in renal allograft recipients in Norway. The importance of immunosuppressive drug regimen and health status before pregnancy. *Acta Obst Gynecol Scand 1994;73:541-546.*

Holemans K, Aerts L, Van Assche FA. Fetal growth restriction and consequences for the offspring in animal models. J *Soc Gynecol Investig 2003;10:392-399.*

Horwood LJ, Darlow BA, Mogridge N. Breast milk feeding and cognitive ability at 7-8 years. *Arch Dis Child Fetal Neonatal Ed 2001:84:F23-F27.*

Hou S. Pregnancy in chronic renal insufficiency and end-stage renal disease. *Am J Kidney Dis 1999;33:235-252.*

Hou S. Pregnancy in renal transplant recipients. *Adv Ren Replace Ther 2003;10:40-47.*

Hughson M, Farris III AB, Douglas-Denton R, Hoy WE, Bertram JF. Glomerular number and size in autopsy kidneys: the relationship to birth weight. *Kidney Int 2003;63:2113-2122.*

Huxley RR, Shiell AW, Law CM. The role of size at birth and postnatal catch-up growth in determining systolic blood pressure: a systematic review of the literature. *J Hypertens 2000;18:815-831.*

Huynh LA, Min DI. Outcomes of pregnancy and the management of immunosuppressive agents to minimize fetal risks in organ transplant patients. *Ann Pharmacother 1994;28:1355-1357.*

Imani S, Jusko WJ, Steiner R. Diltiazem retards the metabolism of oral prednisone with effects on T-cell markers. *Pediatr Transplant 1999;3:126-130.*

Ingelfinger JR, Woods LL. Perinatal programming, renal development, and adult renal function. *Am J Hypertens 2002;15:46S-49S.*

Jain A, Venkataramanan R, Fung JF, Carlton Gartner J, Lever J, Balan V, Warty V, Starzl TE. Pregnancy after liver transplantation under Tacrolimus. *Transplantation 1997;64:559-565.*

Janssen NM, Genta MS. The effects of immunosuppressive and anti-inflammatory medications on fertility, pregnancy, and lactation. *Arch Intern Med 2000;160:610-619.*

Jones TE, Morris RG. Pharmacokinetic interaction between tacrolimus and diltiazem: dose-response relationship in kidney and liver transplant recipients. *Clin Pharmacokinet 2002;41:381-388.*

Kainz A, Harabacz I, Cowlrick IS, Gadgil SD, Hagiwara D. Review of the course and outcome of 100 pregnancies in 84 women treated with tacrolimus. *Transplantation 2000;70:1718-1721.*

Keller G, Zimmer G, Mall G, Ritz E, Amann K. Nephron number in patients with primary hypertension. *N Engl J Med 2003;348:101-108.*

Khedun SM, Moodley J, Naicker T, Maharaj B. Drug management of hypertensive disorders of pregnancy. *Pharmacol Ther 1997;74:221-258.*

Kistner A, Celsi G, Vanpee M, Jacobson SH. Increased blood pressure but normal renal function in adult women born preterm. *Pediatr Nephrol 2000;15:215-220.*

Klebanoff MA, Secher NJ, Mednick BR, Schulsinger C. Maternal size at birth and the development of hypertension during pregnancy. A test of the Barker hypothesis. *Arch Intern Med 1999;159:1607-1612.*

Kohen-Avramoglu R, Theriault A, Adeli K. Emergence of the metabolic syndrome in childhood: an epidemiological overview and mechanistic link to dyslipidemia. *Clin Biochem 2003;36:413-420.*

Konje JC, Bell SC, Morton JJ, de Chazal R, Taylor DJ. Human fetal kidney morphometry during gestation and the relationship between weight, kidney morphometry and plasma active renin concentration at birth. *Clin Sci (Lond) 1996;91:169-175.*

Koslowska-Boszko B, Korczak G, Wierzbicki P, Lis K, Gaciong Z, Lao M, Sicinska J, Gorski A. Pregnancy following kidney transplantation: risk for offsprings. *Transplant Proc 1997;29:262-265.*

Lackland DT, Bendall HE, Osmond C, Egan BM, Barker DJP. Low birth weights contribute to the high rates of early-onset chronic renal failure in the Southern United States. *Arch Intern Med 2000;160:1472-1476.*

Lackland DT, Egan BM, Ferguson PL. Low birth weight as a risk factor for hypertension. *J Clin Hypertens 2003;5:133-136.*

Lamarque V, Leleu MF, Monka C, Krupp P. Analysis of 629 pregnancy outcomes in transplant recipients treated with Sandimmun. *Transplant Proc 1997;29:2480.*

Langley-Evans SC, Langley-Evans AJ, Marchand MC. Nutritional programming of blood pressure and renal morphology. *Arch Physiol Biochem 2003;111:8-16.*

Langley-Evans SC. Fetal programming of cardiovascular function through exposure to maternal undernutrition. *Proc Nutr Soc 2001;60:505-513.*

Langley-Evans SC. Intrauterine programming of hypertension in the rat: nutrient interactions. *Comp Biochem Physiol A Physiol 1996;114:327-333.*

Law CM, de Swiet M, Osmond C, Fayers PM, Barker DJP, Cruddas AM, Fall CH. Initiation of hypertension *in utero* and its amplification throughout life. *BMJ 1993;306:24-27.*

Law CM, Shiell AW, Newsome CA, Syddall HE, Shinebourne EA, Fayers PM, Martyn CN, de Swiet M. Fetal, infant, and childhood growth and adult blood pressure. A longitudinal study from birth to 22 years of age. *Circulation 2002;105:1088-1092.*

Leeson CP, Kattenhorn M, Deanfield JE, Lucas A. Duration of breast feeding and arterial distensibility in early adult life: population based study. *BMJ 2001;322:643-647.*

Lelièvre-Pégorier M, Merlet-Bénichou C. The number of nephrons in the mammalian kidney: environmental influences play a determining role. *Exp Nephrol 2000;8:63-65.*

Liedholm H, Wahlin-Boll E, Hanson A, Ingemarsson I, Melander A. Transplacental passage and breast milk concentrations of hydralazine. *Eur J Clin Pharmacol 1982;21:417-419.*

Lindheimer MD, Davison JM, Katz AI. The kidney and hypertension in pregnancy: twenty exciting years. *Semin Nephrol 2001;21:173-189.*

Lindsay RS, Lindsay RM, Edwards CR, Seckl JR. Inhibition of 11-beta-hydroxysteroid dehydrogenase in pregnant rats and the programming of blood pressure in the offspring. *Hypertension 1996;27:1200-1204.*

Lo Giudice P, Dubourg L, Hadj-Aïssa A, Saïd M-H, Claris O, Audra P, Martin X, Cochat P. Renal function of children exposed to cyclosporin *in utero*. *Nephrol Dial Transplant 2000;15:1575-1579.*

Lucas SRR, Coimbra TM, Zaladek Gil F. Intrauterine food restriction as a determinant of offspring nephrosclerosis. *Nephrol Dial Transplant 2000;15:A52.*

Mackenzie HS, Lawler EV, Brenner BM. Congenital oligonephropathy: the fetal flaw in essential hypertension? *Kidney Int 1996;49:S30-S34.*

Magee LA, Cham C, Waterman EJ, Ohlsson A, von Dadelszen P. Hydralazine for treatment of severe hypertension in pregnancy: meta-analysis. *BMJ 2003;327:955-960.*

Mañalich R, Reyes L, Herrera M, Melendi C, Fundora I. Relationship between weight at birth and the number and size of renal glomeruli in humans: a histomorphometric study. *Kidney Int 2000;58:770-773.*

Manning J, Beutler K, Knepper MA, Vehaskari VM. Upregulation of renal BSC1 and TSC in prenatally programmed hypertension. *Am J Physiol Renal Physiol 2002;283:F202-F206.*

Martin JA, Hamilton BE, Sutton PD, Ventura SJ, Menacker F, Munson ML. Births: final data for 2002. *Natl Vital Stat Rep 2003;52:1-113.*

Martinovic J, Benachi A, Laurent N, Daikha-Dahmane F, Gubler MC. Fetal toxic effects and angiotensin-II-receptor antagonists. *Lancet 2001;358:241-242.*

Martins JPC, Monteiro JC, Paixao ADO. Renal function in adult rats subjected to prenatal dexamethasone. *Clin Exp Pharmacol Physiol 2003;30:32-37.*

McCrabb GJ, Egan AR, Hosking BJ. Maternal undernutrition during mid-pregnancy in sheep. Placental size and its relationship to calcium transfer during late pregnancy. *Br J Nut 1991;65:157-168.*

McTernan CL, Draper N, Nicholson H, Chalder SM, Driver P, Hewison M, Kilby MD, Stewart PM. Reduced placental 11beta-hydroxysteroid dehydrogenase type 2 mRNA levels in human pregnancies complicated by intrauterine growth restriction: an analysis of possible mechanisms. *J Clin Endocrinol Metab 2001;86:4979-4983.*

Merlet-Bénichou C, Gilbert T, Muffat-Joly M, Lelièvre-Pégorier M, Leroy B. Intrauterine growth retardation leads to a permanent nephron deficit in the rat. *Pediatr Nephrol 1994;8:175-180.*

Merlet-Bénichou C, Gilbert T, Vilar J, Moreau E, Freund N, Lelièvre-Pégorier M. Nephron number: variability is the rule. Causes and consequences. *Lab Invest 1999;79:515-527.*

Meyberg R, Boos R, Babajan A, Ertan AK, Schmidt W. Intrauterine growth retardation-perinatal mortality and postnatal morbidity in a perinatal center. *Z Geburtshilfe Neonatol 2000;204:218-23.*

Midtvedt K, Hartmann A, Brekke IB, Lyngdal PT, Nentdal Ø, Haugen G. Successful pregnancies in a combined pancreas and renal allograft recipient and in a renal graft recipient on tacrolimus treatment. *Nephrol Dial Transplant 1997;12:2764-2765.*

Mimran A, Mourad G, Ribstein J, Halimi J-M. Cyclosporine-associated hypertension. *In: Laragh JH, Brenner BM, eds. Hypertension: Pathophysiology, Diagnosis and Management. Second Edition. Raven Press, Ltd., New York, 1995:2459-2469.*

Moore VM, Cockington RA, Ryan P, Robinson JS. The relationship between birth weight and blood pressure amplifies from childhood to adulthood. *J Hypertens 1999;17:883-888.*

Moritz KM, Dodic M, Wintour EM. Kidney development and the fetal programming of adult disease. *BioEssays 2003;25:212-220.*

Mott GE, Lewis DS, Jackson EM, McMahan CA. Preweaning diet programs postweaning plasma thyroxine concentrations in baboons. *Proc Soc Exp Biol Med. 1996;212:342-348.*

Nguyen C, Duhl AJ, Escallon CS, Blakemore KJ. Multiple anomalies in a fetus exposed to low-dose methotrexate in the first trimester. *Obstet Gynecol 2002;99:599-602.*

Norgard B, Pedersen L, Fonager K, Rasmussen SN, Sorensen HT. Azathioprine, mercaptopurine and birth outcome: a population-based cohort study. *Aliment Pharmacol Ther 2003;17:827-834.*

Nyberg G, Haljamäe U, Frisenette-Fich C, Wennergren M, Kjellmer I. Breast-feeding during treatment with cyclosporine. *Transplantation 1998;65:253-255.*

Ocran KW, Plauth M, Mai I, Lochs H. Tacrolimus toxicity due to drug interaction with mibefradil in a patient after liver transplantation. *Z Gastroenterol. 1999;37:1025-1028.*

Ots M, Troy JL, Rennke HG, Mackenzie HS, Brenner BM. Impact of the supplementation of kidney mass on blood pressure and progression of kidney disease. *Nephrol Dial Transplant 2004;19:337-341.*

Pabelick C, Kemmer F, Koletzko B. Befunde bei Neugeborenen nierentransplantierter Mütter. *Monatsschr Kinderheilkd 1991;139:136-140.*

Papatsonis DN, Lok CA, Bos JM, Geijn HP, Dekker GA. Calcium channel blockers in the management of preterm labor and hypertension in pregnancy. *Eur J Obstet Gynecol Reprod Biol. 2001;97:122-140.*

Paruk F, Moodley J. Maternal and neonatal outcome in early- and late-onset pre-eclampsia. *Semin Neonatol 2000;5:197-207.*

Phillips DI, Barker DJ, Fall CH, Seckl JR, Whorwood CB, Wood PJ, Walker BR. Elevated plasma cortisol concentrations: a link between low birth weight and the insulin resistance syndrome? *J Clin Endocrinol Metab 1998;83:757-760.*

Phillips DI, Walker BR, Reynolds RM, Flanagan DE, Wood PJ, Osmond C, Barker DJ, Whorwood CB. Low birth weight predicts elevated plasma cortisol concentrations in adults from 3 populations. *Hypertension 2000;35:1301-1306.*

Phillips DIW. Fetal growth and programming of the hypothalamic-pituitary-adrenal axis. *Clin Exp Pharmacol Physiol 2001;28:967-970.*

Picaud JC, Audra P, Putet G, Belle L, Salle BL. Nouveau-nés de mères transplantées rénales. *Arch Pediatr 1991;48:323-327.*

Piétrement C, Malot L, Santerne B, Roussel B, Motte J, Morville P. Neonatal acute renal failure secondary to maternal exposure to telmisartan, angiotensin II receptor antagonist. *J Perinatol 2003;23:254-255.*

Pilarski LM, Yacyshyn BR, Lazarovits AI. Analysis of peripheral blood lymphocyte populations and immune function from children exposed to cyclosporine or to azathioprine *in utero. Transplantation 1994;57:133-144.*

Prévot A, Martini S, Guignard JP. *In utero* exposure to immunosuppressive drugs. *Biol Neonate 2002(a);81:73-81.*

Prévot A, Mosig D, Guignard JP. The effects of Losartan on renal function in the newborn rabbit. *Pediatr Res 2002(b);51:728-732.*

Prévot A, Semama DS, Justrabo E, Guignard JP, Escousse A, Gouyon JB. Acute cyclosporine A-induced nephrotoxicity: a rabbit model. *Pediatr Nephrol 2000;14:370-375.*

Quinkler M, Stewart PM. Hypertension and the cortisol-cortisone shuttle. *J Clin Endocrinol Metab 2003;88:2384-2392.*

Radomski JS, Ahlswede BA, Jarrell BE, Mannion J, Cater J, Moritz MJ, Armenti VT. Outcomes of 500 pregnancies in 335 female kidney, liver, and heart transplant recipients. *Transplant Proc 1995;27:1089-1090.*

Ramsey-Goldman R, Schilling E. Immunosuppressive drug use during pregnancy. *Rheum Dis Clin North Am 1997;23:149-167.*

Regazzoni BM, Genton N, Pelet J, Drukker A, Guignard J-P. Long-term followup of renal functional reserve capacity after unilateral nephrectomy in childhood. *J Urol 1998;160:844-848.*

Reik W, Walter J. Genomic imprinting: parental influence on the genome. *Nat Rev Genet 2001;2:21-32.*

Relier JP, Bonnet H, Deiber M. Retard de croissance intra-utérin. *In: Relier JP, Laugier J, Salle BL (eds). Médecine Périnatale, Médecine-Sciences Flammarion, 1989, pp 75-82.*

Rezzani R, Rodella L, Bianchi R. Cyclosporine and pregnancy in the rat. *Transplantation 1997;63:164-167.*

Rieu P, Neyrat N, Hiesse C, Charpentier B. Thirty-three pregnancies in a population of 1725 renal transplant patients. *Transplant Proc 1997;29:2459-2460.*

Roberts JM, Pearson G, Cutler J, Lindheimer M. Summary of the NHLBI working group on research on hypertension during pregnancy. *Hypertension 2003;41:437-445.*

Roberts SB. Prevention of hypertension in adulthood by breastfeeding? *Lancet 2001;357:406-407.*

Robinson SM, Barker DJP. Coronary heart disease: a disorder of growth. *Proc Nutr Soc 2002;61:537-542.*

Rose G. Sick individuals and sick populations. *Int J Epidemiol 1985;14:32-38.*

Rostand SG. Oligonephronia, primary hypertension and renal disease: "is the child father to the man?" *Nephrol Dial Transplant 2003;18:1434-1438.*

Sahajpal V, Ashton N. Renal function and angiotensin AT1 receptor expression in young rats following intrauterine exposure to a maternal low-protein diet. *Clin Sci (Lond) 2003;104:607-614.*

Saïd MH, Abokasem A, Hadj-Aïssa A, Claris O, Audra P, Cochat P. Renal function of children born to transplanted women under cyclosporine A. *Pediatr Nephrol 1996;10:C153.*

Saji H, Yamanaka M, Hagiwara A, Ijiri R. Losartan and fetal toxic effects. *Lancet 2001;357:363.*

Salle B, Claris O. Le Prématuré. *In: Relier JP, Laugier J, Salle BL (eds). Médecine Périnatale, Médecine-Sciences Flammarion, 1989, pp 59-73.*

Shaheen FA, al-Sulaiman MH, al-Khader AA. Long-term nephrotoxicity after exposure to cyclosporine *in utero. Transplantation 1993;56:224 225.*

Sharkey LC, McCune SA, Yuan O, Lange C, Fray J. Spontaneous pregnancy-induced hypertension and intrauterine growth restriction in rats. *Am J Hypertens 2001;14:1058-1066.*

Sherman RC, Langley-Evans SC. Early administration of angiotensin-converting enzyme inhibitor captopril, prevents the development of hypertension programmed by intrauterine exposure to a maternal low-protein diet in the rat. *Clin Sci (Lond) 1998;94:373-381.*

Sibai BM. Diagnosis and management of gestational hypertension and preeclampsia. *Obstet Gynecol 2003;102:181-192.*

Silver LE, Decamps PJ, Korst LM, Platt LD, Castro LC. Intrauterine growth restriction is accompanied by decreased renal volume in the human fetus. *Am J Obstet Gynecol 2003;188:1320-1325.*

Singhal A, Cole TJ, Lucas A. Early nutrition in preterm infants and later blood pressure: two cohorts after randomised trials. *Lancet 2001;357:413-419.*

Tendron A, Decramer S, Justrabo E, Gouyon JB, Semama DS, Gilbert T. Cyclosporin A administration during pregnancy induces a permanent nephron deficit in young rabbits. *J Am Soc Nephrol 2003;14:3188-3196.*

Tendron A, Prévot A, Justrabo E, Merlet-Bénichou C, Gouyon J-B, Semama DS, Gilbert T. *In utero* cyclosporine A (CsA) exposure and renal organogenesis in the rabbit. *Schweiz Med Wochenschr 2000; 130 Suppl. 124:10S.*

Thame M, Wilks RJ, McFarlane-Anderson N, Bennett FI, Forrester TE. Relationship between maternal nutritional status and infant's weight and body proportions at birth. *Eur J Clin Nutr 1997; 51: 134-138.*

Thibault C, Levasseur MC. *In: La reproduction chez les Mammifères et l'Homme. INRA-Ellipse, Paris, 1991:378-421.*

Thiru Y, Bateman DN, Coulthard MG. Successful breast feeding while mother was taking cyclosporin. *Br Med J 1997;315:463.*

Tufro-McReddie A, Romano LM, Harris JM, Ferder L, Gomez RA. Angiotensin II regulates nephrogenesis and renal vascular development. *Am J Physiol 1995;269:F110-F115.*

Vickers MH, Breier BH, Cutfield WS, Hofman PL, Gluckman PD. Fetal origins of hyperphagia, obesity, and hypertension and postnatal amplification by hypercaloric nutrition. *Am J Physiol Endocrinol Metab 2000;279:E83-E87.*

Vickers MH, Ikenasio BA, Breier BH. Adult growth hormone treatment reduces hypertension and obesity induced by an adverse prenatal environment. *J Endocrinol 2002;175:615-623.*

Vickers MH, Ikenasio BA, Breier BH. IGF-1 treatment reduces hyperphagia, obesity, and hypertension in metabolic disorders induced by fetal programming. *Endocrinology 2001;142:3964-3973.*

Villar J, Belizan JM. The relative contribution of prematurity and fetal growth retardation to low birth-weight in developing and developed societies. *Am J Obstet Gynecol 1982;143:793-798.*

Vyas S, Kumar A, Piecuch S, Hidalgo G, Singh A, Anderson V, Markell MS, Baqi N. Outcome of twin pregnancy in a renal transplant recipient treated with Tacrolimus. *Transplantation 1999;67:490-492.*

Walker JJ. Pre-eclampsia. *Lancet 2000;356:1260-1265.*

Widdowson EM, McCance RA. A review: new thoughts on growth. *Pediatr Res 1975;9:154-156.*

Widdowson EM, McCance RA. The determinants of growth and form. *Proc R Soc Lond 1974;185:1-17.*

Woods LL, Rasch R. Perinatal Ang II programs adult blood pressure, glomerular number, and renal function in rats. *Am J Physiol 1998;275:R1593-R1599.*

Woods LL. Fetal origins of adult hypertension: a renal mechanism? *Curr Opin Nephrol Hypertens 2000;9:419-425.*

Wyeth Pharmaceuticals. *Rapamune: current prescribing information.*

Young LE. Imprinting of genes and the Barker hypothesis. *Twin Res 2001;4:307-317.*

In: Hypertension: New Research
Editor: Elwood F. Benhagen, pp. 239-262
ISBN: 1-59454-204-X

Chapter IX

MECHANISMS OF STATIN NEPHROPROTECTIVE ACTIONS

Michal Chmielewski* and Boleslaw Rutkowski
Department of Nephrology, Transplantology and Internal Medicine;
Medical University of Gdansk, Poland

ABSTRACT

Cardiac related morbidity and mortality is as much as 20 times higher in patients suffering from chronic renal failure (CRF), when compared to general population. It is mainly due to exacerbation of atherosclerotic processes in this group of patients. Lipid disturbances play a major role in atherosclerosis development. They also compose a constant feature of CRF. Therefore, they are considered as prime risk factors for cardio-vascular related complications in CRF patients, especially in those with hypertension or diabetes mellitus as their primary disease. HMG-CoA reductase inhibitors (statins) are the most potent drugs lowering plasma cholesterol level. They are also capable of decreasing triglycerides concentration. Numerous trials have shown the effectiveness of statins in slowing down the progression of atherosclerosis and in decreasing number of cardio-vascular incidents. However, the beneficial effects of statins go beyond the simple ability to normalize cholesterol level. Results of many recent studies point to the existence of other, cholesterol – independent mechanisms of statins' actions. These, so called pleiotropic effects include: anti-proliferative, anti-inflammatory and anti-thrombotic actvities. It is of special importance in CRF population, since cell proliferation, inflammatory processes and coagulation disturbances contribute significantly to CRF pathogenesis. Statins, therefore seem not only to decrease cardiac related complications in CRF patients, but also to have the abilities to slow down the progression of CRF itself. This chapter aims at presenting studies on pleiotropic activities of statins, with special emphasis on their nephroprotective role.

* Address for correspondence: Michal Chmielewski; Dept of Nephrology, Transplantology and Internal Medicine; Medical University of Gdansk; Ul. Debinki 7; 80-211 Gdansk; Poland. Tel +48 58 3492558; Fax +48 58 3461186; e-mail: chmiel@amg.gda.pl

Introduction

Hypertensive nephrosclerosis (HN) is one of the major causes of end-stage renal disease (ESRD) [1]. Relative risk of developing ESRD is increased over 20 times in severely hypertensive patients, when compared to general population [2]. In United States HN is responsible for 25% of ESRD cases, with only diabetic nephropathy being more common [3]. According to third National Health and Nutrition Examination Survey (NHANES III) an estimated 3.0% (5.6 million) of the civilian US population has elevated serum creatinine levels, 70% of whom are hypertensive [4]. Patients suffering from ESRD are at increased risk of cardiovascular and cerebrovascular complications. Cardiovascular mortality rate is approximately 20 times higher, and cerebrovascular incidents are nearly 10 times more frequent than in the general population [5]. Given these numbers it seems self-evident that suitable treatment of ESRD patients is a major challenge for physicians.

Lipid Disturbances in Renal Diseases

Vascular complications leading to increased morbidity and mortality during ESRD are mainly due to exacerbation of atherosclerotic processes in this group of patients [6]. The primary risk factor for the development of atheroslerosis is dyslipidemia. Lipid disturbances compose a constant feature of ESRD. They consist of both quantitative and qualitative abnormalities in serum lipoproteins. The major change in lipid profile during chronic renal failure (CRF) is hypertriglyceridemia, affecting up to 70% of patients [6]. It is mainly a consequence of impaired plasma triglyceride (TG) removal, but TG overproduction is also present [7]. Hypercholesterolemia is less evident, as it is observed in 20-30% of CRF patients. It results mainly from increased cholesterol biosynythesis [8, 9]. Probably more important than changes in lipid concentrations are disturbances affecting major lipoprotein subclasses. Accumulation of apo-B-containing TG-rich particles, including very low density lipoproteins (VLDL) and intermediate density lipoproteins (IDL) is the main feature of ESRD [10]. Though low density lipoprotein (LDL) cholesterol is usually within normal ranges, LDL particles tend to be smaller, more dense and, therefore more atherogenic in ESRD patients. Furthermore, they are subjected to enhanced oxidative modifications. Vitamin C and E deficiencies, reduced activity of the glutathione system, chronic inflammatory state, bioincompatibility of dialysis membranes and solutions are the major factors leading to increased oxidative stress in ESRD [11]. Expression of scavenger receptors, responsible for oxidized LDL removal is also enhanced in the course of ESRD [12, 13]. This leads to increased foam cell formation and atherosclerotic plaque development. Dialysis, having an ameliorating influence on uremia, doesn't have such an effect on the lipid profile. Lipid abnormalities in hemodialysed patients consist mainly of increased plasma TG level and reduced plasma high density lipoprotein (HDL) cholesterol [14, 15]. Impaired lipid metabolism is also common in patients on peritoneal dialysis. It is, to some extent a consequence of increased absorption of glucose from the dialysate [14]. But it is after renal transplantation when most severe changes in lipid metabolism occur. Cholesterol level begins to rise immediately after transplantation reaching the maximum after 2-3 months from the operation [16, 17]. Cholesterol concentration is increased in all the lipoprotein fractions. In the course of further treatment the level of total cholesterol decreases, still, after six months from the transplantation it exceeds 200 mg/dl in 80% of patients [18]. It is now well acknowledged that the mentioned above complications are caused by the immunosuppresive treatment [19-21].

Lipid disturbances in the course of ESRD are responsible for the increase in cardiovascular and cerebrovascular complications. However, they also lead to the progression of the disease itself. It has been shown by several authors that elevated level of plasma cholesterol is related to accelerated progression of renal insufficiency [22-24]. Hyperlipidemia is also considered a risk factor for chronic rejection after kidney transplantation [17, 25, 26]. Lipids, being indispensable for body homeostasis, when in excess, become nephrotoxic. LDL, as well as TG-rich lipoproteins (VLDL and IDL) promote proliferation of mesangial cells *in vitro* [27]. According to *Kamanna et al.* [28] lipoproteins, especially oxidized LDL stimulate mesangial cell membrane tyrosine receptor phosphorylation, and subsequently MAP kinase signaling cascade leading to cell proliferation. They further enhance glomerular inflammation processes by stimulating monocyte adhesion to the glomerular endothelium, most probably by increasing the expression of principal factors involved in monocyte recruitment: intercellular adhesion molecule-1 (ICAM-1), monocyte chemoattractant protein-1 (MCP-1) and macrophage-colony stimulating factor (M-CSF) [29-31]. The addition of lipoproteins to cultured human mesangial cells enhance the secretion of several cytokines involved in inflammation processes: interleukin-6 (Il-6), platelet-derived growth factor (PDGF), or transforming growth factor-β (TGF-β) [27]. LDL may further promote glomerulosclerosis through the stimulation of mesangial matrix synthesis, as was shown by *Rovin et al.* [31]. It is also well known that lipids augment vascular tension by increasing thromboxane A2 and endothelin synthesis, as well as by decreasing the concentration of L-arginine, precursor of nitric oxide (NO) [32-34]. Finally, some forms of glomerular injury, named lipoprotein glomerulopaties are caused by intraglomerular lipoprotein thrombi [35, 36]. Presented data undrelines, how important it is to treat lipid disturbances in ESRD patients.

Experimental data, as well as histopathological findings in humans demonstrate that atherosclerotic changes in the vessel wall and progressive glomerular lesions possess numerous similar features, suggesting analogous pathobiologic mechanisms [37]. The mechanism of atherosclerotic plaque formation begins with the migration of LDL from plasma into subendothelial space, where LDL are subjected to oxidative modifications [38]. They become unrecognizable to LDL-receptors. Instead, they are removed, mainly by macrophages, through scavenger receptors. In contrast to LDL-receptors, scavenger receptor expression is not inhibited by increased intracellular cholesterol concentration. Therefore, scavenger receptors acquire more and more oxidized LDL particles leading to the formation of cholesterol-engorged foam cells. After the foam cell dies lipid droplets are released, contributing to the development of atherosclerotic lesion's necrotic core [38]. Treatment that would be capable of inhibiting these processes, would also be expected to slow down the progression of both, atherosclerosis and renal insufficiency.

Statins – General Information

3-hydroxy-3-methylglutaryl-CoA reductase inhibitors (statins) are currently the most potent drugs lowering plasma cholesterol concentration. They inhibit endogenous cholesterol synthesis on the level of 3-hydroxy-3-methylglutaryl CoA (HMG-CoA) reductase. Statins bind to this enzyme at nanomolar concentrations, whereas the natural substrate, HMG-CoA binds at micromolar concentrations [39]. This leads to competitive displacement of HMG-CoA and inhibition of the synthesis of cholesterol precursor, mevalonate. Active cholesterol synthesis is a requirement for VLDL assembly and secretion [40]. As VLDL are precursors of IDL and LDL, statins, by inhibiting cholesterol synthesis decrease the concentrations of all these lipoproteins. Further, reduction of intracellular cholesterol concentration by statins leads to activation of compensating mechanisms to assure intracellular lipid homeostasis. Namely, it activates membrane-bound transcription factors called sterol regulatory element binding proteins (SREBPs) that regulate multiple genes involved in cholesterol homeostasis [41]. SREBPs directly stimulate the expression of more than 30 genes dedicated to the synthesis and uptake of cholesterol, fatty acids and TG, among them the LDL-receptor gene. This leads to an increase in the number of LDL-receptors and intensification of LDL clearance from the plasma, providing yet another mechanism, by which statins decrease plasma cholesterol concentration [40]. Lipid lowering properties of statins do not restrict themselves solely to cholesterol. More potent drugs, e.g. atorvastatin or rosuvastatin have been shown to decreaseTG levels by 20-30% [42, 43].

The first drug of the group that became known as "statins" was mevastatin, isolated by *Endo et al.* [44] in 1976 from a fungus, *Penicilium citrinum.* It was withdrawn short after introduction due to its side-effects, but it served as a model for the isolation of other HMG-CoA reductase inhibitors. The first statin to be registered in the US was lovastatin (mevinolin). It was isolated by *Alberts et al.* [45] from another fungus, *Aspergillus tereus.*

All of the currently available statins have a part similar to HMG-CoA, the natural substrate of HMG-CoA reductase. The rest of the molecule varies considerably among particular drugs, determining their pharmacokinetic and pharmacodynamic properties.

Beneficial effects of statins on decreasing the risk of coronary complications and prolonging survival have been documented in many large trials, with thousands of patients participating [46-49]. Statins appear also to have a positive impact on the prevention of other vascular complications, e.g. strokes [50]. Similar results have been obtained in patients with kidney diseases, both in persons with mild chronic renal insufficiency, as well as in ESRD patients [51, 52]. The study on the impact of statins on mortality in ESRD showed that patients treated with statins had a mortality rate of 143/1000 person-years, compared with a rate of 202/1000 person-years for patients not using HMG-CoA reducase inhibitors. Statin use was independently associated with a reduced risk of total mortality as well as cardiovascular-specific mortality [52].

Potential usefulness of statins in treating kidney diseases has been investigated by several authors. *Kasiske et al.* [53] introduced lovastatin in rats with experimental CRF. After 10 weeks of therapy urine albumin excretion was significantly reduced, as compared to the control group. Moreover, the percent of glomeruli with focal glomerulosclerosis was three times smaller in the group treated with the statin. In an experiment by *O'Donnell et al.* [54], after 22 weeks of treating rats with experimental CRF with lovastatin the animals had a 76%

reduction in urine albumin excretion and one-sixth the incidence of focal glomerusclerosis, compared with vehicle-treated control rats. Other experiments dealing with the use of lovastatin in rats with experimental CRF showed decrease in blood urea concentration, mesangial cell proliferation, and in glomeruli sclerosis [55, 56]. Clinical observations provided similarly promising results. *Shoji et al.* [57] used pravastatin in patients with microalbuminuria in the course of diabetic nephropathy. After three months of such treatment they observed decrease in albumin excretion in all patients. In the work by *Rabelink et al.* [58] partial remission of nephrotic syndrome was achieved in all patients after 48 weeks of treatment with simvastatin. These observations, though not related to patients with HN are important, since proteinuria is the predominant clinical sign of HN. However, patient groups were small in these studies.

There is also some clinical evidence that statins may slow down the progression of renal insufficiency [59]. These observations gain more importance in the light of the hypothesis that mechanisms leading to glomerulosclerosis are very similar to those responsible for the development of atherosclerosis [37]. It is particularly true in case of HN, which is often called "hypertensive nephroagiosclerosis" [60].

Pleiotropic Abilities

Knowing that lipoprotein disturbances lead to atherosclerosis, and given the information that they can also have an injurious impact on kidneys, it would seem self-evident, that the mentioned above beneficial effects of statins are related solely to their lipid lowering properties. However, analysis of large clinical trials shows that the advantages of statin use are not associated with the degree of cholesterol reduction [46-49]. In fact, they exceed it by far. Furthermore, a growing number of experimental studies indicates that many actions of HMG-CoA reductase inhibitors are independent from cholesterol lowering. For instance, *Hidaka et al* [61] observed inhibition of the migration of cultured porcine smooth muscle cells stimulated with PDGF by simvastatin. This effect was reversed by the addition of mevalonate to the culture. However, supplementation with LDL was unable to reverse the effect of statin. In another work vascular smooth muscle cell proliferation was inhibited by lovastatin [62]. Addition of mevalonate completely reversed this effect, whereas supplementation with cholesterol had no impact on lovastatin induced action. Similar results were obtained in rat mesangial cells, where exogenous LDL did not prevent lovastatin inhibition of cell proliferation [63]. These investigations, as well as many others, show clearly that some effects of statin use are not related to cholesterol lowering.

It is known, however, that by inhibiting HMG-CoA reductase activity statins influence the biosynthesis of more compounds than merely cholesterol.

Statins and Protein Prenylation

Mevalonate is the direct product of HMG-CoA reductase activity. Not all mevalonate molecules, however, participate in cholesterol formation. Some of them join together to form 15-carbon, and 20-carbon compounds - isoprenoids, named farnesyl pyrophosphate (FPP), and geranylgeranyl pyrophosphate (GGPP), respectively. These two compounds play a major role in a process called protein prenylation [64] (Figure 1). It consists in posttranslational modification of certain proteins by isoprenoids leading to protein activation. Both FPP and GGPP have the ability of covalent addition to cysteine residues at the carboxy-terminus of the proteins. The process is mediated by two enzymes, farnesyl transferase and geranylgeranyl transferase. The enzymes recognize a specific sequence at the carboxy-terminus, named CAAX motif, where C means cysteine, A an aliphatic amino acid, and X stands for the carboxy-terminal amino acid, which determines which isoprenoid is to be added. In situations where X is methionine or serine, preferential protein prenylation occurs via farnesyl transferase, and where X is leucine, GGPP addition occurs. The enzymes catalyze the attachment of isoprenoid to the cysteine residue of the CAAX motif, and the –AAX moiety is removed. It is now known that prenylation is not confined to proteins containing the CAAX motif. Still, in such cases isoprenoids are also attached to cysteine residue at, or very near the carboxy-terminus of the protein [64]. Prenylated protein is translocated to the inner cell membrane or plasma membrane, where isoprenoid serves as an "anchor" to fix the protein on the membrane's surface, thereby activating it (Figure 2).

About 0.5% of the proteins in animal cells are activated through prenylation [65]. The process of prenylation has been most thoroughly investigated on Ras proteins. The Ras superfamily of proteins plays a major role in cell differentiation, proliferation and fibrogenesis [66]. Of particular interest to researchers in the past few years has been p21ras. This protein plays a crucial part in transmitting signals from growth factors and cytokines to the cell nucleus through tyrosine kinase receptor [67]. Numerous growth factors, including PDGF, epidermal growth factor (EGF), insulin-like growth factor-1, and fibroblast growth factor influence cell proliferation through tyrosine kinase cascade. Binding of growth factor to the tyrosine kinase receptor causes receptor autophosphorylation, which leads to activation of a number of proteins that transmit the signal to cell nucleus, enabling specific genes expression, cell growth and proliferation. One of these transmitting proteins is p21ras. It can, however, be activated only when attached with the isoprenoid to inner cell membrane [67] (Figure 3). Therapeutic strategies that aim at prenylation inhibition reduce p21ras activation. This in turn can have a crucial impact on inhibiting cell growth and proliferation. Increased cell proliferation is characteristic predominantly for primary glomerulonephritis, but occurs in HN as well. Myointimal hypertrophy, caused by proliferation of vascular smooth muscle cells is one of the most important pathological features of HN [60]. Fibroblast proliferation is also common. In a study by Vrtovsnik et al. [68] lovastatin inhibited DNA synthesis and proliferation of renal proximal tubular epithelial cells in a concentration-dependent manner. Medium supplementation of LDL-cholesterol did not modify lovastatin-induced inhibition of DNA synthesis. In contrast, both FPP and GGPP significantly reduced the antiproliferative effect of the statin. Further, immunoblot analysis revealed that lovastatin decreased the amount of membrane-bound p21ras in cells stimulated with fetal calf serum. Again, this action was prevented by the addition of mevalonate, as well as isoprenoids. These results confirm that the antiproliferative activity of statins is related, at least in part, to inhibition of p21ras prenylation.

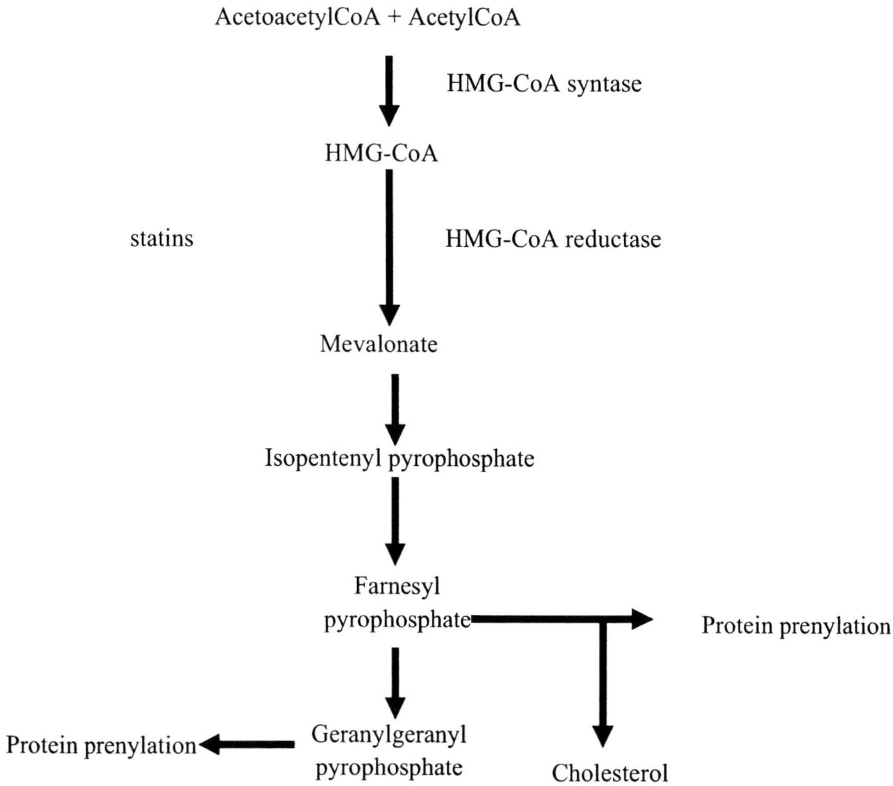

Figure 1. Biosynthesis of farnesyl pyrophosphate (FPP), and geranylogeranyl pyrophosphate (GGPP); (HMG-CoA - 3-hydroxy-methyloglutaryl-coenzymeA)

Ras, however, is not the only prenylated protein involved in cell proliferation. It is known that the progression from phase G1 to phase S of the cell-cycle is dependent on the activity of protein kinases, known as cyclin-dependent kinases (CDK) [69]. One of the major CDK inhibitors is p27kip1 protein. By decreasing CDK activity it inhibits cell-cycle progression. It has been shown that lovastatin increases the concentration of p27kip1 in mesangial cells, but without altering the level of protein's mRNA [70]. It seems, therefore that lovastatin decreases p27kip1 degradation. Indeed, in a set of experiments on rat FRTL-5 cells the half-life of p27kip1 in pravastatin-treated cells was nearly three times as long as its half-life in non-treated ones [71]. Elimination of p27kip1 is facilitated by a class of geranylgeranylated small GTP-binding proteins, termed Rho small GTPases [71]. GGPP promotes the translocation of Rho from the cytoplasm to cell membranes, enabling its activation. By decreasing GGPP formation statins inhibit Rho prenylation, block the elimination of p27kip1, CDK activation and cell-cycle progression (Figure 4). Indeed, it has been demonstrated that pravastatin inhibits the G1 to S phase transition of human mesangial cells stimulated with fetal calf serum [72]. This inhibitory effect of pravastatin was reversed by GGPP. These results indicate that statins act as antiproliferative agents through the inhibition of isoprenoid formation.

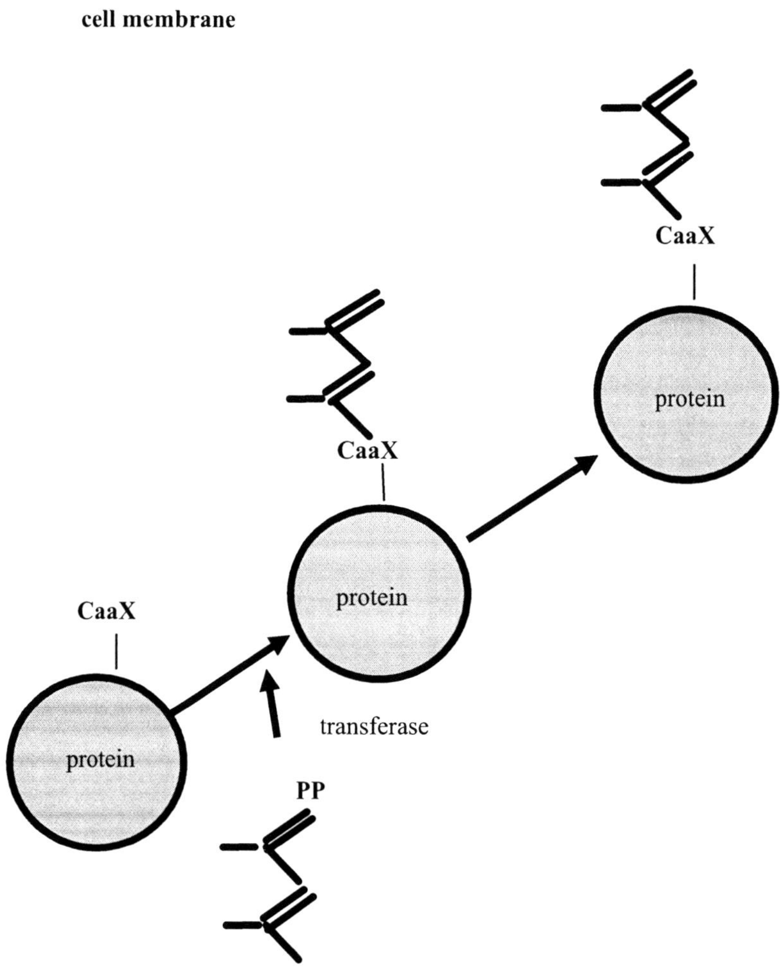

Figure 2. Prenylation of proteins (association of isoprenoid to the cystein residue of the CaaX sequence enables transport of the protein onto the cellular membrane, and, thus, its activation.

Rho has also been found to play an important role in apoptosis [73]. Namely, in an activated state Rho prevents this process. In a study by Guijarro et al. [74] treatment with lipophilic statins enhanced apoptosis of human and rat vascular smooth muscle cells in culture. Addition of isoprenoids, FPP and GGPP fully reversed the pro-apoptotic effects of statins. Further, exposure of rat vascular smooth muscle cells to statins was associated with attenuation of the presence of Rho in the cell membranes. The degree of inhibition of Rho prenylation by different statins closely paralleled their pro-apoptotic effect. In another study, treatment of cultured human peripheral blood monocytes with mevastatin was associated with massisve apoptosis of the cells [75]. It seems, therefore that induction of cell apoptosis, possibly through inhibition of Rho prenylation is yet another mechanism of the antiproliferative action of statins.

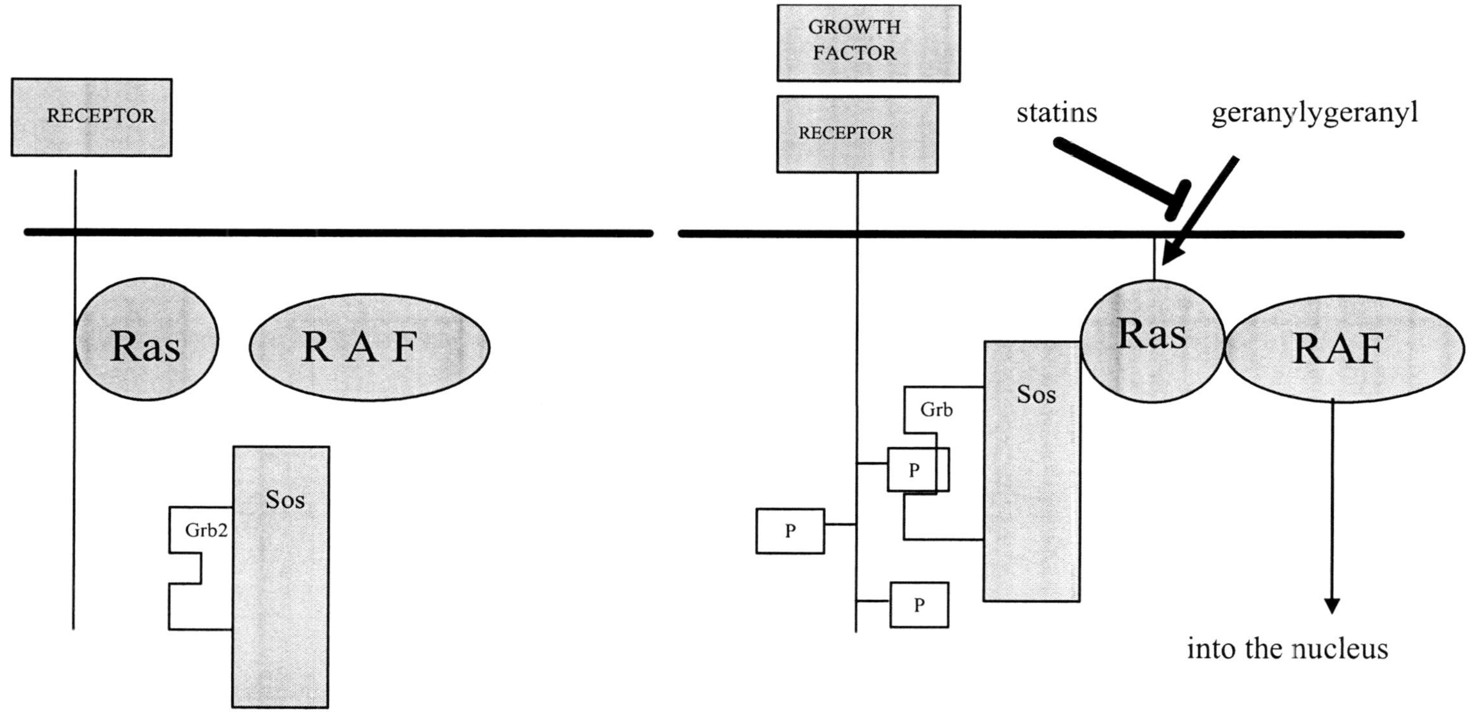

Figure 3. Tyrosine kinase cascade (association of the growth factor to the extracellular domain of the receptor causes autofosforylation of the intracellular domain. That enables the binding of the Grb2-Sos complex, followed by activation of Ras, RAF, and a cascade of kinases, with the Erk 1, and Erk 2 kinases, that transmit the signal to the nucleus, thus influecing gene expresion, and cellular proliferation. This action is prevented by statins. By inhibiting geranylogeranylation of Ras protein they block the signal transmition).

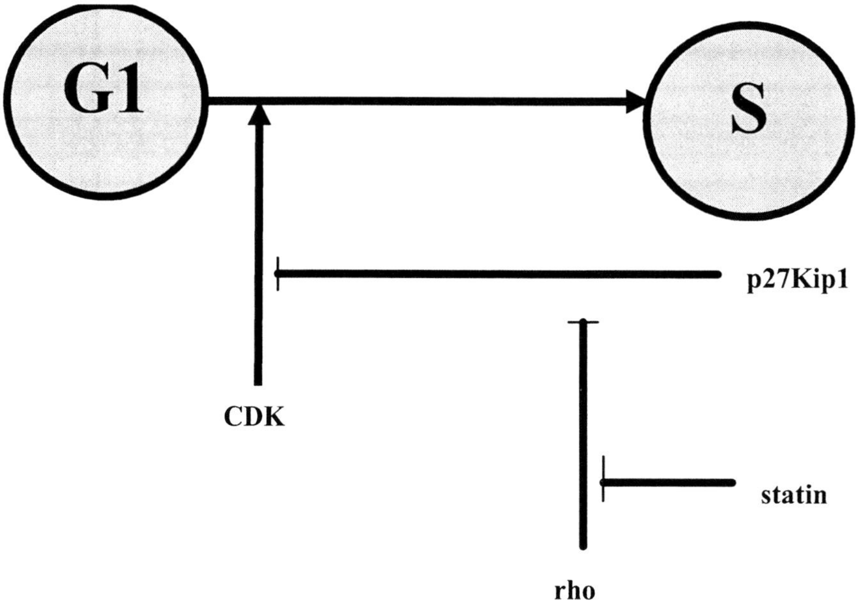

Figure 4. The role of rho protein in progression of the cell cycle (the progression from G1 to S phase of cell cycle is stimulated by cAMP dependant kinases [CDK]; their activity is inhibited by p27Kip1 protein; rho takes part in elimination of p27Kip1, thus enabling activation of CDK, and cell cycle progression).

Anti-Inflammatory Activities of Statins

Cell proliferation is a part of a general inflammatory process which affects kidneys in response to injurious factors, such as arterial hypertension. This process, apart from cellular proliferation includes: release of several adhesion molecules, chemokines, pro-inflammatory cytokines, activation of inflammatory enzymes, oxidative stress, alterations in nitric oxide (NO) synthesis, coagulation disturbances etc. One of the markers of ongoing inflammation is increased plasma concentration of C-reactive protein (CRP). It has also been demonstrated that levels of CRP are associated with increased risk of myocardial infarction and stroke among apparently healthy individuals [76]. The impact of pravastatin on CRP level was evaluated in a group of patients taking part in Cholesterol and Recurrent Events (CARE) trial [76]. After five years patients on pravastatin treatment had median CRP levels 21.6% lower than those on placebo (p=0.007). This effect was, at least to some extent, independent from cholesterol lowering, as the magnitude of CRP reduction associated with pravastatin use did not correlate with the magnitude of LDL reduction. In an interesting study by *Sirken et al.* [77] statin therapy was demonstrated to decrease erythropoietin (EPO) requirements in hemodialysis patients. Increased levels of CRP have been associated with relative erythropoietin resistance in dialysis patients. Therefore the authors suggest that the improvement in EPO responsiveness may be caused by the effect of statins on CRP. These observations raise the possibility that HMG-CoA reductase inhibitors may have clinically important anti-inflammatory actions.

Nuclear factor κB (NF κB) is a family of dimeric proteins which act as gene transactivators for numerous pro-inflammatory compounds [78]. The most common type of NF κB comprises a p50 subunit bound to a p65 subunit. In physiological conditions it is held in cytoplasm bound to an inhibitory protein, I κB. During inflammation cell is influenced by several stimuli including: cytokines, immunoglobulin aggregates, reactive oxygen species and angiotensin II. Cell stimulation results in I κB phosphorylation. Phosphorylated I κB is degraded by proteasomes and released NF κB translocated into the nucleus, where it binds to promoter regions of numerous genes, involved in cellular proliferation and inflammatory processes [78]. This increases the expression of many inflammatory enzymes, chemokines, pro-inflammatory cytokines and adhesion molecules, leading, among others, to glomerular injury and tubulointerstitial fibrosis. In *in vitro* studies the activity of monocyte chemoattractant protein 1 (MCP-1), a major chemokine involved in the recruitment of immune cells into the renal interstitium was shown to be NF κB dependent [79-81]. Other potent mediators of inflammatory process, i.e. IL-1β or TNF-α are also related to NF κB activation in mesangial cells [82, 83]. NF κB was also demonstrated to be activated in an experimental model of glomerulonephritis in rats and hypercholesterolemia [84, 85]. Since NF κB is a common factor for several pro-inflammatory molecules, inhibition of its activity could lead to attenuation of inflammation processes in the kidney. In a work by *Guijarro et al.* [86] cultured human mesangial cells were stimulated with bacterial lipopolisaccharides. It led to an activation of NF κB activity. However, treatment of mesangial cells with lovastatin resulted in a significant reduction of lipopolisaccharide-induced NF κB activation. This inhibitory action of lovastatin was most probably dependent on the decrease in mevalonate production, since in the presence of mevalonate or FPP the lovastatin inhibition of NF κB activation was substantially reversed. This study demonstrates yet another mechanism, by which HMG-CoA reductase inhibitors exhibit their nephroprotective actions.

Statins and Coagulation Disturbances

Coagulation disturbances are among the major risk factors for accelerated atherosclerosis and increased rate of cardio- and cerebrovascular complications. They are a constant feature of CRF. Increase in tissue factor (TF) and factor VII activity, as well as enhanced platelet aggregation constitute the most important coagulation disturbances related to CRF [87-89]. Renal transplantation is also accompanied by fibrynolysis system suppresion and increase in platelet aggregation activity, the latter most possibly due to immunosupression treatment [90, 91]. Statins appear to be capable of attenuating some of these disorders. In patients with end stage renal failure treated with continous ambulatory peritoneal dialysis (CAPD) a six months simvastatin administration resulted in a decrease in platelet aggregation, both in whole blood and platelet-rich plasma [92]. Further, the fibrinolytic activity index increased significantly after simvastatin treatment, reaching values observed in the control group. Similarly promising results were obtained in patients after transplantation. Though the work of *Hölschermann et al.* [93] was conducted on a group of patients after cardiac transplantation, its results can be, to some degree, transfered to kidney transplant population. The authors observed a significant decrease in monocyte TF activity after simvastatin treatment. It paralleled with a reduced TF mRNA expression in monocytes from patients treated with simvastatin. TF, a cell membrane-bound glycoprotein serves as a primary cellular initiator of the coagulation cascade [93]. Correction of the disorders of its activity by statins helps restoring the hemostatic balance in patients with renal diseases.

Statins and Endothelial Functions

Nitric oxide (NO) is a labile free radical, widely distributed in tissues [94]. NO posseses numerous actions, which are crucial for vascular homeostasis. It mediates vascular relaxation induced by some vasodilators, including acetylcholine and bradykinin [95]. It inhibits platelet aggregation, most probably by stimulation of the soluble guanylyl cyclase [96]. Further, NO was shown to inhibit cell proliferation in various cell cultures [97-99]. It also posseses antiadhesive properties for leukocytes [100]. Of interest is that NO inhibits the activation of mentioned above NF κB, and as such is a potent anti-inflammatory compound [101]. NO is synthesized from L-arginine through the action of NO synthase (NOS). Three isoenzymes of NOS are known: two calcium/calmodulin-dependent, and a calcium-idependent, inducible isoenzyme of NOS (iNOS) [102]. Vascular NO is predominantly produced by endothelial cells and vascular smooth muscle cells [102]. Under normal conditions endothelial NO, synthesized by constitutive calcium/calmodulin-dependent NOS isoenzyme is sufficient for maintaining vascular regulation. Vascular smooth muscle cells start producing NO via iNOS activation only under the conditions of endothelial dysfunction. Such conditions are present in the course of CRF [103]. Overproduction of reactive oxygen species, release of pro-inflammatory chemokines and cytokines during CRF causes endothelial injury. Increase in NO production by endothelial cells and vascular smooth muscle cells should be expected. This is, however, not the case in the course of CRF. The total amount of NO is increased, especially in end stage renal failure patients, mainly as a result of the loss of renal clearance [104]. The production of "hemodynamically active" NO is, however, reduced [104, 105]. This is, most probably due to lower activity of NOS in CRF patients, as compared to control population [105]. Numerous factors are indicated, as being responsible for the impairment of NOS activity. In CRF plasma levels of assymentrical dimethylarginine, potent endogenous NOS inhibitor, were being reported to rise [106, 107]. Furthermore, the bioavailability of the NO precursor, L-arginine was found to be decreased in experimental studies on CRF rats [108]. Finally, increased plasma levels of phenylacetic acid, observed in patients with CRF, inhibit the activity of iNOS, reducing NO production [102]. Disturbances of NO availability during CRF contribute to intraglomerular hypertension and increased peripheral vascular resistance [109, 110]. This, in turn, promotes the progression of renal insufficiency and accelerates the development of atherosclerosis.

Since hypercholesterolemia is thought to be involved in the impairment of NO availability, statins, by lowering serum cholesterol level, may promote NO production [111]. This hypothesis is supported by a study demonstrating that a single treatment of LDL apheresis is sufficient to significantly improve endothelium-dependent relaxations in hypercholesterolemic humans [112]. Further, statins were found to prevent oxLDL-mediated downregulation of endothelial NOS mRNA and protein level [94]. However, studies by *Laufs et al.* [113] suggest that HMG-CoA reductase inhibitors have also a direct influence on endothelial NOS. As the effects of statins on endothelial NOS are reversed with GGPP (but not FPP), they may be attributed to the inhibition of Rho prenylation. As documented by

Laufs et al. [114] treatment with mevastatin decreases Rho geranylgeranylation, membrane translocation, and leads to the up-regulation of endothelial NOS expression. Apart from enhancing NOS activity statins improve endothelial function by increasing the expression of tissue-type plasminogen activator, and by inhibiting the expression of endothelin-1 [94, 115]. As these factors are strongly related to blood pressure regulation, one could expect that statins might have some impact on blood pressure levels. Indeed, in experimental studies, both pravastatin and lovastatin significantly decreased mean arterial blood pressure after a few weeks of treatment [116, 117]. In a study on patients treated with angiotensin-converting enzyme (ACE) inhibitors, these additionally receiving statins had a significantly more marked reduction in blood pressure than the group receiving only ACE inhinibitors and dietary intervention [118]. Finally, in a randomized, double-blind crossover trial pravastatin was shown to significantly reduce systolic and diastolic pressure in persons with primary hypercholesterolemia and essential hypertension [119]. Since hypercholesterolemia causes endothelial injury and may contribute to increase in blood pressure, the authors suggest that antihypertensive effects of statins are mediated by lipid reduction. On the other hand blood pressure reduction was not correlated with changes in plasma cholesterol level. This suggests that some other mechanisms, e.g. increase in NO production or endothelin-1 inhibition are important [119]. Regardless of the mechanisms engaged, statins, by improving endothelial function appear to be capable of attenuating atheroslerosis and retarding the progression of renal insufficency.

Immunomodulatory Activities of Statins

The best method of renal replacement therapy in ESRD is kidney transplantation. Transplanted patients have a longer life expectancy, and improved life quality than patients on dialysis. However, transplantation is often accompanied by marked hyperlipidemia [16, 17]. As much as 75%-80% of kidney recepients are affected by this disturbance [120]. It is now well acknowledged that hyperlipidemia after transplantation is caused by immunosupressive treatment [19-21]. It is an imporatant complication, since it constitutes a significant risk factor for cardiovascular complications in this group of patients. Furthermore, lipid disturbances may deteriorate graft function, contributing to accelerated graft insufficiency [18, 121]. Treatment aimed at lowering plasma lipids seems, therefore, advisable in this patient population. However, statins appear to have an additional, cholesterol-independent influence on graft survival. In *in vitro* studies lovastatin decreases the proliferation of mitogen-stimulated T lyphocytes, and inhibits natural killer cells (NKC) cytotoxicity in culture [122, 123]. Results from the study by *Kobashigawa et al.* [124] suggest that pravastatin inhibits NKC cytotoxicity in heart transplaneted recipients. In kidney transplanted patients *Katznelson et al.* [125] observed fewer episodes of biopsy-proven acute rejection in patients treated with pravastatin, as compared to controls. The mechanisms of the above observations are still unclear. It might be a consequence of prenylation inhibition [120]. As described above, this action leads to a decrease in cell proliferation. This also reffers to cells related to immune response: NKC, T-lymphocytes, monocytes etc. The other posssible explanation is that the immunomodulatory effects of statins are secondary to their interactions with cyclosporine [120]. Cyclosporine in plasma is highly bound to lipids. Therefore, statins, by decreasing lipid levels increase cyclosporine bioavailability.

In a randomized multicenter trial by *Holdaas et al.* [126] fluvastatin had no effect on the incidence nor severity of acute rejection following renal transplantation. Therefore, intriguing as they are, immunosuppressive properties of statins need further elucidation.

Safety of Statin Treatment

Taking into consideration all the benefits that can be gained from the use of statins it is tempting to offer these drugs to all the patients with kidney diseases. However, statin treatment is still related to many fears and controversies caused by their side effects. Numerous reports on myopathy, including rhabdomyolysis after statin use are available in the literature [127-130]. It was because of the deaths caused by rhabdomyolysis that cerivastatin was withdrawn from the market in July 2001. This, often fatal complication can appear following high concentrations of statins in blood. Therefore it is either caused by drug overdosage, or while administering statins together with other drugs that possess the same path of metabolism. Renal failure itself can also be responsible for increase in the concentration of statins that are metabolised and excreted by kidneys. In case of lovastatin and simvastatin producers advice lowering the dosage in severe renal failure. Special caution in administering HMG-CoA reductase inhibitors with other drugs is of greatest importance in patients after renal transplantation. Majority of statins are metabolized through the same pathway as cyclosporine, namely through the 3A4 isoenzyme of the cytochrome P450 [131]. Cytochrome P450 is a panel of microsomal enzymes, consisting of many isoforms (CYP) which metabolize drugs in different tissues, in case of statins mainly in liver and intestine. Numerous drugs are metabolized through the cytochrome P450. Additionally, some of them may change the activity of certain isoenzymes (Table 1). Two of cytochrome P450 isoforms are related to statin metabolism. Fluvastatin is metabolized through the CYP 2C9 isoenzyme. Though many drugs influence the activity of this isoenzyme, their concomitant use does not cause significant changes in fluvastatin concentration. Isoenzyme CYP 3A4 is of much greater importance in statin pharmacokinetics. Lovastatin, simvastatin and atorvastatin are metabolized through this pathway. Likewise, cerivastatin, currently withdrawn from the market, is mainly metabolized by this isoenzyme. CYP 3A4 is also the main metabolism path for two imoportant drugs used as immunosuppressive agents in patients after renal transplantation, cyclosporine and tacrolimus. Cyclosporine is additionally a potent inhibitor of CYP 3A4 activity. This has a major impact on concentration of HMG-CoA reductase inhibitors in case of concomitant use with cyclosporine. It can rise up to 20-times in statins for which the 3A4 isoenzyme is the only way of metabolism [132]. In case of lipophilic statins it may cause drug penetration into muscle cells, and rhabdomyolysis. Cytochrome P450 is not the only common point of statin and cyclosporine metabolism. It appears that these drugs may compete on the level of their elimination into the bile. This hypothesis seems to be confirmed by the fact that the concentration of pravastatin, drug which is not metabolized by cytochrome P450 rises in case of concomitant use with cyclosporine [132].

It has to be stressed, however, that statins are safe when administered in adequate doses. This has been proven in many studies, on a significant number of patients [133-136].

Table 1. Substrates, inducers and inhibitors of cytochrome P450

Cytochrome P450	Substrates	Inducers	Inhibitors
CYP2C9	– NSAIDs – angiotensine II receptor inhibitors – fluvastatin – fenytoine – torasemide	– barbiturates – rifampicin	– amiodarone – isoniazid – fluconazole – fluvastatin – cotrimoxazole – metronidazole
CYP3A4	– lidocaine – calcium anatagonists – cyclosporine – tacrolimus – atorvastatin – cerivastatin – lovastatin – simvastatin – cyclophosphamide – erythromycin	– barbiturates – rifampicin – fenytoine	– cyclosporine – diltiazem – erythromycin – fluconazole – ketoconazole – ranitidine – verapamil – grapefruit juice

CONCLUSION

Despite enormous scientific effort we are still far from recognizing all properties, positive as well as negative of HMG-CoA reductase inhibitors. Furher studies are necessary to assess all the benefits and menaces related to the use of statins. However, the ability to normalize lipid profile as well as numerous pleiotropic properties make statins worth considering in patients with kidney diseases.

REFERENCES

[1] Rutkowski B, Tylicki L, Manitius J, and Lysiak-Szydlowska W, Hypertensive nephropathy - an increasing clinical problem. Miner Electrolyte Metab, 1999. 25(1-2): p. 65-68.

[2] Klag MJ, Whelton PK, Randall BL, Neaton JD, Brancati FL, Ford CE, Shulman NB, and Stamler J, Blood pressure and end-stage renal disease in men. N Engl J Med, 1996. 334(1): p. 13-18.

[3] Excerpts from United States Renal Data System 1999 Annual Data Report. Am J Kidney Dis, 1999. 34(2 Suppl 1): p. S1-176.

[4] Coresh J, Wei GL, McQuillan G, Brancati FL, Levey AS, Jones C, and Klag MJ, Prevalence of high blood pressure and elevated serum creatinine level in the United States: findings from the third National Health and Nutrition Examination Survey (1988-1994). Arch Intern Med, 2001. 161(9): p. 1207-1216.

[5] London GM and Drueke TB, Atherosclerosis and arteriosclerosis in chronic renal failure. Kidney Int, 1997. 51(6): p. 1678-1695.

[6] Mathur S, Devaraj S, and Jialal I, Accelerated atherosclerosis, dyslipidemia, and oxidative stress in end-stage renal disease. Curr Opin Nephrol Hypertens, 2002. 11(2): p. 141-147.

[7] Rutkowski B, Szolkiewicz M, Korczynska J, Sucajtys E, Stelmanska E, Nieweglowski T, and Swierczynski J, The role of lipogenesis in the development of uremic hyperlipidemia. Am J Kidney Dis, 2003. 41(3 Suppl 1): p. S84-88.

[8] Chmielewski M, Nieweglowski T, Swierczynski J, Rutkowski B, and Boguslawski W, Diurnal rhythm of cholesterol biosynthesis in experimental chronic renal failure. Mol Cell Biochem, 2001. 228(1-2): p. 33-37.

[9] Chmielewski M, Sucajtys E, Swierczynski J, Rutkowski B, and Boguslawski W, Contribution of increased HMG-CoA reductase gene expression to hypercholesterolemia in experimental chronic renal failure. Mol Cell Biochem, 2003. 246 (1-2): p. 187-191.

[10] Quaschning T, Krane V, Metzger T, and Wanner C, Abnormalities in uremic lipoprotein metabolism and its impact on cardiovascular disease. Am J Kidney Dis, 2001. 38(4 Suppl 1): p. S14-19.

[11] Locatelli F, Canaud B, Eckardt KU, Stenvinkel P, Wanner C, and Zoccali C, Oxidative stress in end-stage renal disease: an emerging threat to patient outcome. Nephrol Dial Transplant, 2003. 18(7): p. 1272-1280.

[12] Ando M, Lundkvist I, Bergstrom J, and Lindholm B, Enhanced scavenger receptor expression in monocyte-macrophages in dialysis patients. Kidney Int, 1996. 49(3): p. 773-780.

[13] Karpati I, Paragh G, Kovacs E, Balogh Z, Szabolcs M, Szabo J, Kakuk G, and Foris G, Disturbed LDL and scavenger receptor functions in monocytes from chronic haemodialysed patients. Nephrol Dial Transplant, 1999. 14(11): p. 2664-2668.

[14] Oda H and Keane WF, Lipid abnormalities in end stage renal disease. Nephrol Dial Transplant, 1998. 13 Suppl 1: p. 45-49.

[15] Król E, Wróblewska M, Rutkowski B, and Badzio T, Classification of lipid disorders in chronic hemodialyzed patients. Miner Electrolyte Metab, 1996. 22: p. 13-15.

[16] Kisielnicka E, Zdrojewski Z, Wroblewska M, Kortas B, and Rutkowski B, Lipid disturbances in a two-year follow-up after successful kidney transplantation. Transplant Proc, 2000. 32(6): p. 1358-1362.

[17] Dimeny E, Wahlberg J, Lithell H, and Fellstrom B, Hyperlipidaemia in renal transplantation--risk factor for long-term graft outcome. Eur J Clin Invest, 1995. 25(8): p. 574-583.

[18] Guijarro C, Massy ZA, and Kasiske BL, Clinical correlation between renal allograft failure and hyperlipidemia. Kidney Int Suppl, 1995. 52: p. S56-59.

[19] Kisielnicka E, Zdrojewski Z, Wroblewska M, Kortas B, Lysiak-Szydlowska W, and Rutkowski B, Does immunosuppressive regimen influence the lipid disturbances in kidney recipients? Am J Nephrol, 2000. 20(5): p. 385-390.

[20] Hilbrands LB, Demacker PN, Hoitsma AJ, Stalenhoef AF, and Koene RA, The effects of cyclosporine and prednisone on serum lipid and (apo)lipoprotein levels in renal transplant recipients. J Am Soc Nephrol, 1995. 5(12): p. 2073-2081.

[21] Raine AE, Carter R, Mann JI, Chapman JR, and Morris PJ, Increased plasma LDL cholesterol after renal transplantation associated with cyclosporine immunosuppression. Transplant Proc, 1987. 19(1 Pt 2): p. 1820-1821.

[22] Hsu CY, Bates DW, Kuperman GJ, and Curhan GC, Diabetes, hemoglobin A(1c), cholesterol, and the risk of moderate chronic renal insufficiency in an ambulatory population. Am J Kidney Dis, 2000. 36(2): p. 272 281.

[23] Washio M, Okuda S, Ikeda M, Hirakata H, Nanishi F, Onoyama K, Yoshimura T, and Fujishima M, Hypercholesterolemia and the progression of the renal dysfunction in chronic renal failure patients. J Epidemiol, 1996. 6(4): p. 172-177.

[24] Krolewski AS, Warram JH, and Christlieb AR, Hypercholesterolemia--a determinant of renal function loss and deaths in IDDM patients with nephropathy. Kidney Int Suppl, 1994. 45: p. S125-131.

[25] Roodnat JI, Mulder PG, Zietse R, Rischen-Vos J, van Riemsdijk IC, JN IJ, and Weimar W, Cholesterol as an independent predictor of outcome after renal transplantation. Transplantation, 2000. 69(8): p. 1704-1710.

[26] Isoniemi H, Nurminen M, Tikkanen MJ, von Willebrand E, Krogerus L, Ahonen J, Eklund B, Hockerstedt K, Salmela K, and Hayry P, Risk factors predicting chronic rejection of renal allografts. Transplantation, 1994. 57(1): p. 68-72.

[27] Nishida Y, Oda H, and Yorioka N, Effect of lipoproteins on mesangial cell proliferation. Kidney Int Suppl, 1999. 71: p. S51-53.

[28] Kamanna VS, Bassa BV, Vaziri ND, and Roh DD, Atherogenic lipoproteins and tyrosine kinase mitogenic signaling in mesangial cells. Kidney Int Suppl, 1999. 71: p. S70-75.

[29] Kamanna VS, Pai R, Ha H, Kirschenbaum MA, and Roh DD, Oxidized low-density lipoprotein stimulates monocyte adhesion to glomerular endothelial cells. Kidney Int, 1999. 55(6): p. 2192-2202.

[30] Kamanna VS, Pai R, Roh DD, and Kirschenbaum MA, Oxidative modification of low-density lipoprotein enhances the murine mesangial cell cytokines associated with monocyte migration, differentiation, and proliferation. *Lab Invest*, 1996. 74(6): p. 1067-1079.

[31] Rovin BH and Tan LC, LDL stimulates mesangial fibronectin production and chemoattractant expression. *Kidney Int*, 1993. 43(1): p. 218-225.

[32] Bath PM and Martin JF, Serum platelet-derived growth factor and endothelin concentrations in human hypercholesterolaemia. *J Intern Med*, 1991. 230(4): p. 313-317.

[33] Davi G, Averna M, Catalano I, Barbagallo C, Ganci A, Notarbartolo A, Ciabattoni G, and Patrono C, Increased thromboxane biosynthesis in type IIa hypercholesterolemia. *Circulation*, 1992. 85(5): p. 1792-1798.

[34] Jeserich M, Munzel T, Just H, and Drexler H, Reduced plasma L-arginine in hypercholesterolaemia. *Lancet*, 1992. 339(8792): p. 561.

[35] Saito T, Oikawa S, Sato H, Sato T, Ito S, and Sasaki J, Lipoprotein glomerulopathy: significance of lipoprotein and ultrastructural features. *Kidney Int Suppl*, 1999. 71: p. S37-41.

[36] Saito T, Sato H, Oikawa S, Kudo K, Kurihara I, Nakayama K, Abe K, Yoshinaga K, and Sakaguchi H, Lipoprotein glomerulopathy. Report of a normolipidemic case and review of the literature. *Am J Nephrol*, 1993. 13(1): p. 64-68.

[37] Diamond JR, Analogous pathobiologic mechanisms in glomerulosclerosis and atherosclerosis. *Kidney Int Suppl*, 1991. 31: p. S29-34.
[38] Lusis AJ, Atherosclerosis. *Nature*, 2000. 407(6801): p. 233-241.
[39] Istvan ES and Deisenhofer J, Structural mechanism for statin inhibition of HMG-CoA reductase. *Science*, 2001. 292(5519): p. 1160-1164.
[40] Aguilar-Salinas CA, Barrett H, and Schonfeld G, Metabolic modes of action of the statins in the hyperlipoproteinemias. *Atherosclerosis*, 1998. 141(2): p. 203-207.
[41] Horton JD, Goldstein JL, and Brown MS, SREBPs: activators of the complete program of cholesterol and fatty acid synthesis in the liver. *J Clin Invest,* 2002. 109(9): p. 1125-1131.
[42] Le NA, Innis-Whitehouse W, Li X, Bakker-Arkema R, Black D, and Brown WV, Lipid and apolipoprotein levels and distribution in patients with hypertriglyceridemia: effect of triglyceride reductions with atorvastatin. *Metabolism*, 2000. 49(2): p. 167-177.
[43] White CM, A review of the pharmacologic and pharmacokinetic aspects of rosuvastatin. *J Clin Pharmacol*, 2002. 42(9): p. 963-970.
[44] Endo A, Tsujita Y, Kuroda M, and Tanzawa K, Inhibition of cholesterol synthesis in vitro and in vivo by ML-236A and ML-236B, competitive inhibitors of 3-hydroxy-3-methylglutaryl-coenzyme A reductase. *Eur J Biochem,* 1977. 77(1): p. 31-36.
[45] Alberts AW, Chen J, Kuron G, Hunt V, Huff J, Hoffman C, Rothrock J, Lopez M, Joshua H, Harris E, Patchett A, Monaghan R, Currie S, Stapley E, Albers-Schonberg G, Hensens O, Hirshfield J, Hoogsteen K, Liesch J, and Springer J, Mevinolin: a highly potent competitive inhibitor of hydroxymethylglutaryl-coenzyme A reductase and a cholesterol-lowering agent. *Proc Natl Acad Sci U S A,* 1980. 77(7): p. 3957-3961.
[46] Randomised trial of cholesterol lowering in 4444 patients with coronary heart disease: the Scandinavian Simvastatin Survival Study (4S). *Lancet*, 1994. 344(8934): p. 1383-1389.
[47] Shepherd J, Cobbe SM, Ford I, Isles CG, Lorimer AR, MacFarlane PW, McKillop JH, and Packard CJ, Prevention of coronary heart disease with pravastatin in men with hypercholesterolemia. West of Scotland Coronary Prevention Study Group. *N Engl J Med*, 1995. 333(20): p. 1301-1307.
[48] Sacks FM, Pfeffer MA, Moye LA, Rouleau JL, Rutherford JD, Cole TG, Brown L, Warnica JW, Arnold JM, Wun CC, Davis BR, and Braunwald E, The effect of pravastatin on coronary events after myocardial infarction in patients with average cholesterol levels. Cholesterol and Recurrent Events Trial investigators. *N Engl J Med,* 1996. 335(14): p. 1001-1009.
[49] Collins R, Armitage J, Parish S, Sleigh P, and Peto R, MRC/BHF Heart Protection Study of cholesterol-lowering with simvastatin in 5963 people with diabetes: a randomised placebo-controlled trial. *Lancet*, 2003. 361(9374): p. 2005-2016.
[50] Corvol JC, Bouzamondo A, Sirol M, Hulot JS, Sanchez P, and Lechat P, Differential effects of lipid-lowering therapies on stroke prevention: a meta-analysis of randomized trials. *Arch Intern Med,* 2003. 163(6): p. 669-676.
[51] Tonelli M, Moye L, Sacks FM, Kiberd B, and Curhan G, Pravastatin for secondary prevention of cardiovascular events in persons with mild chronic renal insufficiency. *Ann Intern Med,* 2003. 138(2): p. 98-104.

[52] Seliger SL, Weiss NS, Gillen DL, Kestenbaum B, Ball A, Sherrard DJ, and Stehman-Breen CO, HMG-CoA reductase inhibitors are associated with reduced mortality in ESRD patients. *Kidney Int,* 2002. 61(1): p. 297-304.

[53] Kasiske BL, O'Donnell MP, Garvis WJ, and Keane WF, Pharmacologic treatment of hyperlipidemia reduces glomerular injury in rat 5/6 nephrectomy model of chronic renal failure. *Circ Res,* 1988. 62(2): p. 367-374.

[54] O'Donnell MP, Kasiske BL, Katz SA, Schmitz PG, and Keane WF, Lovastatin but not enalapril reduces glomerular injury in Dahl salt- sensitive rats. *Hypertension*, 1992. 20(5): p. 651-658.

[55] O'Donnell MP, Kasiske BL, Kim Y, Schmitz PG, and Keane WF, Lovastatin retards the progression of established glomerular disease in obese Zucker rats. *Am J Kidney Dis,* 1993. 22(1): p. 83-89.

[56] Harris KP, Purkerson ML, Yates J, and Klahr S, Lovastatin ameliorates the development of glomerulosclerosis and uremia in experimental nephrotic syndrome. *Am J Kidney Dis*, 1990. 15(1): p. 16-23.

[57] Shoji T, Nishizawa Y, Toyokawa A, Kawagishi T, Okuno Y, and Morii H, Decreased albuminuria by pravastatin in hyperlipidemic diabetics. *Nephron*, 1991. 59(4): p. 664-665.

[58] Rabelink AJ, Hene RJ, Erkelens DW, Joles JA, and Koomans HA, Partial remission of nephrotic syndrome in patient on long-term simvastatin. *Lancet*, 1990. 335(8696): p. 1045-1046.

[59] Tonelli M, Moye L, Sacks FM, Cole T, and Curhan GC, Effect of pravastatin on loss of renal function in people with moderate chronic renal insufficiency and cardiovascular disease. *J Am Soc Nephrol*, 2003. 14(6): p. 1605-1613.

[60] Tylicki L, Rutkowski B, and Horl WH, Multifactorial determination of hypertensive nephroangiosclerosis. *Kidney Blood Press Res*, 2002. 25(6): p. 341-353.

[61] Hidaka Y, Eda T, Yonemoto M, and Kamei T, Inhibition of cultured vascular smooth muscle cell migration by simvastatin (MK-733). *Atherosclerosis*, 1992. 95(1): p. 87-94.

[62] Munro E, Patel M, Chan P, Betteridge L, Clunn G, Gallagher K, Hughes A, Schachter M, Wolfe J, and Sever P, Inhibition of human vascular smooth muscle cell proliferation by lovastatin: the role of isoprenoid intermediates of cholesterol synthesis. *Eur J Clin Invest*, 1994. 24(11): p. 766-772.

[63] O'Donnell MP, Kasiske BL, Kim Y, Atluru D, and Keane WF, Lovastatin inhibits proliferation of rat mesangial cells. *J Clin Invest,* 1993. 91(1): p. 83-87.

[64] Zhang FL and Casey PJ, Protein prenylation: molecular mechanisms and functional consequences. *Annu Rev Biochem*, 1996. 65: p. 241-269.

[65] Marshall CJ, Protein prenylation: a mediator of protein-protein interactions. *Science*, 1993. 259(5103): p. 1865-1866.

[66] Khwaja A, O'Connolly J, and Hendry BM, Prenylation inhibitors in renal disease. *Lancet*, 2000. 355(9205): p. 741-744.

[67] O'Donnell MP, Kasiske BL, Massy ZA, Guijarro C, Swan SK, and Keane WF, Isoprenoids and Ras: potential role in chronic rejection. *Kidney Int Suppl*, 1995. 52: p. S29-33.

[68] Vrtovsnik F, Couette S, Prie D, Lallemand D, and Friedlander G, Lovastatin-induced inhibition of renal epithelial tubular cell proliferation involves a p21ras activated, AP-1-dependent pathway. *Kidney Int*, 1997. 52(4): p. 1016-1027.

[69] Hengst L and Reed SI, Translational control of p27Kip1 accumulation during the cell cycle. *Science*, 1996. 271(5257): p. 1861-1864.

[70] Terada Y, Inoshita S, Nakashima O, Yamada T, Kuwahara M, Sasaki S, and Marumo F, Lovastatin inhibits mesangial cell proliferation via p27Kip1. *J Am Soc Nephrol*, 1998. 9(12): p. 2235-2243.

[71] Hirai A, Nakamura S, Noguchi Y, Yasuda T, Kitagawa M, Tatsuno I, Oeda T, Tahara K, Terano T, Narumiya S, Kohn LD, and Saito Y, Geranylgeranylated rho small GTPase(s) are essential for the degradation of p27Kip1 and facilitate the progression from G1 to S phase in growth-stimulated rat FRTL-5 cells. *J Biol Chem,* 1997. 272(1): p. 13-16.

[72] Nishimura M, Tanaka T, Yasuda T, Kurakata S, Kitagawa M, Yamada K, Saito Y, and Hirai A, Effect of pravastatin on type IV collagen secretion and mesangial cell proliferation. *Kidney Int Suppl,* 1999. 71: p. S97-100.

[73] Bobak D, Moorman J, Guanzon A, Gilmer L, and Hahn C, Inactivation of the small GTPase Rho disrupts cellular attachment and induces adhesion-dependent and adhesion-independent apoptosis. *Oncogene*, 1997. 15(18): p. 2179-2189.

[74] Guijarro C, Blanco-Colio LM, Massy ZA, O'Donnell MP, Kasiske BL, Keane WF, and Egido J, Lipophilic statins induce apoptosis of human vascular smooth muscle cells. *Kidney Int Suppl,* 1999. 71: p. S88-91.

[75] Vamvakopoulos JE and Green C, HMG-CoA reductase inhibition aborts functional differentiation and triggers apoptosis in cultured primary human monocytes: a potential mechanism of statin-mediated vasculoprotection. *BMC Cardiovasc Disord,* 2003. 3(1): p. 6.

[76] Ridker PM, Rifai N, Pfeffer MA, Sacks F, and Braunwald E, Long-term effects of pravastatin on plasma concentration of C-reactive protein. The Cholesterol and Recurrent Events (CARE) Investigators. *Circulation*, 1999. 100(3): p. 230-235.

[77] Sirken G, Kung SC, and Raja R, Decreased erythropoietin requirements in maintenance hemodialysis patients with statin therapy. *Asaio J,* 2003. 49(4): p. 422-425.

[78] Massy ZA, Guijarro C, O'Donnell MP, Kim Y, Kashtan CE, Egido J, Kasiske BL, and Keane WF, The central role of nuclear factor-kappa B in mesangial cell activation. *Kidney Int Suppl,* 1999. 71: p. S76-79.

[79] Viedt C, Dechend R, Fei J, Hansch GM, Kreuzer J, and Orth SR, MCP-1 induces inflammatory activation of human tubular epithelial cells: involvement of the transcription factors, nuclear factor-kappaB and activating protein-1. *J Am Soc Nephrol,* 2002. 13(6): p. 1534-1547.

[80] Sung FL, Zhu TY, Au-Yeung KK, Siow YL, and O K, Enhanced MCP-1 expression during ischemia/reperfusion injury is mediated by oxidative stress and NF-kappaB. *Kidney Int*, 2002. 62(4): p. 1160-1170.

[81] Wang Y, Rangan GK, Goodwin B, Tay YC, and Harris DC, Lipopolysaccharide-induced MCP-1 gene expression in rat tubular epithelial cells is nuclear factor-kappaB dependent. *Kidney Int*, 2000. 57(5): p. 2011-2022.

[82] Satriano J and Schlondorff D, Activation and attenuation of transcription factor NF-kB in mouse glomerular mesangial cells in response to tumor necrosis factor-alpha, immunoglobulin G, and adenosine 3':5'-cyclic monophosphate. Evidence for involvement of reactive oxygen species. *J Clin Invest*, 1994. 94(4): p. 1629-1636.

[83] Tetsuka T, Srivastava SK, and Morrison AR, Tyrosine kinase inhibitors, genistein and herbimycin A, do not block interleukin-1 beta-induced activation of NF-kappa B in rat mesangial cells. *Biochem Biophys Res Commun*, 1996. 218(3): p. 808-812.

[84] Sakurai H, Hisada Y, Ueno M, Sugiura M, Kawashima K, and Sugita T, Activation of transcription factor NF-kappa B in experimental glomerulonephritis in rats. *Biochim Biophys Acta*, 1996. 1316(2): p. 132-138.

[85] Wilson SH, Caplice NM, Simari RD, Holmes DR, Jr., Carlson PJ, and Lerman A, Activated nuclear factor-kappaB is present in the coronary vasculature in experimental hypercholesterolemia. *Atherosclerosis,* 2000. 148(1): p. 23-30.

[86] Guijarro C, Kim Y, Schoonover CM, Massy ZA, O'Donnell MP, Kasiske BL, Keane WF, and Kashtan CE, Lovastatin inhibits lipopolysaccharide-induced NF-kappaB activation in human mesangial cells. *Nephrol Dial Transplant*, 1996. 11(6): p. 990-996.

[87] Zemanova P, Opatrny Jr K, Opatrna S, Vit L, Sefrna F, and Racek J, Tissue factor, its pathway inhibitor, and metabolic disturbances in long-term peritoneal dialysis. *Kidney Blood Press Res*, 2003. 26(5-6): p. 368-375.

[88] Kario K, Matsuo T, Yamada T, Nakao K, Shimano C, and Matsuo M, Factor VII hyperactivity in chronic dialysis patients. *Thromb Res,* 1992. 67(1): p. 105-113.

[89] Zdrojewski Z, Lizakowski S, Raszeja-Specht A, Skibowska A, and Rutkowski B, Influence of spontaneous platelet aggregation on progression of glomerular disease. *Nephron*, 2002. 92(1): p. 36-42.

[90] Hryszko T, Malyszko J, Malyszko JS, Brzosko S, Pawlak K, and Mysliwiec M, A possible role of thrombin-activatable fibrinolysis inhibitor in disturbances of fibrinolytic system in renal transplant recipients. *Nephrol Dial Transplant,* 2001. 16(8): p. 1692-1696.

[91] Malyszko J, Malyszko JS, Takada A, and Mysliwiec M, Effects of immunosuppressive drugs on platelet aggregation in vitro. *Ann Transplant*, 2002. 7(1): p. 55-68.

[92] Malyszko J, Malyszko JS, Hryszko T, and Mysliwiec M, Influence of simvastatin on aspects of thrombogenesis in CAPD patients. *Perit Dial Int,* 2003. 23(3): p. 260-266.

[93] Holschermann H, Hilgendorff A, Kemkes-Matthes B, Schonburg M, Bauer EP, Tillmanns H, and Haberbosch W, Simvastatin attenuates vascular hypercoagulability in cardiac transplant recipients. *Transplantation*, 2000. 69(9): p. 1830-1836.

[94] Hernandez-Perera O, Perez-Sala D, Navarro-Antolin J, Sanchez-Pascuala R, Hernandez G, Diaz C, and Lamas S, Effects of the 3-hydroxy-3-methylglutaryl-CoA reductase inhibitors, atorvastatin and simvastatin, on the expression of endothelin-1 and endothelial nitric oxide synthase in vascular endothelial cells. *J Clin Invest,* 1998. 101(12): p. 2711-2719.

[95] Moncada S, Palmer RM, and Higgs EA, The discovery of nitric oxide as the endogenous nitrovasodilator. *Hypertension*, 1988. 12(4): p. 365-372.

[96] Moro MA, Russel RJ, Cellek S, Lizasoain I, Su Y, Darley-Usmar VM, Radomski MW, and Moncada S, cGMP mediates the vascular and platelet actions of nitric oxide: confirmation using an inhibitor of the soluble guanylyl cyclase. *Proc Natl Acad Sci U S A,* 1996. 93(4): p. 1480-1485.

[97] Garg UC and Hassid A, Nitric oxide-generating vasodilators inhibit mitogenesis and proliferation of BALB/C 3T3 fibroblasts by a cyclic GMP-independent mechanism. *Biochem Biophys Res Commun*, 1990. 171(1): p. 474-479.

[98] Garg UC and Hassid A, Nitric oxide-generating vasodilators and 8-bromo-cyclic guanosine monophosphate inhibit mitogenesis and proliferation of cultured rat vascular smooth muscle cells. *J Clin Invest,* 1989. 83(5): p. 1774-1777.

[99] Garg UC and Hassid A, Inhibition of rat mesangial cell mitogenesis by nitric oxide-generating vasodilators. *Am J Physiol,* 1989. 257(1 Pt 2): p. F60-66.

[100] Gaboury J, Woodman RC, Granger DN, Reinhardt P, and Kubes P, Nitric oxide prevents leukocyte adherence: role of superoxide. *Am J Physio*l, 1993. 265(3 Pt 2): p. H862-867.

[101] Katsuyama K, Shichiri M, Marumo F, and Hirata Y, NO inhibits cytokine-induced iNOS expression and NF-kappaB activation by interfering with phosphorylation and degradation of IkappaB-alpha. *Arterioscler Thromb Vasc Biol*, 1998. 18(11): p. 1796-1802.

[102] Jankowski J, van der Giet M, Jankowski V, Schmidt S, Hemeier M, Mahn B, Giebing G, Tolle M, Luftmann H, Schluter H, Zidek W, and Tepel M, Increased plasma phenylacetic acid in patients with end-stage renal failure inhibits iNOS expression. *J Clin Invest*, 2003. 112(2): p. 256-264.

[103] Annuk M, Zilmer M, and Fellstrom B, Endothelium-dependent vasodilation and oxidative stress in chronic renal failure: impact on cardiovascular disease. *Kidney Int Suppl*, 2003(84): p. S50-53.

[104] Schmidt RJ and Baylis C, Total nitric oxide production is low in patients with chronic renal disease. *Kidney Int*, 2000. 58(3): p. 1261-1266.

[105] Wever R, Boer P, Hijmering M, Stroes E, Verhaar M, Kastelein J, Versluis K, Lagerwerf F, van Rijn H, Koomans H, and Rabelink T, Nitric oxide production is reduced in patients with chronic renal failure. *Arterioscler Thromb Vasc Biol,* 1999. 19(5): p. 1168-1172.

[106] MacAllister RJ, Rambausek MH, Vallance P, Williams D, Hoffmann KH, and Ritz E, Concentration of dimethyl-L-arginine in the plasma of patients with end-stage renal failure. *Nephrol Dial Transplant*, 1996. 11(12): p. 2449-2452.

[107] Vallance P, Leone A, Calver A, Collier J, and Moncada S, Accumulation of an endogenous inhibitor of nitric oxide synthesis in chronic renal failure. *Lancet*, 1992. 339(8793): p. 572-575.

[108] Bouby N, Hassler C, Parvy P, and Bankir L, Renal synthesis of arginine in chronic renal failure: in vivo and in vitro studies in rats with 5/6 nephrectomy. *Kidney Int,* 1993. 44(4): p. 676-683.

[109] Bagi Z, Hamar P, Antus B, Rosivall L, and Koller A, Chronic renal failure leads to reduced flow-dependent dilation in isolated rat skeletal muscle arterioles due to lack of NO mediation. *Kidney Blood Press Res,* 2003. 26(1): p. 19-26.

[110] Aiello S, Remuzzi G, and Noris M, Nitric oxide/endothelin balance after nephron reduction. *Kidney Int Suppl*, 1998. 65: p. S63-67.

[111] Liao JK, Shin WS, Lee WY, and Clark SL, Oxidized low-density lipoprotein decreases the expression of endothelial nitric oxide synthase. *J Biol Chem,* 1995. 270(1): p. 319-324.

[112] Tamai O, Matsuoka H, Itabe H, Wada Y, Kohno K, and Imaizumi T, Single LDL apheresis improves endothelium-dependent vasodilatation in hypercholesterolemic humans. *Circulation*, 1997. 95(1): p. 76-82.

[113] Laufs U, La Fata V, Plutzky J, and Liao JK, Upregulation of endothelial nitric oxide synthase by HMG CoA reductase inhibitors. *Circulation*, 1998. 97(12): p. 1129-1135.
[114] Laufs U and Liao JK, Post-transcriptional regulation of endothelial nitric oxide synthase mRNA stability by Rho GTPase. *J Biol Chem*, 1998. 273(37): p. 24266-24271.
[115] Essig M, Nguyen G, Prie D, Escoubet B, Sraer JD, and Friedlander G, 3-Hydroxy-3-methylglutaryl coenzyme A reductase inhibitors increase fibrinolytic activity in rat aortic endothelial cells. Role of geranylgeranylation and Rho proteins. *Circ Res*, 1998. 83(7): p. 683-690.
[116] Wilson TW, Alonso-Galicia M, and Roman RJ, Effects of lipid-lowering agents in the Dahl salt-sensitive rat. *Hypertension,* 1998. 31(1 Pt 2): p. 225-231.
[117] Jiang J and Roman RJ, Lovastatin prevents development of hypertension in spontaneously hypertensive rats. *Hypertension,* 1997. 30(4): p. 968-974.
[118] Sposito AC, Mansur AP, Coelho OR, Nicolau JC, and Ramires JA, Additional reduction in blood pressure after cholesterol-lowering treatment by statins (lovastatin or pravastatin) in hypercholesterolemic patients using angiotensin-converting enzyme inhibitors (enalapril or lisinopril). *Am J Cardiol,* 1999. 83(10): p. 1497-1499, A1498.
[119] Glorioso N, Troffa C, Filigheddu F, Dettori F, Soro A, Parpaglia PP, Collatina S, and Pahor M, Effect of the HMG-CoA reductase inhibitors on blood pressure in patients with essential hypertension and primary hypercholesterolemia. *Hypertension*, 1999. 34(6): p. 1281-1286.
[120] Katznelson S and Kobashigawa JA, Dual roles of HMG-CoA reductase inhibitors in solid organ transplantation: lipid lowering and immunosuppression. *Kidney Int Suppl,* 1995. 52: p. S112-115.
[121] Carvalho MF and Soares V, Hyperlipidemia as a risk factor of renal allograft function impairment. *Clin Transplant*, 2001. 15(1): p. 48-52.
[122] Chakrabarti R and Engleman EG, Interrelationships between mevalonate metabolism and the mitogenic signaling pathway in T lymphocyte proliferation. *J Biol Chem*, 1991. 266(19): p. 12216-12222.
[123] Cutts JL, Scallen TJ, Watson J, and Bankhurst AD, Role of mevalonic acid in the regulation of natural killer cell cytotoxicity. *J Cell Physiol*, 1989. 139(3): p. 550-557.
[124] Kobashigawa JA, Katznelson S, Laks H, Johnson JA, Yeatman L, Wang XM, Chia D, Terasaki PI, Sabad A, Cogert GA, and et al., Effect of pravastatin on outcomes after cardiac transplantation. *N Engl J Med,* 1995. 333(10): p. 621-627.
[125] Katznelson S, Wilkinson AH, Kobashigawa JA, Wang XM, Chia D, Ozawa M, Zhong HP, Hirata M, Cohen AH, Teraski PI, and et al., The effect of pravastatin on acute rejection after kidney transplantation--a pilot study. *Transplantation,* 1996. 61(10): p. 1469-1474.
[126] Holdaas H, Jardine AG, Wheeler DC, Brekke IB, Conlon PJ, Fellstrom B, Hammad A, Holme I, Isoniemi H, Moore R, Rowe PA, Sweny P, Talbot DA, Wadstrom J, and Ostraat O, Effect of fluvastatin on acute renal allograft rejection: a randomized multicenter trial. *Kidney Int,* 2001. 60(5): p. 1990-1997.
[127] Sica DA and Gehr TW, 3-Hydroxy-3-methylglutaryl coenzyme A reductase inhibitors and rhabdomyolysis: considerations in the renal failure patient. *Curr Opin Nephrol Hypertens*, 2002. 11(2): p. 123-133.

[128] Stirling CM and Isles CG, Rhabdomyolysis due to simvastatin in a transplant patient: Are some statins safer than others? *Nephrol Dial Transplant*, 2001. 16(4): p. 873-874.
[129] Weise WJ and Possidente CJ, Fatal rhabdomyolysis associated with simvastatin in a renal transplant patient. *Am J Med,* 2000. 108(4): p. 351-352.
[130] Rodriguez ML, Mora C, and Navarro JF, Cerivastatin-induced rhabdomyolysis. *Ann Intern Med,* 2000. 132(7): p. 598.
[131] Bottorff M and Hansten P, Long-term safety of hepatic hydroxymethyl glutaryl coenzyme A reductase inhibitors: the role of metabolism-monograph for physicians. *Arch Intern Med,* 2000. 160(15): p. 2273-2280.
[132] Olbricht C, Wanner C, Eisenhauer T, Kliem V, Doll R, Boddaert M, O'Grady P, Krekler M, Mangold B, and Christians U, Accumulation of lovastatin, but not pravastatin, in the blood of cyclosporine-treated kidney graft patients after multiple doses. *Clin Pharmacol Ther,* 1997. 62(3): p. 311-321.
[133] Newman CB, Palmer G, Silbershatz H, and Szarek M, Safety of atorvastatin derived from analysis of 44 completed trials in 9,416 patients. *Am J Cardiol,* 2003. 92(6): p. 670-676.
[134] Schrama YC, Hene RJ, de Jonge N, Joles JA, Van Rijn HJ, Bar DR, Ververs TF, Van Tol A, and Koomans HA, Efficacy and muscle safety of fluvastatin in cyclosporine-treated cardiac and renal transplant recipients: an exercise provocation test. *Transplantation*, 1998. 66(9): p. 1175-1181.
[135] Holdaas H, Hartmann A, Stenstrom J, Dahl KJ, Borge M, and Pfister P, Effect of fluvastatin for safely lowering atherogenic lipids in renal transplant patients receiving cyclosporine. *Am J Cardiol,* 1995. 76(2): p. 102A-106A.
[136] Vanhaecke J, Van Cleemput J, Van Lierde J, Daenen W, and De Geest H, Safety and efficacy of low dose simvastatin in cardiac transplant recipients treated with cyclosporine. *Transplantation,* 1994. 58(1): p. 42-45.

In: Hypertension: New Research
Editor: Elwood F. Benhagen, pp. 263-284
ISBN: 1-59454-204-X

Chapter X

HYPERTENSIVE NEPHROPATHY-PATHOGENETIC AND CLINICAL CONSIDERATIONS

Bolesław Rutkowski and Leszek Tylicki
Department of Nephrology, Transplantology and Internal Medicine;
Medical University of Gdansk, Poland

ABSTRACT

Essential hypertension is a world-wide disease affecting nowadays approximately 30-40% population in Western countries. The modern medicine limited cardiovascular complications and death rate in this population, and in turn, the mean life time of these patients was prolonged. Otherwise, the systematically increasing rate of kidney injury, another organ complication is observed.

The specific lesion of nephroangiosclarosis affects the medium and small-sized arteries up to the interlobular arteries. Arteriolosclerosis denotes lessions of the afferent and/or the efferent glomerular arterioles. The arcuate and interlobular arteries show myointimal hypertrophy, reduplication of the internal elastic lamina and hypertrophy of the media. The arterial/arteriolar wall is also thickened by hyaline, eosinophilic, PAS-positive deposites. In these places smooth muscle cells are atrophic. Intimal and media hypertrophy seems to play the most important role as far as the patient outcome is considered. In morphometric studies, it was demonstrated that glomerulosclerosis, interstitial volume, and creatinine clearance correlated with the presence of arterial muscular hypertrophy, but not with arterial/arteriolar. Along with arterial changes, glomeruli are usally ischaemic, with thickened and folded capillary walls. Numerous glomeruli are completely sclerotic presenting global glomerulosclerosis.

Possible pathways to transduce these forces into biochemical signals include ion channels, integrin interaction between cells and extracellular matrix, and activation of tyrosine kinases. In turn, synthesis of growth factors or mitogenic agonists is increased, among which angiotensin II, transforming growth factor (TGF) beta-1, and plasminogen-activator inhibitor type 1 (PAI 1) play the most important roles. Oxidative stress is also involved in this process where reactive oxygen species serve as signaling molecules.

According to this hypothesis the vascular injury leads to the development of progressive damage of subsequent kidney structures such as glomeruli, tubules and interstitium.

Essential hypertension is a world-wide disease affecting nowadays approximately 30-40% population in Western countries. The modern medicine limited cardiovascular complications and death rate in this population, and in turn, the mean life time of these patients was prolonged. Otherwise, the systematically increasing rate of kidney injury, another organ complication is observed [1]. The possibility that renal scaring and contraction may be the consequence of arterial hypertension was originally proposed by Frederick A. Mahomed from Guys Hospital in 1897 [2]. Some decades later Theodor Fahr detailed described this renal pathology as `benign nephrosclerosis` [3]. As this term stresses only interstitial fibrosis, a more detailed name `hypertensive nephroangiosclerosis` has been later suggested to indicate that renal arteries, the most important and specific component for this nephropathy, are involved. The clinical syndrome used to describe this condition has been termed `hypertensive nephropathy` (HN) or 'hypertensive kidney disease'. More recently, analysis of the impact of systolic hypertension among 334,000 men screened for the Multiple Risk Factor Intervention Trial (MRFIT) revealed that systolic blood pressure was an independent risk factor for all-cause ESRD [4]. Other studies such as Hypertension Detection and Follow Up Program (HDFP) [5], the Systolic Hypertension in the Elderly Program (SHEP) [6] report that systolic blood pressure is an independent risk factor for ESRD attributed to hypertension.

Histological Features

The specific lesion of nephroangiosclarosis affects the medium and small-sized arteries up to the interlobular arteries. Arteriolosclerosis denotes lessions of the afferent and/or the efferent glomerular arterioles. The previous are common but not obligatory in nephrosclerosis. The arcuate and interlobular arteries show myointimal hypertrophy, reduplication of the internal elastic lamina and hypertrophy of the media. They may display fibroelastic thickening. The arterial/arteriolar wall is also thickened by hyaline, eosinophilic, PAS-positive deposites. In these places smooth muscle cells are atrophic. Although the nature of the hyaline material has not been unequivocally established, immunofluorescence and electron microscopic findings favor it to be insudation of plasma into the arterial/arteriolar wall. The vascular lumen is narrowed. Intimal and media hypertrophy seems to play the most important role as far as the patient outcome is considered. In morphometric studies, it was demonstrated that glomerulosclerosis, interstitial volume, and creatinine clearance correlated with the presence of arterial muscular hypertrophy, but not with arterial/arteriolar hyalinosis or intimal thickening. Renal vascular lesion can be seen yet after 5 years of hypertension and occur in other arteries and arterioles in the body, but are most severe in the kidneys [7,8].

Along with arterial changes, glomeruli are usally ischaemic, with thickened and folded capillary walls. Numerous glomeruli are completely sclerotic presenting global glomerulosclerosis. The histological picture of focal glomerulosclerosis is also observed in some glomeruli as a consequence of increased intraglomerular pressure [7,8]. Some findings point to the racial differences in glomerular changes between Caucasians and African Americans. The later manifest significant increased percent of solidified glomeruli in the absence of the collagenous changes in the capsular space. In contrast, the percent of obsolescent glomeruli in which Bowman's space is occupied by collagenous, and the tuft is retracted is not usually different between African Americans and Caucasians. Whether these phenotypic differences might reflect differing mechanisms of tissue injury needs to be clarified. [9].

Table 1 . Morphological features of hypertensive nephropathy

structure	Changes
Kidneys	1 / kidney contraction 2 / granular kidney surface 3 / adhesion capsule to kidney surface 4 / thinner cortex
Arteries and arterioles Arterie interlobulares Arterie arcuate Afferent arterioles	1 / hyaline, eosinophilic deposits in arterial and arteriolar wall (under endothelium and in media). Degradation of smooth muscle cells in this place. 2 / reduplication of internal elastic lamina, myointimal hypertrophy, fibrous intimal thickening 3 / media hypertrophy
Interstitium	1 / increase fibrous connective tissue 2 / infiltration by lymphocytes and plasma cells
Tubules	1 / tubular atrophy 2 / thickening of the tubular basement membrane 2 / hyaline casts in the lumen
Glomeruli	The changes derived from intraglomerular hypertension (focal, segmental glomerulosclerosis) 1/ swelling of endothelial and visceral epithelial cells 2/ widening of the basement membrane 3/ fibrosis of capsule 4 / increase of mesangial matrix The changes derived from ischaemia (global glomerulosclerosis) 1/ collapse of the glomerular tuft 2/ wrinkling of the basement membrane 3/ decrease of mesangial cells 4/ increase of extracellular matrix

Many biopsy specimens exhibit focal tubular atrophy. Atrophic and microcystic tubules contain hyaline casts. In advanced stage of benign nephroangioslclerosis, extensive interstitial fibrosis is observed. The fibrotic interstitium is interspersed with inflammatory cells and the interstitial volume can increase even up to 60% of the renal cortex [7,8].

PATHOGENESIS

Non-immunological vascular injury is regarded classically as the initial tissue injury in hypertensive nephropathy. Mechanical forces related with blood flow, such as stretch and shear stress, may contribute to this process [10,11]. Possible pathways to transduce these forces into biochemical signals include ion channels, integrin interaction between cells and extracellular matrix, and activation of tyrosine kinases [11-13]. In turn, synthesis of growth factors or mitogenic agonists is increased, among which angiotensin II, transforming growth factor (TGF) beta-1, and plasminogen-activator inhibitor type 1 (PAI 1) play the most important roles. Oxidative stress is also involved in this process where reactive oxygen species serve as signaling molecules [14-19]. According to this hypothesis the vascular injury leads to the development of progressive damage of subsequent kidney structures such as glomeruli, tubules and interstitium.

Vascular injury may lead to progressive kidney damage via two possible pathways, ie. ischeamia and increased glomerular pressure. Ischaemia derives from the myointimal hypertrophy and fibroelastic changes in preglomerular vessels. Increased glomerular pressure and subsequent hyperfiltration is a result of disturbances in the mechanisms of intrarenal autoregulation due to lesion of myocytes of afferent arterioles that in turn leads to the transmittion of increased systemic blood pressure to glomerular capillary tuft. In addition, as a consequence of progressive loss of nephrons, compensatory glomerular hyperfiltration per nephron develops that in turn intensifies existing disturbances [20].

The mentioned-above paradigm is challenged by hypothesis suggesting that tubulo-interstitial compartment constitute the initial site of kidney injury. In two-kidney one clip rats Mai at al demonstrated that interstitial injury occurs early before glomerular changes become evident [21]. In hypertensive rats others observed increased lipid peroxidation in renal tubules but not in the vascular compartment much earlier than proteinuria or loss of renal function could be detected [22]. In this regard, we have recently shown increased urine excretion of tubular damage markers in patients with untreated primary hypertension without clinical signs of vascular and glomerular injury [23]. It could be supposed that tubulointerstitial inflammation yields cytokines, growth factors, vasoactive molecules and free oxygen radicals that contribute to development of arteriolar and glomerular lesions. Some authors go further and extend this hypothesis, assuming that subtle interstitial injury is not so much the manifestation of hypertensive kidney disease but rather the underlying reason for hypertension [24].

The hypothesis known as a perinatal programming is also taken into account. According to this intrauterine and perinatal events resulted in decrease of birth weight which may further predispose to development of essential hypertension as well as renal injury (reviewed in [25]). It is postulated that growth retarding influences, such as poor nutrition during pregnancy, may impact on the renal development. Reduction of nephron number, which was shown to be present in humans with low birth weight [26], may be followed by increase of single nephron glomerular pressure and glomerular filtration rate. Where this increase within single nephron is sustained, focal glomerusclerosis may occur, resulting in nephron loss [27]. Rats exposed to either high-level or low-level intrauterine food restriction exhibit reduced nephron number, increased glomerular diameter and early onset of glomerulosclerosis [28,29]. In the human study of Australian aborigines, an inverse association between birth weight and albuminuria, surrogate marker of early kidney involvement in numerous kidney diseases, including HN, was demonstrated [30]. Whether the programming is implicated in the pathogenesis of HN remains yet in the area of speculations. The findings reporting that African Americans, a population particularly predisposed to the primary hypertension and HN, have smaller kidney and larger glomerular volume seem to support this concept [31].

Risk Factors

The pathogenesis of HN and hypertensive ESRD is not completely clear also from another point of view. It was observed that some hypertensive patients show a decline in renal function despite adequate blood pressure control [32,33]. Additionally, pathological reports have revealed renal vascular changes familiar to HN in normotensive subjects [34,35]. Moreover, it remains to be elucidated why only some patients with hypertension develops progressive kidney damage. It could be that other factors than blood pressure contribute to the development of renal complications in the course of essential hypertension (reviewed in [36,37]).

Table 2. Factors involved in the development and progression of hypertensive nephroangiosclerosis

Risk factors
Black race
Age
Smoking
Genetic susceptibility
Hypothetical risk factors
Gender (male)
Metabolic disturbances:
Hyperlipidemia
Insulin resistance
Hyperuricemia
Hyperhomocysteinemia
Hantavirus infection
Heavy metals toxicity
Ochratoxin A
Cocaine abuse
Dietary salt intake
Nonsteroidal anti-inflammatory drugs abuse
Perinatal programming

The prevalence of HN and ESRD attributed to essential hypertension is higher in **black** than in white individuals [38]. Further, a greater histological severity of HN is usually observed in African Americans as compared to Caucasians [39]. Importantly, this relationship is independent from the time point of the biopsy, i.e. stage of nephropathy, and age of the patients. Further, several studies have shown that these racial differences could not be explained by the higher prevalence and greater severity of hypertension in African Americans, nor by socioeconomic status or decreased access to health care [40,41]. The excess renal scarring in blacks may be associated with genetic susceptibility and/or environmental amplification of mechanisms involved in the pathogenesis of HN.

Bleyer at al. evaluated clinical correlates of hypertensive ESRD [42]. **Age** was the factor most closely associated with this diagnosis among white patients. The incidence of HN as a cause of ESRD is greater in patients over 64 years old, reaching 31% as compared to 19.2% in younger patients [43]. Interestingly, the aging process affects the kidney similarly to the hypertension-related injury. Sclerosis and hyalinosis of arterial walls, glomerulosclerosis, atrophy of tubular epithelium and interstitial fibrosis are common morphologic lesions in the kidneys of elderly individuals [44].

Whether **gender** may be another risk factor for HN still remains matter of the debate. HN is more common in males [39,45,46]. Moreover, the incidence of impaired renal function is greater in males than in females despite adequate blood pressure control [5,32]. Unfortunately, many studies did not address gender as a risk factors for HN, other studies failed to confirm a relationship [47-49]. Conversely, an association between female gender and increased risk of hypertensive ESRD has been observed among blacks [37]. Despite a role for the androgens in mediating renal injury in renin-dependent hypertension was recently suggested [37], this issue needs to be evaluated in future studies

Strong evidence associating **cigarette smoking** and hypertensive kidney injury is available. The prevalence of microalbuminuria, an early marker of hypertension-related kidney involvement, is almost double in smoking as compared to nonsmoking lean patients with primary hypertension [50]. In a study of 442 patients with primary hypertension, smoking was the strongest predictor for microalbuminuria as well [37]. Regaldo et al. demonstrated that smoking is an independent risk factor for the decline of renal function in patients with severe hypertension [51]. Finally the strong association between smoking and hypertensive ESRD prevalence was confirmed [42]. How cigarette smoking induces renal injury and renal function impairment is still unclear. Hemodynamic and nonhemodynamic mechanisms are believed to be involved in this process. Stimulation of sympathetic nerve activity [52], intrarenal stimulation of endothelin-1 synthesis [53], disturbances of endothelial control of vascular tone and the release of endothelial-derived relaxing factors seem to play important roles in functional changes [54], i.e. increased renal vascular resistance and diminished renal plasma flow. Cigarette smoking also promotes development of atherosclerosis, which may enhance hypertensive renal injury. The mechanisms of smoking-related atherosclerosis include structural injury of endothelial cells [55], mitogenic influence of nicotine on the arterial smooth muscle cells [56], induction of the hypercoagulable state derived from increased platelet aggregation and fibrinogen plasma level [57]. Smoking-induced induction of the atherogenic lipoprotein profile was shown in animals [58]. Oxidative stress is probably another major player in the genesis of this process [59].

Development of HN parallels with systemic atherosclerosis. Tracy et al. observed a strong correlation between atherosclerotic vascular alterations and renal arteriolar hyalinosis [60]. Others confirmed close relationship between atherosclerosis and development of hypertensive ESRD [42]. It is hypothesized that factors known to promote atherosclerosis may also enhance the progression of hypertensive vascular damage at the kidney level. Insulin resistance, lipid and purine metabolic disturbances are **metabolic disturbances** frequently associated with primary hypertension in the cluster of abnormalities named syndrome X [61].

Lipid abnormalities seem to be really important risk factor for chronic kidney diseases [62,63]. There is a possible synergy between the elevated blood pressure and lipid abnormalities on hypertensive-related renal injury [64-66]. In the ARIC study, hypertrigliceridemia and low plasma levels of high-density lipoprotein were associated with the onset of hypertensive renal disease. Hypercholesterolemia was associated with the development of ESRD in the MRFIT [47]. In addition, hypercholesterolemia correlates with global glomerulosclerosis in patients with biopsy-proven hypertensive. The mechanisms of lipid-related renal injury include not only the promotion of glomerulosclerosis but also the development of interstitial inflammation and fibrosis [67]. Hyperlipidemia may also impair both arterial and arteriolar endothelial function, namely the production of a number potent vascular vasoactive substances [68,69].

Insulin resistance may also modulate the development of hypertension-related renal injury. This is indirectly suggested by the fact that hypertensive patients with hyperinsulinemia excrete greater amounts of urinary albumin [70,71]. Insulin may increase blood pressure through a variety of mechanisms, including enhancement of sympathetic activity and increased renal sodium retention [72,73]. Insulin may also induce glomerular hyperfiltration, tubular scaring and direct injury and dysfunction of endothelial cells [23,74,75].

Another possible risk factor is **hyperuricemia**. Meserli et al. have shown more severe renal vessels damage in hypertensive patients presenting with hyperuricemia than in those with normal uric acid serum concentration [76]. The presence of hyperuricemia is believed to influence on the development of proteinuria and a worse renal outcome in hypertensives [77]. In addition, a direct deleterious impact of purine metabolism abnormalities on tubulointerstitial compartments is also postulated. Morphological, post-mortem examination of kidneys obtained from patients with hypertension demonstrated interstitial uric acid deposits similar to those observed in gouty kidneys [78]. Moreover, even the subtle alterations of purine metabolism may affect tubular injury in patients with essential hypertension [23].

Hyperhomocysteinemia is commonly present in patients with essential hypertension and suggested to contribute to the development and progression of HN, independently of arterial pressure [79,80]. In this regard homocysteine-induced development of glomerulosclerosis has been observed both in Dahl salt-sensitive hypertensive rats, and in normotensive Sprague-Dawley rats [81]. The precise mechanism linking homocysteine with vascular damage is not fully understood. Direct influence of homocysteine on endothelial injury [82], endothelial dysfunction [83,84], smooth muscle cells proliferation [85], and enhancement of vascular monocyte adhesion may be involved [86].

Other possible factors contributing to the development of hypertension-related renal complications include exposure to heavy metals (ie. lead, cadmium) [87,88], fungal metabolite ochratoxin A [89,90], increase salt intake [50,91], abuse of nonsteroidal anti-inflammatory drugs and cocaine [92-94]. There is also an interesting hypothesis suggesting a possible causal association between asymptomatic infection with **Hantavirus** and development of HN. To verify this assumption, three distinct Baltimore populations, totaling

8,080 persons have been evaluated: healthy subjects, ESRD patients on maintenance hemodialysis therapy, and patients with proteinuria but normal renal function [95]. Patients with proteinuria were more commonly Hantavirus seropositive than the healthy group. Similarly, immunological markers of past Hantavirus infection among hemodialyzed patients were more common than in healthy persons. Strikingly, all the seropositive hemodialysis patients clustered among the 40% patients with HN. None were found among the other diagnoses. Hantaviruses are known to infect and injure vascular endothelial cells [96,97], and renal tubular cells [98]. Vascular dysfunction leading to severe vasodilatation and hypotension is believed as one of the most important renal deleterious effect exerted by these viruses, directly or indirectly related to immunological mechanisms [99].

Genetic Susceptibility

Genetic factors are believed to be at least partially responsible for renal complications of essential hypertension. Animal studies have documented that genetic factors could determine susceptibility to hypertension-related renal damage. The kidney of the Brown Norway rat (BNR) is much more susceptible to hypertension-induced damage than is the kidney of the spontaneously hypertensive rat (SHR). When the kidney of a normotensive BNR was transplanted to replace one kidney of SHR, the BNR kidney developed progressive glomerulosclerosis in response to hypertension even though the native SHR kidney was unaffected [100]. The transfer of chromosome 1 from BNR to SHR causes a significantly greater extent of renal vascular injury due to hypertension in comparison to the SHR progenitor strain [101]. Finally, a susceptibility gene for HN in the rat has been mapped [102].

There are also data which suggest that a genetic susceptibility exists also in humans. As compared to Caucasians, hypertension in African-Americans occurs earlier, is more severe, and more often causes ESRD even after adjustment for severity of hypertension [4,43]. Importantly, increased risk of hypertension-related ESRD in African-Americans persists even after statistical correction for environmental co-factors [4]. Finally, familial clustering of hypertensive ESRD has been demonstrated both in African-Americans [103] and in Caucasians [104] supporting the concept of renal susceptibility genes. Nevertheless, to data no gene or group of genes has been unequivocally linked to the development and progression of HN.

Genes of Renin-Angiotensin System

Candidate genes involved in the pathogenesis of progressive renal damage include the genes linked to the renin-angiotensin system. A few genes of this system have been examined [105-107], but only angiotensin-1 converting enzyme (ACE) insertion/deletion (I/D) polymorphism is believed to be clearly associated with increased risk of renal complications of essential hypertension. In a study of 45 patients with biopsy proven HN and two control groups with a total of 27,908 individuals, the proportion of subjects with the D allele (64%) was higher in the sample of studied patients than that in the control (54%) [108]. DD and DI genotypes were also more prevalent in the group with HN than in the control groups. Association of DD genotype with histopathologic-proven HN in Caucasian was also reported by others [109]. The physiological importance of these findings relies on the fact that the DD genotype is believed to be linked to increased circulating [110] and tissue [111] ACE levels.

Other Genes

Other possible candidate genes encode paracrine and autocoid agents that influence endothelial and smooth muscle response to increased pressure and blood flow in the afferent arterioles. In this way, renal ischemia may be enhanced or elevated blood pressure may be transferred to the glomeruli. Genes for kallikrein [112], nitric oxide synthase [113,114] and endothelins [115] are examples. A second group contains genes for cytokines and other factors that have been implicated in the inflammatory and fibrotic processes that occurr in the nephrosclerotic kidneys. Transforming growth factors, platelet-derived growth factor, epidermal growth factor, tumor necrosis factor and plasminogen-activator inhibitor type-1 are examples [116-118]. Polymorphism of the gene for the cytoskeleton protein adducin is currently of interest as well [119].

In the near future, the spectrum of evaluation may extend to genes connected with redox homeostasis. The total plasma antioxidant status seems to be under strong genetic control, especially among smokers [120], whereas it is well known that oxidative stress contributes in the molecular pathogenesis of HN [18]. Genetic abnormalities of programmed cell death may also determine development of HN [121]. It is likely that multiple genes of different systems are involved in the predisposition to renal inury in hypertenisves, and the future studies should identify such association.

CLINICAL COURSE

Patients with HN present with a long-lasting essential hypertension. Their family history on this point is also significant. They commonly present no complaints. The physical examination, with the exception of increased systemic blood pressure is usually unremarkable. Laboratory studies reveal normal urine sediment and proteinuria, most often in non-nephrotic range. Other hypertensive organ damage processes such as left ventricular hypertrophy and hypertensive retinopathy are observed as well [122].

In the absence of antihypertensive treatment, renal involvement was very frequent in primary hypertension. Perera described that proteinuria was present in 42%, and chronic renal failure in 18% of a series of 5000 patients followed until death [123]. With the advent of antihypertensive therapy the renal prognosis of hypertensive patients improved dramatically. Although the histopathological abnormalities of HN is present in hypertensives commonly [124], only very few patients (< 2%) develop progressive renal failure [125]. In addition the rate of progression of HN is relatively slow. The rate of decline in GFR is 1-2 ml/min/year that is the slowest value among common renal disease such as diabetic nephropathy (5-6 ml/min/year) and proteinuric nondiabetic nephropathies (6-8 ml/min), and may be additionally decrease by appropriate pharmacological management [126]. Nevertheless, data collected in the Figure 1 are showing that hypertensive nephropathy became really relevant clinical problem. In many countries nearly or even more than 1/3 of dialysed patients developed ESRD during the course of the primary hypertension [127]. This problem is especially characteristic to the group of elderly people. It is possible to draw a hypothesis that appearance of the increased number of patients with hypertensive nephropathy is the paradoxical effect of the successful antihypertensive therapy during last 10-15 years. Significantly diminished number of ischaemic heart disease and stroke cases was observed in USA in this period of time [128]. So those patients lived longer enough in order to develop hypertensive nephropathy. It is also obvious that in elderly patients presenting many factors able to induce renal injury additionally.

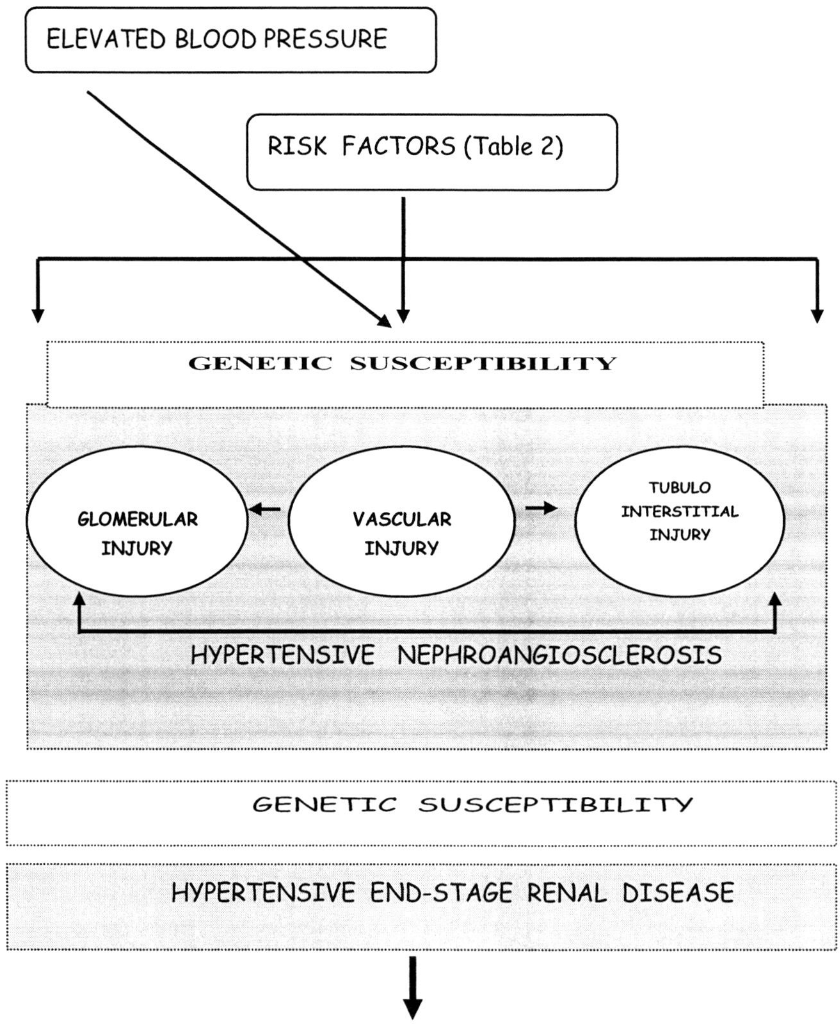

Figure 1. Diagram showing our impression on pathogenesis of hypertensive nephropathy

One should take into account, however, that so high percentage of hypertensive kidney disease as an underlying reason of ESRD in many national registries may be a little overestimated. In most reports the diagnosis of hypertensive nephrosclerosis is made on exclusively clinical grounds, without renal biopsy or any effective demonstration that hypertension preceded renal injury. Moreover, the insidious manifestation of hypertensive nephrosclerosis may well mimic those entities such as oligosymptomatic primary renal disease, renal atherosclerotic disease, cholesterol microembolization, and unnoticed episodes of malignant hypertension. A few large biopsy-based studies have addressed this problem. Zucchelli and Zuccala have shown "true" HN in 40-50% of patients clinically diagnosed as such [129,130]. Fogo et al. [45] have observed an 85% agreement between clinical diagnosis and histological diagnosis of HN in African Americans. Even if HN is misdiagnosed in some cases and its true incidence rate is smaller than reported, the consequent demand for replacement therapy is considerable given the high prevalence of hypertension. As such, it probably will tend to increase as patient survival improves.

Diagnosis

There is no rigorous definition of HN. Usually, this renal pathology is defined as nondiabetic chronic kidney disease associated with chronic hypertension, with or without moderate proteinuria, and with a pathologic picture characterized by arteriosclerosis, arteriolosclerosis, glomerulosclerosis, and interstitial fibrosis in the absence if immune deposites [20,126]. By definition, the diagnosis of HN should rest on histology, however, it is usually based solely on clinical grounds. Since the majority of HN patients are elderly and proteinuria, the predominant clinical sign, is commonly less than 0.5 g/24 h, a renal biopsy is usually not performed. A careful past history, family history, search for signs for target organ damage, such as left-ventricular hypertrophy and hypertensive retinal changes, careful urine microcopy, measurement of 24-hour urinary protein and performance of renal ultrasound should established the diagnosis, with additional tests for glomerulonephritis or vasculitic diseases if indicated [20,122]. The most commonly used clinical criteria for diagnosis is derived from Schlessinger et al. and includes (i) family history of hypertension (first degree relative), (ii) left ventricular hypertrophy, (iii) proteinuria (<500 mg/24h), (iv) long-lasting hypertension (systolic blood pressure $\geq$ 140 mmHg and/or diastolic blood pressure $\geq$ 90 mmHg) preceding any evidence of renal disease, and (v) absence of nephrotoxin exposure, congenital or intrinsic renal disease, or systemic illness associated with renal disease [131]. Renal biopsy should be considered in all doubt cases, e.g., when patients do not have accelerated hypertension or a long history of hypertension preceding the onset of proteinuria and whose 24-h urine protein excretion exceeds 1.5 g/24h. Unfortunately, in cases in which the patient is seen initially with hypertension and advanced chronic renal failure, the differential diagnosis can be difficult or even impossible [132].

During differential diagnosis a particular attention should be drawn on the exclusion of primary renal diseases and systemic diseases affecting kidneys. One should point to such pathological entities as glomerulopathies, interstitial nephritis and atherosclerotic renal disease, which may mimic clinical course of HN. In these cases kidney injury may occur independently on essential hypertension, otherwise, hypertension may be secondary to processes of renal damage. In Table 3 the main confounding diagnoses are listed and the appropriate diagnostic approach is recommended to differentiate these entities [122,132].

Treatment

There is no specific therapy of hypertensive nephropathy. The management consists of the treatment of elevated systemic blood pressure. Clinical trials on management of hypertensive nephropathy are few. Only the AASK study prospectively examined the impact of clinical management on renal outcomes in patients with HN [133]. This study enrolling patients with a clinical diagnosis of HN followed for up to 5 years revealed no significant difference between conventional and aggressive blood pressure lowering strategy on the rate of decline in glomerular filtration. Nevertheless, patients with chronic kidney diseases are at high cardiovascular risk and these both aspects should be taken into account when the therapeutic strategy is considered. The current recommendations derive from the 7th Report of Joint National Committee on Prevention Detection and Management of Hypertension and Guidelines on Management of Hypertension elaborated by WHO and International Society of Hypertension in 2003 [134,135]. Considering a hypertensive nephropathy as an organ damage, patients with such diagnosis belong to the group of high or very-high cardiovascular risk. Therefore, the antihypertensive pharmacological therapy should be commenced without any delay along with standard nonpharmacological management including life-style modifying approaches such as smoking cessation, weight reduction, dietary fat and sodium restriction, physical activity program (physical exercise minimum 30 minutes per day), and introduction to the diet more fruits, vegetables and fishes. The target blood pressure in patients with proteinuria greater than 1 g/24 hours should be less than 125/75 mmHg, otherwise less than 130/80 mmHg. The patients with renal failure should be treated even yet when the high normal blood pressure is diagnosed (130-140/85-90) to the target blood pressure less than 130/80.

Table 3. Differential diagnosis of hypertensive nephropathy

Glomerulonephritis	- greater proteinuria, nephrotic syndrome - erythrocyturia, urine blood casts **[diagnosis is based on renal biopsy]**
Interstitial nephritis	- leucocyturia, urine leucocyte casts - deformity of renal calyxes, cicatrisation of renal cortex - positive urine culture **[diagnosis is based on imaging examination or renal biopsy]**
Atherosclerotic renal disease	- clinical signs of atherosclerosis in other organs - asymmetry of kidney size **[diagnosis is based on imaging examination - doppler ulrasonography, arteriography]**
Cholesterol embolisation	- history of vascular intervention, fibrinolytic therapy **[diagnosis is based on skin/muscle/kidney biospy]**

There is no doubt that blood pressure lowering leads to slower rate of decline in renal function independently on the antihypertensive medication class was used. The increasing body of evidence suggests, however, that agents inhibiting renin-angiotensin system such as angiotensin converting enzyme inhibitors retard the progressive course of chronic kidney diseases much more effectively than antihypertensive medications from other classes [136]. The renoprotective efficacy of angiotensin-converting enzyme inhibitors (ACEIs) has been demonstrated both in diabetic and non-diabetic renal diseases [137,138]. The AASK was the first study that demonstrated that ACEIs should be antihypertensive drugs of choice also in patients with hypertensive nephropathy [139]. The study showed that therapy with ramipril, as compared to amlodipine, leads to a 38% risk reduction for the combined outcome of rapidly declining GFR, ESRD and death, and a 22% risk reduction as compared to metoprolol. This beneficial renal outcome is determined by several specific hemodynamic and non-hemodynamic properties of ACEIs, such as preferential dilatation of renal efferent arterioles that reduces intraglomerular pressure, the improvement of glomerular barrier permselectivity and the inhibition of local inflammation process [136]. One may hypothesize that angiotensin II type 1 receptor antagonists, another class of drugs inhibiting renin-angiotensin system at the level of receptor possesses the similar properties. Their renoprotective potential was also considered but yet proved only in patients with diabetic nephropathy [140]. The fact that ACEIs and ARAs antagonize the RAS at different levels, synthesis and receptor, suggests that these agents used in combination may have additive effects that result in even greater renoprotection when used in combination. Indeed, in patients with non-diabetic renal disease, the combination treatment with concomitant use of agents from both classes was recently proven to have a higher renoprotective efficacy than monotherapy with either drug alone (COOPERATE Study) [141].

It is necessary to mention that there are also studies underlying renoprototective properties of statins in subjects with HN [142,143]. Detailed information in this regard are shpown in special chapter of this issue.

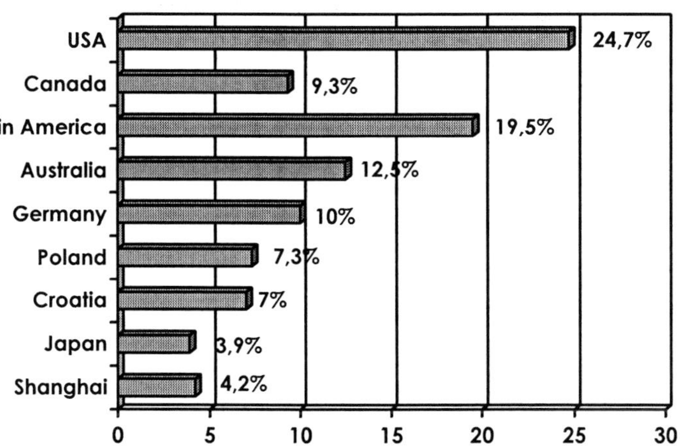

Figure 2. Hypertensive nephropathy as an underlying reason of end-stage renal disease among patients treated with dialysis in different parts of the world [144].

REFERENCES

[1] Rutkowski B, Tylicki L, Debska-Slizien A: Pathogenetic and epidemiological aspects of hypertenisve nephropathy. *Pol Arch Med Wewn* 2003;110:1167-1171

[2] Cameron JS, Hicks J: Frederick Akbar Mohamed and his role in the description of hypertension at Guy's Hospital. *Kidney Int* 1996;49:1488

[3] Fahr T: Über Nephrosklerose. *Virchows Arch* 1919;26:119-178

[4] Klag MJ, Whelton PK, Randall BL, Neaton JD, Brancati FL, Stamler J: End-stage renal disease in African-American and white men. 16-year MRFIT findings. *JAMA* 1997;277:1293-1298

[5] Shulman NB, Ford CE, Hall WD, Blaufox MD, Simon D, Langford HG, Schneider KA: Prognostic value of serum creatinine and effect of treatment of hypertension on renal function. Results from the hypertension detection and follow-up program. The Hypertension Detection and Follow-up Program Cooperative Group. *Hypertension* 1989;13:I80-93

[6] Young JH, Klag MJ, Muntner P, Whyte JL, Pahor M, Coresh J: Blood pressure and decline in kidney function: findings from the Systolic Hypertension in the Elderly Program (SHEP). *J Am Soc Nephrol* 2002;13:2776-2782

[7] Tracy RE, Ishii T: What is 'nephrosclerosis'? Lessons from the US, Japan, and Mexico. *Nephrol Dial Transplant* 2000;15:1357-1366

[8] Takebayashi S, Kiyoshi Y, Hisano S, Uesugi N, Sasatomi Y, Meng J, Sakata N: Benign nephrosclerosis: incidence, morphology and prognosis. *Clin Nephrol* 2001;55:349-356

[9] Fogo A: Hypertensive risk factors in kidney disease in African Americans. *Kidney Int Suppl* 2003*;63* (Suppl. 83):S17-S21

[10] Lehoux S, Tedgui A: Signal transduction of mechanical stresses in the vascular wall. *Hypertension* 1998;32:338-345

[11] Davis MJ, Donovitz JA, Hood JD: Stretch-activated single-channel and whole cell currents in vascular smooth muscle cells. *Am J Physiol* 1992;262:C1083-1088

[12] Muller JM, Chilian WM, Davis MJ: Integrin signaling transduces shear stress--dependent vasodilation of coronary arterioles. *Circ Res* 1997;80:320-326

[13] Reusch HP, Chan G, Ives HE, Nemenoff RA: Activation of JNK/SAPK and ERK by mechanical strain in vascular smooth muscle cells depends on extracellular matrix composition. *Biochem Biophys Res Commun* 1997;237:239-244

[14] Suzuki H, DeLano FA, Parks DA, Jamshidi N, Granger DN, Ishii H, Suematsu M, Zweifach BW, Schmid-Schonbein GW: Xanthine oxidase activity associated with arterial blood pressure in spontaneously hypertensive rats. *Proc Natl Acad Sci U S A* 1998;95:4754-4759

[15] Ruiz-Ortega M, Bustos C, Hernandez-Presa MA, Lorenzo O, Plaza JJ, Egido J: Angiotensin II participates in mononuclear cell recruitment in experimental immune complex nephritis through nuclear factor-kappa B activation and monocyte chemoattractant protein-1 synthesis. *J Immunol* 1998;161:430-439

[16] Oikawa T, Freeman M, Lo W, Vaughan DE, Fogo A: Modulation of plasminogen activator inhibitor-1 in vivo: a new mechanism for the anti-fibrotic effect of renin-angiotensin inhibition. *Kidney Int* 1997;51:164-172

[17] Tummala PE, Chen XL, Sundell CL, Laursen JB, Hammes CP, Alexander RW, Harrison DG, Medford RM: Angiotensin II induces vascular cell adhesion molecule-1 expression in rat vasculature: A potential link between the renin-angiotensin system and atherosclerosis. *Circulation* 1999;100:1223-1229

[18] Trolliet MR, Rudd MA, Loscalzo J: Oxidative stress and renal dysfunction in salt-sensitive hypertension. *Kidney Blood Press Res* 2001;24:116-123

[19] Laursen JB, Rajagopalan S, Galis Z, Tarpey M, Freeman BA, Harrison DG: Role of superoxide in angiotensin II-induced but not catecholamine-induced hypertension. *Circulation* 1997;95:588-593

[20] Luke RG: Hypertensive nephrosclerosis: pathogenesis and prevalence. Essential hypertension is an important cause of end-stage renal disease. *Nephrol Dial Transplant* 1999;14:2271-2278

[21] Mai M, Geiger H, Hilgers KF, Veelken R, Mann JF, Dammrich J, Luft FC: Early interstitial changes in hypertension-induced renal injury. *Hypertension* 1993;22:754-765

[22] Bapat S, Post J, Braam B, Goldschmeding R, Koomans H, Verkleij A, Joles J: Visualizing tubular lipid peroxidation in intact renal tissue in hypertensive rats. *J Am Soc Nephrol* 2002;12:2990-2996

[23] Tylicki L, Manitius J, Lysiak-Szydlowska W, Rutkowski B: Tubular injury - the first symptom of hypertensive kidney involvement? *Med Sci Monit* 2003;9:CR135-CR141

[24] Johnson R, Herrera-Acosta J, Schreiner G, Rodriguez-Iturbe B: Subtle acquired renal injury as a mechanism of salt-sensitive hypertension. *N Engl J Med* 2002;346:913-923

[25] Marchand M, Langley-Evans S: Intrauterine programming of nephron number: the fetal flaw revisited. *J Nephrol* 2001;14:327-331

[26] Manalich R, Reyes L, Herrera M, Melendi C, Fundora I: Relationship between weight at birth and the number and size of renal glomeruli in humans: a histomorphometric study. *Kidney Int* 2000;58:770-773

[27] McGraw M, Poucell S, Sweet J, Baumal R: The significance of focal segmental glomerulosclerosis in oligomeganephronia. *Int J Pediatr Nephrol* 1984;5:67-72

[28] Lucas R, Miraglia SM, Zaladek Gil F, Machado Coimbra T: Intrauterine food restriction as a determinant of nephrosclerosis. *Am J Kidney Dis* 2001;37:467-476

[29] Langley-Evans S, Welham S, Jackson A: Fetal exposure to a maternal low protein diet impairs nephrogenesis and promotes hypertension in the rat. *Life Sci* 1999;64:965-974

[30] Hoy W, Mathews J, McCredie D, Pugsley D, Hayhurst B, Rees M, Kile E, Walker K, Wang Z: The multidimensional nature of renal disease: rates and associations of albuminuria in an Australian Aboriginal community. *Kidney Int* 1998;54:1296-1304

[31] Pesce C, Schmidt K, Fogo A, Okoye M, Kim R, Striker L, Striker G: Glomerular size and the incidence of renal disease in African Americans and Caucasians. *J Nephrol* 1994;7:355-358

[32] Rostand SG, Brown G, Kirk KA, Rutsky EA, Dustan HP: Renal insufficiency in treated essential hypertension. *N Engl J Med* 1989;320:684-688

[33] Toto RD, Mitchell HC, Smith RD, Lee HC, McIntire D, Pettinger WA: "Strict" blood pressure control and progression of renal disease in hypertensive nephrosclerosis. *Kidney Int* 1995;48:851-859

[34] Fisher ER, Pirog J: Renal arteriolar obstruction without hypertension. *Nephron* 1976;16:433-438

[35] Kim HS, Krege JH, Kluckman KD, Hagaman JR, Hodgin JB, Best CF, Jennette JC, Coffman TM, Maeda N, Smithies O: Genetic control of blood pressure and the angiotensinogen locus. *Proc Natl Acad Sci U S A* 1995;92:2735-2739

[36] Tylicki L, Rutkowski B, Horl W: Multifactorial determination of hypertensive nephroangiosclerosis. *Kidney Blood Press Res* 2002;25:241-353

[37] Bleyer AJ, Appel RG: Risk factors associated with hypertensive nephrosclerosis. *Nephron* 1999;82:193-198

[38] Tracy R, Bhandaru S, Oalmann M, Guzman M, Newman W: Blood pressure and nephrosclerosis in black and white men and woman aged 25-54. *Mod Pathol* 1991;4:602-609

[39] Marcantoni C, Ma LJ, Federspiel C, Fogo AB: Hypertensive nephrosclerosis in African Americans versus Caucasians. *Kidney Int* 2002;62:172-180

[40] Whittle JC, Whelton PK, Seidler AJ, Klag MJ: Does racial variation in risk factors explain black-white differences in the incidence of hypertensive end-stage renal disease? *Arch Intern Med* 1991;151:1359-1364

[41] Freedman BI, Spray BJ, Tuttle AB, Buckalew VM, Jr.: The familial risk of end-stage renal disease in African Americans. *Am J Kidney Dis* 1993;21:387-393

[42] Bleyer AJ, Chen R, D'Agostino RB, Jr., Appel RG: Clinical correlates of hypertensive end-stage renal disease. *Am J Kidney Dis* 1998;31:28-34

[43] System EfUSRD: 1999 Annual Data Report. *Am J Kidney Dis* 1999;34:S1-176

[44] Moritz A, Oldt M: Arteriolar sclerosis in hypertensive and non-hypertensive individuals. *Am J Pathol* 1937;13:679-728

[45] Fogo A, Breyer JA, Smith MC, Cleveland WH, Agodoa L, Kirk KA, Glassock R: Accuracy of the diagnosis of hypertensive nephrosclerosis in African Americans: a report from the African American Study of Kidney Disease (AASK) Trial. AASK Pilot Study Investigators. *Kidney Int* 1997;51:244-252

[46] Caetano ER, Zatz R, Saldanha LB, Praxedes JN: Hypertensive nephrosclerosis as a relevant cause of chronic renal failure. *Hypertension* 2001;38:171-176

[47] Klag MJ, Whelton PK, Randall BL, Neaton JD, Brancati FL, Ford CE, Shulman NB, Stamler J: Blood pressure and end-stage renal disease in men. *N Engl J Med* 1996;334:13-18

[48] Perry HM, Jr., Miller JP, Fornoff JR, Baty JD, Sambhi MP, Rutan G, Moskowitz DW, Carmody SE: Early predictors of 15-year end-stage renal disease in hypertensive patients. *Hypertension* 1995;25:587-594

[49] Schmieder RE, Veelken R, Gatzka CD, Ruddel H, Schachinger H: Predictors for hypertensive nephropathy: results of a 6-year follow-up study in essential hypertension. *J Hypertens* 1995;13:357-365

[50] Mimran A, Ribstein J, DuCailar G, Halimi JM: Albuminuria in normals and essential hypertension. *J Diabetes Complications* 1994;8:150-156

[51] Regalado M, Yang S, Wesson DE: Cigarette smoking is associated with augmented progression of renal insufficiency in severe essential hypertension. *Am J Kidney Dis* 2000;35:687-694

[52] Benowitz NL, Kuyt F, Jacob P, 3rd: Influence of nicotine on cardiovascular and hormonal effects of cigarette smoking. *Clin Pharmacol Ther* 1984;36:74-81

[53] Gambaro G, Verlato F, Budakovic A, Casara D, Saladini G, Del Prete D, Bertaglia G, Masiero M, Checchetto S, Baggio B: Renal impairment in chronic cigarette smokers. *J Am Soc Nephrol* 1998;9:562-567

[54] Celermajer DS, Adams MR, Clarkson P, Robinson J, McCredie R, Donald A, Deanfield JE: Passive smoking and impaired endothelium-dependent arterial dilatation in healthy young adults. *N Engl J Med* 1996;334:150-154

[55] Bylock A, Bondjers G, Jansson I, Hansson HA: Surface ultrastructure of human arteries with special reference to the effects of smoking. *Acta Pathol Microbiol Scand* [A] 1979;87A:201-209

[56] Carty C, Huribal M, Marsan B, Ricotta J, Dryjski M: Nicotine and its metabolite cotinine are mitogenic for human vascular smooth muscle cells. *J Vasc Surg* 1997;25:682-688

[57] Kannel WB, D'Agostino RB, Belanger AJ: Fibrinogen, cigarette smoking, and risk of cardiovascular disease: insights from the Framingham Study. *Am Heart J* 1987;113:1006-1010

[58] Cluette-Brown J, Mulligan J, Doyle K, Hagan S, Osmolski T, Hojnacki J: Oral nicotine induces an atherogenic lipoprotein profile. *Proc Soc Exp Biol Med* 1986;182:409-413

[59] Heitzer T, Just H, Munzel T: Antioxidant vitamin C improves endothelial dysfunction in chronic smokers. *Circulation* 1996;94:6-9

[60] Tracy RE, Strong JP, Newman WP, 3rd, Malcom GT, Oalmann MC, Guzman MA: Renovasculopathies of nephrosclerosis in relation to atherosclerosis at ages 25 to 54 years. *Kidney Int* 1996;49:564-570

[61] Zavaroni I, Bonini L, Fantuzzi M, Dall`Aglio E, Passeri M, Reaven G: Hyperinsulinaemia, obesity, and syndrome X. *J Intern Med* 1994;235:51-56

[62] Moorhead JF, Chan MK, El-Nahas M, Varghese Z: Lipid nephrotoxicity in chronic progressive glomerular and tubulo-interstitial disease. *Lancet* 1982;2:1309-1311

[63] Keane WF, Kasiske BL, O'Donnell MP, Kim Y: Hypertension, hyperlipidemia, and renal damage. *Am J Kidney Dis* 1993;21:43-50

[64] Tolins JP, Stone BG, Raij L: Interactions of hypercholesterolemia and hypertension in initiation of glomerular injury. *Kidney Int* 1992;41:1254-1261

[65] Kasiske B, O'Donnell M, Cowardin W, Keane W: Lipids and the kidney. *Hypertension* 1990;15:443-450

[66] Grone HJ, Walli A, Grone E, Niedmann P, Thiery J, Seidel D, Helmchen U: Induction of glomerulosclerosis by dietary lipids. A functional and morphologic study in the rat. *Lab Invest* 1989;60:433-446

[67] Eddy AA: Interstitial inflammation and fibrosis in rats with diet-induced hypercholesterolemia. *Kidney Int* 1996;50:1139-1149

[68] Kugiyama K, Kerns SA, Morrisett JD, Roberts R, Henry PD: Impairment of endothelium-dependent arterial relaxation by lysolecithin in modified low-density lipoproteins. *Nature* 1990;344:160-162

[69] Yamamoto H, Bossaller C, Cartwright J, Jr., Henry PD: Videomicroscopic demonstration of defective cholinergic arteriolar vasodilation in atherosclerotic rabbit. *J Clin Invest* 1988;81:1752-1758

[70] Bianchi S, Bigazzi R, Valtriani C, Chiapponi I, Sgherri G, Baldari G, Natali A, Ferrannini E, Campese VM: Elevated serum insulin levels in patients with essential hypertension and microalbuminuria. *Hypertension* 1994;23:681-687

[71] Bianchi S, Bigazzi R, Quinones Galvan A, Muscelli E, Baldari G, Pecori N, Ciociaro D, Ferrannini E, Natali A: Insulin resistance in microalbuminuric hypertension. Sites and mechanisms. *Hypertension* 1995;26:789-795

[72] Christensen NJ, Gundersen HJ, Hegedus L, Jacobsen F, Mogensen CE, Osterby R, Vittinghus E: Acute effects of insulin on plasma noradrenaline and the cardiovascular system. *Metabolism* 1980;29:1138-1145

[73] DeFronzo RA, Cooke CR, Andres R, Faloona GR, Davis PJ: The effect of insulin on renal handling of sodium, potassium, calcium, and phosphate in man. *J Clin Invest* 1975;55:845-855

[74] Dengel DR, Goldberg AP, Mayuga RS, Kairis GM, Weir MR: Insulin resistance, elevated glomerular filtration fraction, and renal injury. *Hypertension* 1996;28:127-132

[75] Pedrinelli R, Giampietro O, Carmassi F, Melillo E, Dell'Omo G, Catapano G, Matteucci E, Talarico L, Morale M, De Negri F, et al.: Microalbuminuria and endothelial dysfunction in essential hypertension. *Lancet* 1994;344:14-18

[76] Messerli FH, Frohlich ED, Dreslinski GR, Suarez DH, Aristimuno GG: Serum uric acid in essential hypertension: an indicator of renal vascular involvement. *Ann Intern Med* 1980;93:817-821

[77] Ruilope LM, Alcazar JM, Hernandez E, Moreno F, Martinez MA, Rodicio JL: Does an adequate control of blood pressure protect the kidney in essential hypertension? *J Hypertens* 1990;8:525-531

[78] Cannon PJ, Stason WB, Demartini FE, Sommers SC, Laragh JH: Hyperuricemia in primary and renal hypertension. *N Engl J Med* 1966;275:457-464

[79] Lip GY, Edmunds E, Martin SC, Jones AF, Blann AD, Beevers DG: A pilot study of homocyst(e)ine levels in essential hypertension: relationship to von Willebrand factor, an index of endothelial damage. *Am J Hypertens* 2001;14:627-631

[80] Mendis S, Athauda SB, Naser M, Takahashi K: Association between hyperhomocysteinaemia and hypertension in Sri Lankans. *J Int Med Res* 1999;27:38-44

[81] Li N, Chen YF, Zou AP: Implications of hyperhomocysteinemia in glomerular sclerosis in hypertension. *Hypertension* 2002;39:443-448

[82] Starkebaum G, Harlan JM: Endothelial cell injury due to copper-catalyzed hydrogen peroxide generation from homocysteine. *J Clin Invest* 1986;77:1370-1376

[83] Celermajer DS, Sorensen K, Ryalls M, Robinson J, Thomas O, Leonard JV, Deanfield JE: Impaired endothelial function occurs in the systemic arteries of children with homozygous homocystinuria but not in their heterozygous parents. *J Am Coll Cardiol* 1993;22:854-858

[84] Rolland PH, Friggi A, Barlatier A, Piquet P, Latrille V, Faye MM, Guillou J, Charpiot P, Bodard H, Ghiringhelli O, et al.: Hyperhomocysteinemia-induced vascular damage in the minipig. Captopril-hydrochlorothiazide combination prevents elastic alterations. *Circulation* 1995;91:1161-1174

[85] Buemi M, Marino D, Di Pasquale G, Floccari F, Ruello A, Aloisi C, Corica F, Senatore M, Romeo A, Frisina N: Effects of homocysteine on proliferation, necrosis, and apoptosis of vascular smooth muscle cells in culture and influence of folic acid. *Thromb Res* 2001;104:207-213

[86] Koga T, Claycombe K, Meydani M: Homocysteine increases monocyte and T-cell adhesion to human aortic endothelial cells. *Atherosclerosis* 2002;161:365-374

[87] Batuman V, Landy E, Maesaka JK, Wedeen RP: Contribution of lead to hypertension with renal impairment. *N Engl J Med* 1983;309:17-21

[88] Umemura T: Experimental reproduction of itai-itai disease, a chronic cadmium poisoning of humans, in rats and monkeys. *Jpn J Vet Res* 2000;48:15-28

[89] Schaaf GJ, Nijmeijer SM, Maas RF, Roestenberg P, de Groene EM, Fink-Gremmels J: The role of oxidative stress in the ochratoxin A-mediated toxicity in proximal tubular cells. *Biochim Biophys Acta* 2002;1588:149

[90] Gekle M, Silbernagl S: Mechanism of ochratoxin A-induced reduction of glomerular filtration rate in rats. *J Pharmacol Exp Ther* 1993;267:316-321

[91] Messerli FH, Schmieder RE, Weir MR: Salt. A perpetrator of hypertensive target organ disease? *Arch Intern Med* 1997;157:2449-2452

[92] Toto RD, Anderson SA, Brown-Cartwright D, Kokko JP, Brater DC: Effects of acute and chronic dosing of NSAIDs in patients with renal insufficiency. *Kidney Int* 1986;30:760-768

[93] Fogo A, Superdock KR, Atkinson JB: Severe arteriosclerosis in the kidney of a cocaine addict. *Am J Kidney Dis* 1992;20:513-515

[94] Norris KC, Thornhill-Joynes M, Tareen N: Cocaine use and chronic renal failure. *Semin Nephrol* 2001;21:362-366

[95] Glass GE, Watson AJ, LeDuc JW, Kelen GD, Quinn TC, Childs JE: Infection with a ratborne hantavirus in US residents is consistently associated with hypertensive renal disease. *J Infect Dis* 1993;167:614-620

[96] Pensiero MN, Sharefkin JB, Dieffenbach CW, Hay J: Hantaan virus infection of human endothelial cells. *J Virol* 1992;66:5929-5936

[97] Hautala T, Sironen T, Vapalahti O, Paakko E, Sarkioja T, Salmela PI, Vaheri A, Plyusnin A, Kauma H: Hypophyseal hemorrhage and panhypopituitarism during Puumala Virus Infection: Magnetic Resonance Imaging and detection of viral antigen in the hypophysis. *Clin Infect Dis* 2002;35:96-101

[98] Kim S, Kang ET, Kim YG, Han JS, Lee JS, Kim YI, Hall WC, Dalrymple JM, Peters CJ: Localization of Hantaan viral envelope glycoproteins by monoclonal antibodies in renal tissues from patients with Korean hemorrhagic fever H. *Am J Clin Pathol* 1993;100:398-403

[99] Park J, Kim S, Lee J, Lee M: Circulating immune complexes in Korean hemorrhagic fever. *Seoul J Med* 1986;26:143-153

[100] Churchill PC, Churchill MC, Bidani AK, Griffin KA, Picken M, Pravenec M, Kren V, St Lezin E, Wang JM, Wang N, Kurtz TW: Genetic susceptibility to hypertension-induced renal damage in the rat. Evidence based on kidney-specific genome transfer. *J Clin Invest* 1997;100:1373-1382

[101] St Lezin E, Griffin KA, Picken M, Churchill MC, Churchill PC, Kurtz TW, Liu W, Wang N, Kren V, Zidek V, Pravenec M, Bidani AK: Genetic isolation of a chromosome 1 region affecting susceptibility to hypertension-induced renal damage in the spontaneously hypertensive rat. *Hypertension* 1999;34:187-191

[102] Brown DM, Provoost AP, Daly MJ, Lander ES, Jacob HJ: Renal disease susceptibility and hypertension are under independent genetic control in the fawn-hooded rat. *Nat Genet* 1996;12:44-51

[103] Freedman BI, Soucie JM, McClellan WM: Family history of end-stage renal disease among incident dialysis patients. *J Am Soc Nephrol* 1997;8:1942-1945

[104] O'Dea DF, Murphy SW, Hefferton D, Parfrey PS: Higher risk for renal failure in first-degree relatives of white patients with end-stage renal disease: a population-based study. *Am J Kidney Dis* 1998;32:794-801

[105] Fernandez-Llama P, Poch E, Oriola J, Botey A, Rivera F, Revert L: Angiotensinogen gene M235T and T174M polymorphisms in essential hypertension: relation with target organ damage. *Am J Hypertens* 1998;11:439-444

[106] Chaves FJ, Pascual JM, Rovira E, Armengod ME, Redon J: Angiotensin II AT1 receptor gene polymorphism and microalbuminuria in essential hypertension. *Am J Hypertens* 2001;14:364-370

[107] Pontremoli R, Sofia A, Tirotta A, Ravera M, Nicolella C, Viazzi F, Bezante GP, Borgia L, Bobola N, Ravazzolo R, Sacchi G, Deferrari G: The deletion polymorphism of the angiotensin I-converting enzyme gene is associated with target organ damage in essential hypertension. *J Am Soc Nephrol* 1996;7:2550-2558

[108] Mallamaci F, Zuccala A, Zoccali C, Testa A, Gaggi R, Spoto B, Martorano C, Curatola A, Misefari V, Cuzzola F, Romeo G, Zucchelli P: The deletion polymorphism of the angiotensin-converting enzyme is associated with nephroangiosclerosis. *Am J Hypertens* 2000;13:433-437

[109] Fernandez-Llama P, Poch E, Oriola J, Botey A, Coll E, Darnell A, Rivera F, Revert L: Angiotensin converting enzyme gene I/D polymorphism in essential hypertension and nephroangiosclerosis. *Kidney Int* 1998;53:1743-1747

[110] Rigat B, Hubert C, Alhenc-Gelas F, Cambien F, Corvol P, Soubrier F: An insertion/deletion polymorphism in the angiotensin I-converting enzyme gene accounting for half the variance of serum enzyme levels. *J Clin Invest* 1990;86:1343-1346

[111] Danser AH, Schalekamp MA, Bax WA, van den Brink AM, Saxena PR, Riegger GA, Schunkert H: Angiotensin-converting enzyme in the human heart. Effect of the deletion/insertion polymorphism. *Circulation* 1995;92:1387-1388

[112] Yu H, Song Q, Freedman BI, Chao J, Chao L, Rich SS, Bowden DW: Association of the tissue kallikrein gene promoter with ESRD and hypertension. *Kidney Int* 2002;61:1030-1039

[113] Asakimori Y, Yorioka N, Yamamoto I, Okumoto S, Doi S, Hirai T, Taniguchi Y: Endothelial nitric oxide synthase intron 4 polymorphism influences the progression of renal disease. *Nephron* 2001;89:219-223

[114] Wang Y, Kikuchi S, Suzuki H, Nagase S, Koyama A: Endothelial nitric oxide synthase gene polymorphism in intron 4 affects the progression of renal failure in non-diabetic renal diseases. *Nephrol Dial Transplant* 1999;14:2898-2902

[115] Freedman BI, Yu H, Anderson PJ, Roh BH, Rich SS, Bowden DW: Genetic analysis of nitric oxide and endothelin in end-stage renal disease. *Nephrol Dial Transplant* 2000;15:1794-1800

[116] Freedman BI, Yu H, Spray BJ, Rich SS, Rothschild CB, Bowden DW: Genetic linkage analysis of growth factor loci and end-stage renal disease in African Americans. *Kidney Int* 1997;51:819-825

[117] Gardemann A, Lohre J, Katz N, Tillmanns H, Hehrlein FW, Haberbosch W: The 4G4G genotype of the plasminogen activator inhibitor 4G/5G gene polymorphism is associated with coronary atherosclerosis in patients at high risk for this disease. *Thromb Haemost* 1999;82:1121-1126

[118] Eriksson P, Kallin B, van 't Hooft FM, Bavenholm P, Hamsten A: Allele-specific increase in basal transcription of the plasminogen-activator inhibitor 1 gene is associated with myocardial infarction. *Proc Natl Acad Sci U S A* 1995;92:1851-1855

[119] Nicod J, Frey BM, Frey FJ, Ferrari P: Role of the alpha-adducin genotype on renal disease progression. *Kidney Int* 2002;61:1270-1275

[120] Wang XL, Rainwater DL, VandeBerg JF, Mitchell BD, Mahaney MC: Genetic contributions to plasma total antioxidant activity. *Arterioscler Thromb Vasc Biol* 2001;21:1190-1195
[121] Ying WZ, Wang PX, Sanders PW: Induction of apoptosis during development of hypertensive nephrosclerosis. *Kidney Int* 2000;58:2007-2017
[122] Tylicki L, Rutkowski B: Hypertensive nephropathy: pathogenesis, diagnosis and treatment. *Pol Merkuriusz Lek* 2003;14:168-173
[123] Perera G: Hypertensive vascular disease. *J Chronic Dis* 1995;1:33-42
[124] Bohle A, Wehrmann M, Greschniok A, Junghans R: Renal morphology in essential hypertension: analysis of 1177 unselected cases. *Kidney Int Suppl* 1998;67:S205-206
[125] Madhavan S, Stockwell D, Cohen H, Alderman M: Renal function during antihypertensive treatment. *Lancet* 1995;345:749-751
[126] Toto RD: Hypertensive nephrosclerosis in African Americans. *Kidney Int* 2003;64:2331-2341
[127] Rutkowski B, Tylicki L, Manitius J, Lysiak-Szydlowska W: Hypertensive nephropathy - an increasing clinical problem. *Miner Electrolyte Metab* 1999;25:65-68
[128] Dustan HP, Roccella EJ, Garrison HH: Controlling hypertension. A research success story. *Arch Intern Med* 1996;156:1926-1935
[129] Zucchelli P, Zuccala A: Can we accurately diagnose nephrosclerosis? *Nephrol Dial Transplant* 1995;10:2-5
[130] Zucchelli P, Zuccala A: Progression of renal failure and hypertensive nephrosclerosis. *Kidney Int Suppl* 1998;68:S55-59
[131] Schlessinger SD, Tankersley MR, Curtis JJ: Clinical documentation of end-stage renal disease due to hypertension. *Am J Kidney Dis* 1994;23:655-660
[132] Rutkowski B, Tylicki L, Krupa-Wojciechowska B: Diagnosis and treatment of hypertensive nephropathy; in: Rutkowski B, Czekalski S, eds): Standards of diagnosis and therapeutic procedures in kidney diseases. *Gdansk*, MAK-med, 2001
[133] Wright J, Jr, Bakris G, Greene T, Agodoa L, Appel L, Charleston J, Cheek D, Douglas-Baltimore J, Gassman J, Glassock R, Hebert L, Jamerson K, Lewis J, Phillips R, Toto R, Middleton J, Rostand S: African American Study of Kidney Disease and Hypertension Study Group. Effect of blood pressure lowering and antihypertensive drug class on progression of hypertensive kidney disease: results from the AASK trial. *JAMA* 2002;288:2421-2431
[134] Chobanian AV, Bakris GL, Black HR, Cushman WC, Green LA, Izzo JL, Jr., Jones DW, Materson BJ, Oparil S, Wright JT, Jr., Roccella EJ: The Seventh Report of the Joint National Committee on Prevention, Detection, Evaluation, and Treatment of High Blood Pressure: the JNC 7 report. *Jama* 2003;289:2560-2572
[135] 2003 World Health Organization (WHO)/International Society of Hypertension (ISH) statement on management of hypertension. *J Hypertens* 2003;21:1983-1992
[136] Taal M, Brenner B: Renoprotective benefits of RAS inhibition: from ACEI to angiotensin II antagonists. *Kidney Int* 2000;57:1803-1817
[137] Ruggenenti P, Perna A, Gheradi G, Garini G, Zoccali C, Salvadori M, Scolari F, Schena F, Remuzzi G: Renoprtective properties of ACE-inhibition in non-diabetic nephropathies with non-nephrotic proteinuria. *Lancet* 1999;354:359-364

[138] Lewis E, Hunsicker L, Clarke W, et al.: Collaborative Study Group. The effect of angiotensin-converting-enzyme inhibition on diabetic nephropathy. *N Eng J Med* 1993;329:1462-1465

[139] Douglas JG, Agodoa L: ACE inhibition is effective and renoprotective in hypertensive nephrosclerosis: the African American Study of Kidney Disease and Hypertension (AASK) trial. *Kidney Int Suppl* 2003;S74-76

[140] Lewis E, Hunsicker L, Clarke W, Berl T, Pohl M, Lewis J, Ritz E, Atkins R, Rohde R, Raz I: Collaborative Study Group. Renoprotective effect of the angiotensin-receptor antagonist irbesartan in patients with nephropathy due to type 2 diabetes. *N Eng J Med* 2001;345:851-860

[141] Nakano N, Yoshimura A, Morita H, Takada M, Kayano T, Ideura T: Combination treatment of angiotensin-II receptor blocker and angiotesin-converting-enzyme inhibitor in non-diabetic renal disease (COOPERATE): a randomised controlled trial. *Lancet* 2003;361:117-124

[142] Yamashita T, Kawashima S, Miwa Y, Ozaki M, Namiki M, Hirase T, Inoue N, Hirata K, Yokoyama M: A 3-hydroxy-3-methylglutaryl co-enzyme A reductase inhibitor reduces hypertensive nephrosclerosis in stroke-prone spontaneously hypertensive rats. *J Hypertens* 2002;20:2465-2473

[143] O'Donnell MP, Kasiske BL, Katz SA, Schmitz PG, Keane WF: Lovastatin but not enalapril reduces glomerular injury in Dahl salt-sensitive rats. *Hypertension* 1992;20:651-658

[144] Rutkowski B: Epidemiology of end-sage renal disease (ESRD). *Ann Acad Med Gedan* 2001;31(Supp. 1):73-82

In: Hypertension: New Research
Editor: Elwood F. Benhagen, pp. 285-298
ISBN: 1-59454-204-X

Chapter XI

PROSTACYCLINS – EFFECTIVE IN TREATMENT OF PULMONARY HYPERTENSION

Árpád Pereszlényi Jr.
Department of Thoracic and Vascular Surgery,
Centre for Pneumology and Thoracic Surgery, Coswig, Germany

ABSTRACT

Pulmonary hypertension is a rare disease the characteristic of which is a treacherous progressive course, which almost always leads to a sudden death. It mainly affects middle and younger middle age group. The treatment of this disease is difficult as the actual underlying disorder has not yet been identified into details.

After using all the traditional intensive conservative means of treatment, lung/ heart-lung transplantation often remained the only possibility to improve the quality of patient's life.

Prostacyclins represent a newest and most important therapeutic approach in treatment of pulmonary hypertension nowadays. Prostacyclin PGI2 (Epoprostenol) is the strongest pulmonary vasodilator with potent aggregation-inhibitory, anti-inflammatory and anti-proliferative properties. Lately more and more reports about successful application of prostacyclin PGI2 in pulmonary hypertension treatment appear in the specialized literature.

The objective of this paper is to offer a review on the current activities and results of pulmonary hypertension treatment by means of prostacyclins, and to introduce Epoprostenol to experts.

Key words: Prostacyclins, Epoprostenol, Primary Pulmonary Hypertension, Secondary Pulmonary Hypertension, Lung Transplantation, Heart-Lung Transplantation.

ABBREVIATIONS

PPH	Primary Pulmonary Hypertension

SPH	Secondary Pulmonary Hypertension
PVR	Pulmonary Vascular Resistance
PAP	Pulmonary Artery Pressure
mPAP	Mean Pulmonary Artery Pressure
CO	Cardiac Output
CI	Cardiac Index
TK	Systemic Arterial Pressure
PG	Prostaglandins
TX	Thromboxane
ARDS	Adult Respiratory Distress Syndrome
NO	Nitric Oxide
paO_2	Partial Arterial Oxygen Pressure
$paCO_2$	Partial Arterial Carbondioxide Pressure
KATP	Potassium-Adenosine Triphosphate-Channel
KCa	Potassium-Calcium-Channel
TEA	Chronic Thromboembolic Disease
NIH	National Institute of Health

Introduction

Pulmonary hypertension is a rare, but treacherous disease affecting lungs and heart. Pulmonary vessels narrowing causes pressure increase in the pulmonary artery. The final consequence of this increase results in dis-balance in pulmonary circulation, reduction in gas exchange and overload of the right ventricle, which leads to its failure [1,2].

A lot of drugs and treatment modalities are still on the level of clinical testing and are the subject of a number of tests, and a topic for discussions. For many patients and their attending physicians the only remaining possibility is to perform lung or heart-lung transplantation [2,3,4].

The objective of this paper is to offer a review on the current activities and results of pulmonary hypertension treatment by means of prostacyclins, and to introduce Epoprostenol to experts.

Definition, Treatment of Pulmonary Hypertension

The term Pulmonary Hypertension indicates an increase of mean pulmonary artery pressure above 2,67 kPa (20 mmHg) in lying position at rest [1,2,5].

This disease is characterized by pathologically increased pulmonary vascular resistance and elevated pulmonary artery pressure, which can be explained neither intra vitam nor post mortem by lungs or heart disease, or systemic disease respectively, which could cause pathological changes in pulmonary vessels [1].

The basic hemodynamic sign of pulmonary hypertension is an increased vascular resistance without any proved reason. The pulmonary vascular resistance is almost 18 times higher as the standard one. Systolic pressure in pulmonary artery is often more than 13 kPa (100 mmHg). With exercise the pressures further increase, while pulmonary vascular resistance does not change. Cardiac index is often reduced. Pressure in left atrium is normal. As a consequence of the reduced cardiac index, systemic pressure is generally more likely to be reduced. The end-diastolic pressure in the right ventricle is elevated. Blood oxygen saturation is moderately reduced and pCO_2 is also reduced as a consequence of hyperventilation [1,2,5].

The classical treatment described in the Internal Medicine textbook consisted of infusion of acetylcholine, tolasoline, and isoproterenol. By long-term supply of peroral hydralasine the pulmonary vascular resistance was expected to decrease. Favorable results after sublingual application of isoproterenol and peroral supply of phentolamine were expected, too. In several cases cardiac output was increased by vasodilatation, but pulmonary artery pressure did not decrease. No expected success was reached by anticoagulation treatment [1,2].

Prostacyclin and Lung Transplantation

Recently more and more reports about successful treatment of pulmonary hypertension (primary, secondary) by intravenous prostacyclin - epoprostenol application can be found in the specialized literature [2,6,7]. As it was already mentioned in the introduction, up to the recent times only lung or heart-lung transplantation seemed to be the unique possible (successful) solution for the affected patients [2,3,4,8].

Table 1. Guidelines for Timing referral

COPD (+alfa 1 – antitrypsin deficiency emphysema)
FEV 1 < 25 % predicted
Clinically significant hypoxemia
Hypercapnia
Secondary pulmonary hypertension
Clinical course: rapid rate of decline of FEV 1 or life-threatening exacerbations
CYSTIC FIBROSIS
FEV 1 < 30 % predicted
or FEV 1 > 30 % with rapidly declining lung function
Hypercapnia
Clinical course: increasing frequency and severity of exacerbations, progressive weight loss
IDIOPATHIC PULMONARY FIBROSIS
VC, TLC < 60 – 65 % predicted
Symptomatic disease unresponsive to medical therapy
Secondary pulmonary hypertension
Clinical, radiografic, or physiologic progression on medical therapy
PRIMARY PULMONARY HYPERTENSION
NYHA functional class III or IV
Mean right atrial pressure > 10 mm Hg
Mean pulmonary arterial pressure > 50 mm Hg
Cardiac index < 2,5 $L/min/m^2$
Failure of intensive medical therapy (especially intravenous epoprostenol)

After introduction of prostacyclin into the pulmonary hypertension treatment and numerous promising reports, references about the successful treatment by this drug, indication, timing of lung transplantation, respectively had changed, too. According to the latest guidelines [4,9,10], lung transplantation is indicated for patients with pulmonary hypertension after the failure of intensive medical therapy - especially after the failure of intravenous epoprostenol. TAB.1

Whether this treatment has a long-term therapeutic effect, or it serves as the so-called bridging during the demanding pre-transplantation period, it was generally accepted, that this treatment (or prostacyclin test, respectively) must be performed. So, it is a pre-condition, that at patients before putting them onto the waiting list, the possibility of prostacyclin treatment must be carried out.

Now, a brief overview about the use and application of prostacyclin will be presented. Before that, however, it is needed to mention several patophysiological comments concerning prostaglandins.

Chemical Structure, Clinical Effects of Prostaglandins

Chemically prostaglandins are cyclic derivatives of polyunsaturated 20 carbonate fatty acids - linoleic, linolenic and arachidonic. Arachidonic acid (eikosatetraenic acid) is present in phospholipids of cell membranes. From binding in phospholipids it releases with the effect of phospholipase A2 and thus becomes a fundamental compound for biosynthesis of prostaglandins. Fig.1. [11]. Oxygenation is the following step in biosynthesis of prostaglandins (PG), during which endoperoxide PGG2 origins first. By peroxidase effect PGH2 origins from PGG2. These intermediate products - PGG2 and PGH2 - with effect of PG-isomerase, comprise the so-called "classical prostaglandins": PGA2, PGB2, PGC2, PGD2, PGE2. (The number 2 in the index means the number of double bindings in the chain, and the letters indicate the sort and the position of substitutes in 5-carbonate circle).

Prostacyclin PGI2 is created from endoperoxide PGH2 with the effect of PG-I-isomerase enzyme, thromboxane A2 (TXA2) is created with the effect of PG-thromboxane-A-isomerase. Fig.1. [11].

Prostaglandins are being created in several organs and their physiological effect is very colorful. Prostaglandins increase blood pressure, cause vasodilatation or, on the contrary, vasoconstriction. PG also stimulates stomach secretion, contractility of uterus, inhibits lipolysis, affects the process of coagulation, phagocytosis, etc.

The most of prostaglandins are synthesized in the kidneys. There are fatty inclusions in the interstitial cells of the medulla of the kidneys, which contain arachidonic acid; and this acid is the main precursor of prostaglandins. Recently it was proved that prostaglandins originate in the kidney cortex, i.e. in the walls of vessels, a more rarely in tubules.

Prostaglandins, as it was mentioned above, are vasoactive agents, which have effects on: the kidney blood flow, sodium excretion, water resorption and rennin release. They participate in the intrarenal re-distribution of blood into kidney medulla and thus they reduce water resorption. They inhibit the active transport of sodium in the renal tubules and increase natriuresis. The main meaning of prostaglandins in kidneys is not their direct effect, but their mediation, influence and correction of the effects of other vasoactive hormones, and thus they intervene into renal circulation.

Nowadays it seems that prostacyclin PGI2 is the main agent responsible for the renal effects. This product is unstable and origins in vessel walls. Prostacyclin increases sodium, potassium and water excretion and stimulates rennin secretion. It is evident that it is the most important prostaglandin of the kidney cortex.

PGE2, which originates not only in interstitial cells, but also in vessels and in the nephron, is the most important prostaglandin of kidney medulla. PGE2 and PGI1 have vasodilatation effects. PGF2α, which has even contra, i.e. vasoconstriction effects, also belongs among the important renal prostaglandins. Predominance of the effective prostaglandins decides about the character of vasoactivity in the given case.

Further prostaglandins of E-group are being created in monocytes and macrophages, where they can influence various functions, e.g. phagocytosis.

PGF2 prostaglandin plays very important role during delivery of a child - it is produced by placenta and effects the contraction readiness of uterus.

Thromboxane A2 is produced by thrombocytes and has an important role in the process of coagulation - with its proaggregate and strong vasoconstriction effect [6,12].

Brief Overview of Prostacyclin in Literature

In 1987 Jones DK et al. published a paper – a group of 10 PPH patients, where he compares the results after the application of intravenous prostacyclin (epoprostenol, PGI2) with the results, where peroral vasodilators and anticoagulants (conventional treatment) were used. At all these patients at the same time heart-lung transplantation was indicated. The authors proved that the short term administration of intravenous epoprostenol (mean dose 5.5 ng/kg/min) increased the mean cardiac index (CI), improved pulmonary artery oxygen saturation from 48% to 57%, and increased calculated tissue oxygen delivery from 10 to 11.8 ml/kg/min. The mean pulmonary artery pressure (mPAP) and the mean system pressure decreased. Continued intravenous infusion of epoprostenol for 1 – 25 months was associated with subjective and clinical improvement. Two patients died on treatment, three have undergone heart-lung transplantation, and in five the treatment was not finished during the time when the article was published [13].

In 1989 in the "Chest" journal the same author (Jones DK) reports about a group of 23 patients with similar results as in his previous paper. It must be mentioned that in this case it was not a homogeneous PPH group, there were also secondary pulmonary hypertension (SPH) patients included [14].

Pascual JMS et al. reports about a successful prostacyclin pulmonary hypertension therapy developed after heart transplantation. At 9 patients (from 50), who underwent heart transplantation, a dramatic state of right ventricular failure developed. Prostacyclin was started, and the dose increased from 0.5 to 5.0 ng/kg/min, which led to reach the desired hemodynamic effect (increase of CI, reduction of mPAP). The use of prostacyclin enabled the weaning of other drugs within a 48-hour period with no side effects and no worsening of the hemodynamic conditions after discontinuation of prostacyclin. All the patients with right ventricular failure treated by the above-described mode were successfully managed [15].

Rubin LJ et al. in 1990 reports about the results of a prospective, randomized trial, where 24 PPH patients underwent continuous intravenous prostacyclin treatment. 19 patients successfully completed the study, 4 patients died during the study and 1 was excluded from the study due to the severe side effect – pulmonary edema (as it was stated in the study protocol). The most significant contribution of this study was that continuous intravenous prostacyclin was administered for the first time by portable infusion pump during a period of 18 months [7].

In 1992 the same author – Lewis J.Rubin from the University of Maryland, Baltimore, in the journal "Drugs" introduced prostacyclin in details as a potent pulmonary vasodilatative agent, pointed out the possibility of its application even during the period of several years, and for the first time talked about prostacyclin treatment as "bridging" to lung transplantation [5].

In 1992 Schranz et al. published a prospective cohort study, where 14 infants (2 to 12 months old) after cardiac surgery were successfully treated by tolazoline and/or prostacyclin. According to the protocol tolazoline was administered as a bolus of 0.5 mg/kg for treatment of persistent pulmonary hypertension or acute pulmonary hypertensive crisis. If its effectiveness was proved after 30 mins by hemodynamic measurements, continuous iv infusion of 0.5 mg/kg/hr was established. If tolazoline treatment did not fulfill the criteria for pulmonary vasodilatation, prostacyclin was given by continuous iv infusion at a starting rate of 5 ng/kg/min, followed by 10-15 ng/kg/min. From the total 14 patients, 13 were successfully treated. The authors also described that transient withdrawal of prostacyclin in 5 infants led to significant worsening of hemodynamic parameters [16].

The objective of another prospective study published in 1993 was to determine whether epoprostenol (prostacyclin, PGI2) or heart–lung transplantation (HLT), or both improves survival of patients with severe pulmonary hypertension. Forty four patients were studied; 25 among them received continuous epoprostenol over a four year period. The patients were tested each third month by 12 minutes walking test. The patients, where prostacyclin was not applied, were treated with anticoagulants and nifedipine (<20 mg) or dilthiazem (> 120 mg) three times a day. The patients of both groups were further being prepared for the transplantation. When physical disability occurred, the patient (of prostacyclin group) was urgently listed for transplantation. The results of successful therapeutic intervention (epoprostenol, HLT), which led to improve survival, were compared with the results of survival in Mayo clinic (120 patients). One-year survival was better in the prostacyclin group, however, after two years the survival in both groups was identical. Most of the benefit was conferred by epoprostenol, which prolonged survival twofold from median time of 8 to 17 months and thus doubled the chances of obtaining organ for transplantation [17].

In 1993 Walmrath D et al. published a paper about the positive effect of prostacyclin in ARDS treatment (Adult Respiratory Distress Syndrome). The importance of this study is in the proof of selective effect of aerosolized prostacyclin on pulmonary perfusion and ventilation. Prostacyclin applied this way lowered the mean pulmonary artery pressure (mPAP), pulmonary vascular resistance fell by 30%, systemic arterial pressure decreased slightly from 76.8 to 74.5 mmHg [18].

In 1996 Olschewski H et al. continued in studying the effects of aerosolized prostacyclin. The objective of his study was to compare the effects of aerosolization of prostacyclin and its stable analogue iloprost with those of nasal oxygen, inhaled nitric oxide (NO) and intravenous prostacyclin on hemodynamics and gas exchange in patients with severe pulmonary hypertension. Results: aerosolized prostacyclin decreased pulmonary artery pressure in 6 patients from (mean +/- SE) 62.3 +/- 4.1 mm Hg to 50.8 +/- 5.5 mm Hg and reduced pulmonary vascular resistance from 1721 +/- 253 dyne /s cm^{-5} to 1019 +/- 203 dyne /s cm^{-5}, and increased cardiac output from 2.75 +/- 0.21 L/min to 4.11 +/- 0.54 L/min, mixed venous oxygen saturation from 51.1% +/- 3.4% to 66.3% +/- 4.1% and arterial oxygen saturation from 90.6% +/- 2.7% to 93.8% +/- 23% ($P<0.05$ for all changes). Mean systemic arterial pressure was only slightly affected. The responses lasted from 10 to 13 minutes after inhalation was terminated. Aerosolized iloprost had an identical efficacy profile but was associated with a longer duration of the pulmonary vasodilatory effect (60 min to 120 min). In comparison, intravenous prostacyclin reduced pulmonary vascular resistance, slightly reduced systemic artery pressure, however no clinically significant decrease in pulmonary artery pressure was recorded. Nitric oxide and oxygen were less potent pulmonary dilators in these patients. In one patient, one year of therapy with aerosolized iloprost (100µg/d in six aerosol doses) resulted in sustained efficacy of the inhaled vasodilator regimen and clinical improvement [19].

In this connection it is necessary to point out to a further work of Warren JB and Higenbottam T published in 1996. This was actually a letter to editor with a specific regard to caution when Nitric Oxide is applied. The authors warned on the lack of standard guidelines when using this gas, on lack of storage information and lack of further technical matters. They also pointed out that the products of gas fragmentation contain toxic and potential cancerogen elements. This article also deals with the known “rebound phenomenon” with a severe stage of pulmonary hypertension after gas dose reduction [20].

The increased resistance in pulmonary vasculary bed as a consequence of endothelium damage is a reason of pulmonary hypertension at patients with systemic sclerosis. Rolla et al assumed that the reason of this damage is NO production and releasing failure (NO is being produced by different cells of respiratory system, mainly by pulmonary vessels endothelium). At patients, affected by systemic sclerosis and pulmonary hypertension, lower concentration of NO in expired air was proved. Measuring of NO concentration in the expired air after medicamentous stimulation offers a new possibility of non-invasive function test of endothelium. According to this, then, it could have been possible to enable identification of such patients who profit from vasodilatative treatment. The authors in two patients with systemic sclerosis and pulmonary hypertension tested this hypothesis. The NO concentration in the expired air in both cases was 2.8 and 3.4 ppb, respectively. Later both patients were applied L-Arginine (precursor of NO) and on the second day Glycerin nitrate was applied for 20 minutes. At one patient 30 minutes later the NO concentration in the expired air was 6.3 and 8.2 ppb, respectively. After infusion of physiologic solution no such effect was registered. At the second patient no change of NO concentration in the expired air had been discovered. In the next part of the test an aerosolized iloprost (20µg) was compared to the physiological solution (applied as aerosolium). 30 minutes after iloprost inhalation the authors recorded significant increase of NO concentration in the expired air at the first patient (from 2.2 to 9.5 ppb). Arterial partial pressure O_2 (paO_2) increased from the original 65 to 80 mmHg and pulmonary artery pressure decreased from 54 to 29 mmHg. No changes in heart frequency and arterial systemic pressure were recorded. No significant changes were recorded at the second patient (where physiological solution was applied as control). An increase of NO concentration in expired air after pharmacological stimulation is a clear proof of the smooth muscle of pulmonary vessels` respond to vasodilator iloprost stimulation. The non-increase of NO concentration here is generally being explained with the missing vasodilatative reaction to inhaled iloprost. It is not probable that pulmonary vessels` vasodilatation (in first patient) depends ONLY on the increased expired NO concentration, because similar NO concentration increase had been already recorded also after L-Arginine or Glyceryl-Trinitrate infusions, despite that after their application no influence on pulmonary artery pressure was observed. The relaxation effect of iloprost (as it was proved in the experiment on isolated perfusion of a rat's lung) is realized through KATP and KCa channels and only seldom also by NO release. On the basis of good results of the above-mentioned test the first patient was treated by aerosolized iloprost (100 μg/d in five doses). Three months later significant improvement of hemodynamic parameters in pulmonary circulation was observed. Following the results authors recommended to apply a pharmacological stimulation test for potential respondent identification [21].

Higgenbottam et al. in 1998 compared the effect of prostacyclin (epoprostenol PGI2) with its analogue - iloprost in treatment of severe pulmonary hypertension in eight patients (5 patients with PPH and 3 patients with chronic thromboembolic pulmonary hypertension /TEA/). All patients underwent right heart catheterisation. The results of this exam were: mean (SEM) right atrial pressure was 9.9 (2.2) mmHg, mPAP=67.4 (3.0) mmHg, CI =1.75 (0.13) l/min/m^2 and mixed venous oxygen saturation was 59.1 (3.1) %. Continuous intravenous epoprostenol or iloprost was given for phase I (three to six weeks); the patients then were crossed over to receive the alternative drug in an equivalent phase II. Exercise tolerance was measured at baseline and at the end of phase I and II with a 12-minute walk. Distance covered, rest period, percentage drop in arterial oxygen saturation (delta Sao2%) and percentage rise in heart rate (delta HR%) were also measured. Results: a walking distance covered rose from {mean /SEM/} 407.5 (73) to 591(46) m with PGI2 and to 602.5 (60) m while on iloprost. Rest period decreased from 192 (73) seconds at baseline to 16 (16) seconds with PGI2 and to 58 (34) seconds with iloprost. Delta HR% was 37.5 (6) % at baseline, 35 (3) % on PGI2 , and 24 (6) % on iloprost. It must be concluded that the results from the point of view of statistics were highly significant [22].

In 1998 Olschewski et al. reported on a 45 year old female patient with PPH, pneumonia, decompensated right heart failure (ascites, pleural effusion), circulatory shock and commencing renal and hepatic failure, despite maximum therapy including the use of catecholamines. Iloprost (150 μg/d) and NO were added to the therapy. After this treatment the following parameters improved: mPAP decreased from 65 to 61 mmHg, CI increased from 1.25 to 1.85 l/min/m^2 , PVR decreased from 2416 to 1549 dyn/s/cm^5 . Both methods increased the arterial pO_2 but did not change the systemic arterial pressure. During repeated inhalations with iloprost, the baseline hemodynamics and gas exchange improved dramatically, renal and liver functions normalized. During one year of continued therapy, the clinical status improved very much, concomitant with improved hemodynamics, and the patient has been taken off the transplantation list [23].

Here finally the results of the controlled randomized multicentric trial after application of the inhaled Iloprost, which were published in 2002 at The New England Journal of Medicine (by H. Olschewski et al for the Aerosolized Iloprost Randomized Study Group) must be mentioned. On the large multicentric series of patients in controlled randomized trial it was unambiguously proved that the inhaled iloprost is an effective therapy for the patients with severe pulmonary hypertension [24].

Among the experimental papers, the study of Kleen from Munich University, Germany (1998) is of specific interest. The authors compared the effect of inhaled prostacyclin PGI2 with the effect of prostaglandin PGE1 in aerosolized and intravenous forms. The aerosolized form of PGI2 had a significant effect to the decrease of mPAP and pulmonary vascular resistance. Such an effect after PGE1 application was observed neither after its aerosolized nor after its intravenous forms of application [25].

EPOPROSTENOL, PROSTACYCLIN PGI2

From everything mentioned above, it is evident that epoprostenol, prostacyclin PGI2 represents a new, potent pulmonary vasodilatative agent, and that is why we would like to briefly introduce this product in the following lines.

Flolan®, epoprostenol sodium - an original product of Glaxo-Smithkline co., is a sterile sodium salt formulated for intravenous administration.

Flolan has been proved as a potent drug for a long-term treatment for patients with primary pulmonary hypertension and patients with pulmonary hypertension associated with the scleroderma spectrum of disease in NYHA functional class III and IV, who do not respond adequately to conventional therapy. Epoporostenol (as it was already described above) produces symptomatic improvement and prolonged survival in patients with primary pulmonary hypertension.

Flolan is administered by continuous intravenous infusion via a central venous catheter using an ambulatory infusion pump. During initiation of treatment, Flolan may be administered peripherally. Temporary peripheral intravenous infusion may be used until central access is established.

Chronic infusion of Flolan should be initiated at 2 ng/kg/min and increased in increments of 2 ng/kg/min every 15 minutes or longer until dose-limiting pharmacological effects are elicited or until a tolerance limit to the drug is established and further increases in the infusion rate are not clinically warranted. If the initial infusion rate of 2ng/kg/min is not tolerated, a lower dose, which is tolerated by the patient, should be identified.

Dosage adjustments should be based on persistence, recurrence, or worsening of the patient's symptoms of pulmonary hypertension and the occurrence of adverse events due to excessive doses of Flolan. In general, upward dosage titration from the initial chronic dose should be expected. Increments in dose should be considered if symptoms of pulmonary hypertension persist or recur after improving. The infusion should be increased by 1 to 2 ng/kg/min increments at intervals sufficient to allow assessment of clinical response; these intervals should be at least 15 minutes. In clinical trials, incremental increases in dose occurred at intervals of 24 to 48 hours or longer. Following establishment of a new chronic infusion rate, patient should be observed, and standing and supine blood pressure and heart rate monitored for several hours to ensure that the new dose is tolerated.

During chronic infusion, the occurrence of dose-limiting pharmacological events may necessitate a decrease in infusion rate, but the adverse event may occasionally resolve without dosage adjustment. Dosage decreases should be made gradually in 2 ng/kg/min decrements every 15 minutes or longer until the dose-limiting effects resolve. Abrupt withdrawal of Flolan or sudden large reductions in infusion rates should be avoided. Except in life-threatening situations (e.g. unconsciousness, collapse, etc.), infusion rates of Flolan should be adjusted only under the direction of a physician.

Flolan is contraindicated in patients with known hypersensitivity to this drug or to structurally related compounds, as well, as in patients with severe left ventricular dysfunction.

Patients with following diagnoses should receive Flolan with special care under intensive monitoring (hemodynamics and coagulation parameters):

- patients with higher risk of bleeding (gastroduodenal ulcers, intracranial vessels)
- severe arteriosclerosis of coronary vessels
- instable angina pectoris
- hepatic dysfunction
- severe systemic hyper- or hypotension.

Flolan should be used only by clinicians experienced in the diagnosis and treatment of pulmonary hypertension. The diagnosis of PPH or SPH should be carefully established. Flolan is a potent pulmonary and systemic vasodilator. Dose initiation with Flolan must be performed in a setting with adequate personnel and equipment for physiologic monitoring and emergency care. Dose initiation in controlled PPH clinical trials was performed during right heart cathetrization. In uncontrolled PPH and controlled SPH trials, dose initiation was performed without cardiac cathetrization. The risk of cardiac cathetrization in patients with pulmonary hypertension should be carefully weighed against the potential benefits. During dose initiation, asymptomatic increases in pulmonary artery pressure coincident with increases in cardiac output occurred rarely. In such cases, dose reduction should be considered, but such an increase does not imply that chronic treatment is contraindicated.

During chronic use, Flolan is delivered continuously on an ambulatory basis through a permanent indwelling central venous catheter. Unless contraindicated, anticoagulant therapy should be administered to these patients receiving Flolan to reduce the risk of pulmonary thromboembolism or systemic embolism through a patent foramen ovale. In order to reduce the risk of infection, aseptic technique must be used in the reconstitution and administration of Flolan as well as in routine catheter care. Because Flolan is metabolized rapidly, even brief interruptions in the delivery of Flolan may result in symptoms associated with rebound pulmonary hypertension including dyspnea, dizziness, and asthenia. The decision to initiate therapy with Flolan should be based upon the understanding that there is a high likelihood that intravenous therapy with Flolan will be needed for prolonged periods, possible years, and the patient's ability to accept and care for a permanent intravenous catheter and infusion pump should be carefully considered. Dosage of Flolan during chronic use should be adjusted at the first sign of recurrence or worsening of symptoms attributable to pulmonary hypertension or the occurrence of adverse events associated with Flolan. Following dosage adjustments, standing and supine blood pressure and heart rate should be monitored closely for several hours.

Hemodynamic Effects: Acute intravenous infusion of Flolan for up to 15 minutes in patients with PPH and SPH produce dose-related increases in cardiac index (CI) and stroke volume (SV), and dose-related decreases in pulmonary vascular resistance (PVR) and mean systemic arterial pressure (mSAP). Chronic hemodynamic effects after chronic intravenous infusion (12 weeks) to those above-mentioned effects includes a decrease of mPAP, decrease of right atrial pressure, increase in blood arterial oxygen saturation.

Flolan is infused continuously through a permanent indwelling central venous catheter via a small, portable infusion pump. Thus, therapy with Flolan requires commitment by the patient to drug reconstitution, drug administration, and care of the permanent central venous catheter. Sterile technique must be adhered to in preparing the drug and in the care of the catheter, and even brief interruptions in the delivery of Flolan may result in rapid symptomatic deterioration. A patient's decision to receive Flolan should be based upon the understanding that there is a high likelihood that therapy with Flolan will be needed for prolonged periods, possible years. The patient's ability to accept and care for a permanent intravenous catheter and infusion pump should also be carefully considered.

Drug Interactions: Additional reductions in blood pressure may occur when Flolan is administered with diuretics, antihypertensive agents, or other vasodilators. When other antiplatelet agents or anticoagulants are used concomitantly, there is the potential for Flolan to increase the risk of bleeding. However, patients receiving infusions of Flolan in clinical trials were maintained on anticoagulants without evidence of increased bleeding. In clinical trials, Flolan was used with digoxin, diuretics, anticoagulants, oral vasodilators, and supplemental oxygen. Patients on digoxin may show elevations of digoxin concentrations after initiation of therapy with Flolan, which may be clinically significant in patients prone to digoxin toxicity.

Adverse Effects: During dose initiation and escalation in clinical trials, the most common dose-limiting adverse events, occurring in = 1.0% of patients were: nausea, vomiting, headache, hypotension, flushing, chest pain, anxiety, dizziness, bradykardia, dyspnoe, abdominal pain, musculoskeletal pain, and tachykardia. Adverse effects related to chronic Flolan infusions are headache, jaw pain, flushing, diarrhea, nausea, vomiting, flu-like symptoms, and anxiety/ nervousness.

Interpretation of adverse events is complicated by the clinical features of PPH, which are similar to some of the pharmacological effects of Flolan (e.g., dizziness, syncope). Adverse events likely related to the underlying disease include dyspnea, fatigue, chest pain, right ventricular failure, and pallor. Signs and symptoms suggestive of excessive doses of Flolan are the expected dose-limiting pharmacological effects of Flolan including flushing, headache, hypotension, tachykardia, nausea, vomiting, and diarrhea.

Overdosage: Signs and symptoms of excessive doses of Flolan during clinical trials are the expected dose-limiting pharmacological effects of Flolan, including flushing, headache, hypotension, tachycardia, nausea, vomiting, and diarrhea. Treatment will ordinarily require dose reduction of Flolan.

Clinical Pharmacology (also see Chapter on Chemical structure, clinical effects of prostaglandins): Epoprostenol (prostacyclin PGI2), a metabolite of arachidonic acid (Fig.1), is a naturally occurring prostaglandin with two major pharmacological actions:

1. direct vasodilatation of pulmonary and systemic arterial vascular beds, and
2. inhibition of platelet aggregation.

The vasodilatory effects reduce right and left ventricular afterload and increase cardiac output and stroke volume. The effect of epoprostenol on heart rate in animals varies with dose. At low doses, there is vagally mediated bradycardia, but at higher doses, epoprostenol causes reflex tachycardia in response to direct vasodilatation and hypotension.

Pharmacokinetics: Epoprostenol is extremely unstable and undergoes rapid hydrolysis at physiologic pH in blood and is also subject to enzymatic degradation. Epoprostenol is metabolized to two primary metabolites: 6-keto-prostaglandin F1a (PGF1a) /formed by spontaneous degradation/ and 6,15-diketo-13,14-dihydro-PGF1a /enzymatically formed/, both of which have pharmacological activity orders of magnitude less than epoprostenol in animal test systems. The vascular effects of epoprostenol terminate within 2-3 minutes of discontinuation of infusion. Due to the short duration of action, epoprostenol should be administered by chronic intravenous infusion [26].

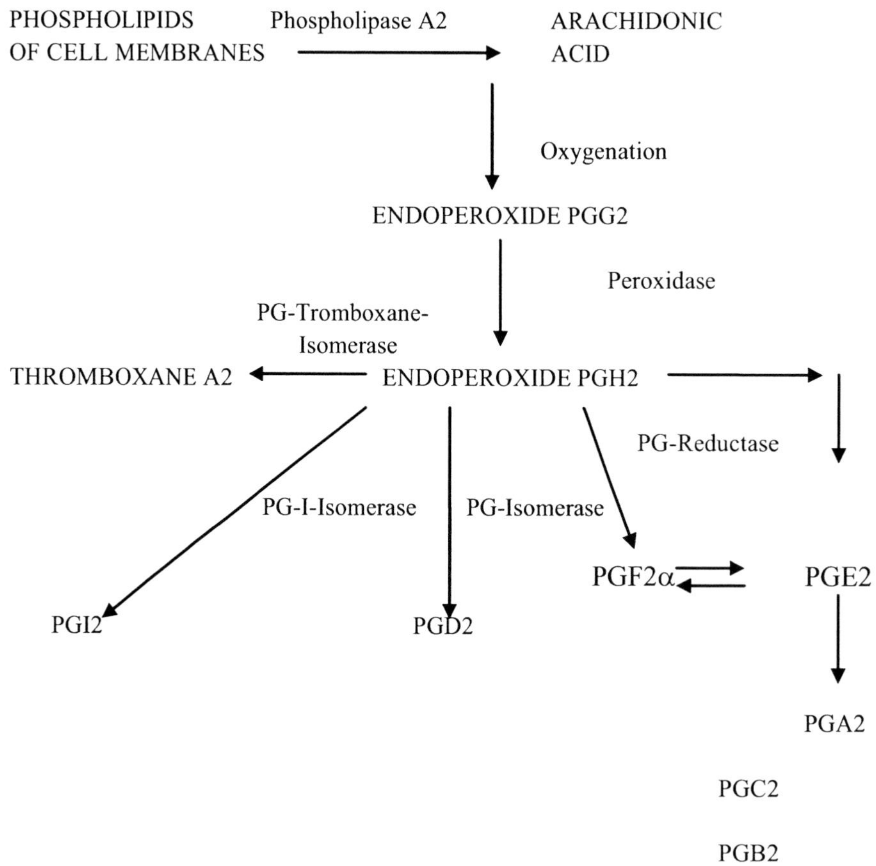

Figure 1. Scheme of prostaglandins' biosynthesis

Conclusion

As it was already mentioned in the introduction, pulmonary hypertension is a serious life-threatening treacherous disease. According to the National Institute of Health (NIH) registry these patients` average survival is 2.5 years [2,27].

According to the other statistics of this Institute, 5 years` survival rate among patients (in New York Heart Association classes III and IV), who were treated with epoprostenol (54%), was twice that of matched historical control patients (27%) [7].

In the future a long-term therapy with stable prostacyclin analogues (in inhaled, transdermal, or oral form) or with inhaled Nitric Oxide appears to be a promising solution to treat this disease. In order to identify molecular mechanisms responsible for pulmonary hypertension, research of heredity and genetic materials is given a great hope [2,28,29,30].

Lungs or heart-lung transplantation, respectively, has its irreplaceable position after the failure of conservative treatment of pulmonary hypertension [3,4]. The development in this area follows less invasive operating techniques and uses newer treatment procedures – e.g. extracorporeal membrane oxygenation already during the lung transplantation procedure [3,8]. Only the future and extensive multi-centric studies will show the legitimacy and will bring perfection to these techniques.

REFERENCES

[1] Dieška D. a kol.: *Textbook of Internal Medicine*, Martin, Osveta publ.1990, 496 p.

[2] Rubin LJ.: Primary pulmonary hypertension. *N Engl J Med* 1997; 336(2):111-117.

[3] Pereszlényi jr., Á., Lang G., Steltzer H., Hetz H., Kocher A., Neuhauser P., Wisser W., Klepetko W.: Bilateral lung transplantation with intra- and postoperatively prolonged ECMO support in patients with pulmonary hypertension. *Eur J Cardio-thorac Surg* 2002;21(5);858-863.

[4] Pereszlényi jr., Á., Haruštiak S., Taghavi S., Birsan T., Huber E., Deviatko E., Klepetko W.: Lung Transplantation Today. *Bratisl Lek Listy* 2000;101(2):63-70.

[5] Rubin LJ.: Primary pulmonary hypertension. Practical therapeutic recommendations. *Drugs* 1992; 43: 37-43.

[6] Galie N., Manes A., Branzi A.: Medical therapy of pulmonary hypertension. The prostacyclins. *Clin Chest Med 2001*;22(3):529-537.

[7] Rubin LJ, Mendoza J, Hood M, McGoon M, Barst R, Williams WB, Diehl JH, Crow J, Long W.: Treatment of primary pulmonary hypertension with continuous prostacyclin (epoprostenol): results of a randomized trial. *Ann Intern Med* 1990;112(7):485-491.

[8] Pereszlényi jr., Á., Haruštiak S., Klepetko W.: Extracorporeal membrane oxygenation in lung transplantation. *Bratisl Lek Listy* 2002;103(1):34-38.

[9] Arcasoy SM, Kotloff RM. Lung Transplantation. *N Engl J Med* 1999;340:1081-1091.

[10] Trulock, EP. Recipient Selection. *Chest Surg Clin North Am* 1993;3:1-18.

[11] Duchoň J et al. *Textbook of medical chemistry and biochemistry*, Martin, Osveta publ.1988, 752 p.

[12] Trojan S et al. *Textbook of physiology*. Prague, Avicenum publ.1987, 1058 p.

[13] Jones DK, Higenbottam TW, Walwork J.: Treatment of primary pulmonary hypertension intravenous epoprostenol (prostacyclin). *Br Heart J* 1987;57(3):270-278.

[14] Jones DK, Higenbottam TW, Walwork J.: Pulmonary vasodilatation with prostacyclin in primary and secondary pulmonary hypertension. *Chest* 1989; 96(3): 784-789.

[15] Pascual JM, Fiorelli AI, Bellotti GM, Stolf NA, Jatene AD.: Prostacyclin in the management of pulmonary hypertension after heart transplantation. *J Heart Transplant* 1990;9(6):644-651.

[16] Schranz D, Zepp F, Iversen S, Wippermann C, Huth R, Zimmer B, Jungst BK, Oelert H.: Effects of tolazoline and prostacyclin on pulmonary hypertension in infants after cardiac surgery. *Crit Care Med* 1992;20(9):1243-1249.

[17] Higenbottam TW, Spiegelhalter D, Scott JP, Fuster V, Dinh-Xaun AT, Caine N, Walwork J. Prostacyclin (epoprostenol) and heart-lung transplantation as treatments for severe pulmonary hypertension. *Br Heart J* 1993;70(4):366-370.

[18] Walmrath D, Schneider T, Pilch J, Grimminger F, Seeger W.: Aerosolised prostacyclin in adult respiratory distress syndrome. *Lancet* 1993; 342(8877): 961-962.

[19] Olschewski H, Walmrath D, Schermuly R, Ghofrani A, Grimminger F, Seeger W.: Aerosolized prostacyclin and iloprost in severe pulmonary hypertension. *Ann Intern Med* 1996;124(9):820-824.

[20] Warren JB, Higenbottam T.: Caution with use of inhaled nitric oxide. *Lancet* 1996;348(9028):629-630.

[21] Rolla G, Colagrande P, Brussino L, Bucca C, Bertero MT, Caligaris-Cappio F.: Exhaled nitric oxide and pulmonary response to iloprost in systemic sclerosis with pulmonary hypertension. *Lancet* 1998;351(9114):1491-1492.

[22] Higenbottam TW, Butt AY, Dinh-Xaun AT, Takao M, Cremona G, Akamine S.: Treatment of pulmonary hypertension with the continuous infusion of a prostacyclin analogue. *Heart* 1998;79(2):175-179.

[23] Olschewski H, Ghofrani HA, Walmrath D, Temmesfeld-Wollbruck B, Grimminger F, Seeger W.: Recovery from circulatory shock in severe pulmonary hypertension (PPH) with aerosolization of iloprost. *Intensive Care Med* 1998;24(6):631-634.

[24] Olschewski H, Simonneau G, Galie N, Higenbottam T, Naeije R, Rubin LJ, Nikkho S, Speich R, Hoeper MM, Behr J, Winkler J, Sitbon O, Popov W, Ghofrani HA, Manes A, Kiely DG, Ewert R, Meyer A, Corris PA, Delcroix M, Gomez-Sanchez M, Siedentop H, Seeger W for the Aerosolized Iloprost Randomized Study Group.: Inhaled iloprost for severe pulmonary hypertension. *N Engl J Med* 2002;347:322-9.

[25] Kleen M, Habler O, Hofstetter C, Pusch R, Mueller M, Welte M, Zwissler B.: Efficacy of inhaled prostanoids in experimental pulmonary hypertension. *Crit Care Med* 1998;26(6):1103-1109.

[26] Product Information for *Flolan® (epoprostenol sodium). GlaxoSmithKline* co.1999.

[27] D'Alonzo GE, Barst RJ, Ayers SM, et al.: Survival in patients with primary pulmonary hypertension: results from a national prospective registry. *Ann Intern Med* 1991;115:343-349.

[28] Saji T, Ozawa Y, Ishikita T, Matsuura H, Matsuo N.: Short-term hemodynamic effect of a new oral PGI2 analogue, betaprost, in primary pulmonary hypertension. *Am J Cardiol* 1996;78:244-247.

[29] Snell GI, Salamonsen RF, Bergin P, Esmore DS, Khan S, Williams TJ.: Inhaled nitric oxid used as a bridge to heart-lung transplantation in a patient with end-stage pulmonary hypertension. *Am J Respir Crit Care Med* 1995;151:1263-1266.

[30] *Therapeutic Applications of Iloprost.* Perspectives for the new millenium. An International Symposium, Dorint Hotel Schweizerhof, Berlin, Germany, February 18-19, 2000.

INDEX

A

B

C

F

G

H

M

N

O

P

T

U

V

W

X

Y

Z